Surgery

CLINICAL CASES UNCOVERED

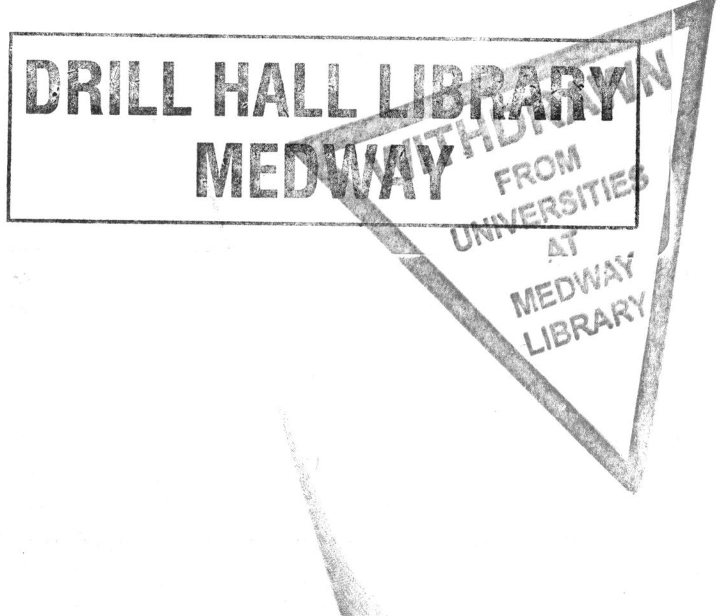

Surgery

CLINICAL CASES UNCOVERED

Harold Ellis
CBE, MCh, FRCS
Clinical Anatomist
Guy's Campus
University of London

Christopher Watson
MA, MD, FRCS
Reader in Surgery and Honorary Consultant Surgeon
Department of Surgery
University of Cambridge School of Clinical Medicine
Addenbrooke's Hospital
Cambridge

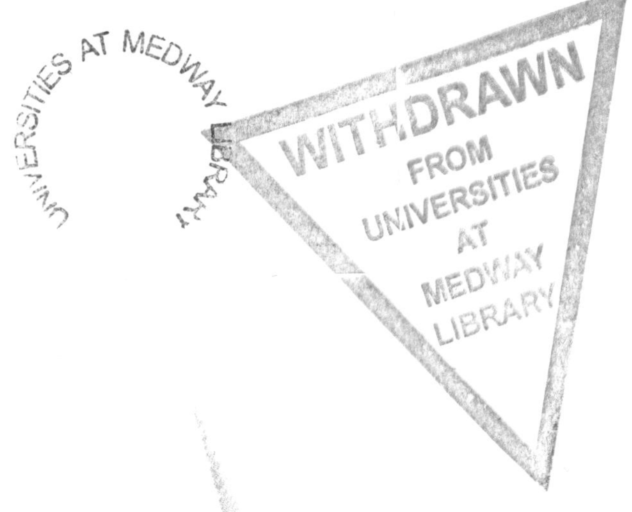

WILEY-BLACKWELL
A John Wiley & Sons, Ltd., Publication

Blackwell Publishing was acquired by John Wiley & Sons in February 2007. Blackwell's publishing program has been merged with Wiley's global Scientific, Technical and Medical business to form Wiley-Blackwell.

Registered office: John Wiley & Sons Ltd, The Atrium, Southern Gate, Chichester, West Sussex, PO19 8SQ, UK

Editorial offices: 9600 Garsington Road, Oxford, OX4 2DQ, UK
The Atrium, Southern Gate, Chichester, West Sussex, PO19 8SQ, UK
111 River Street, Hoboken, NJ 07030-5774, USA

For details of our global editorial offices, for customer services and for information about how to apply for permission to reuse the copyright material in this book please see our website at www.wiley.com/wiley-blackwell

Library of Congress Cataloguing-in-Publication Data

Ellis, Harold, 1926–
Surgery : clinical cases uncovered / Harold Ellis, Christopher Watson.
p. ; cm.
Includes indexes.
ISBN 978-1-4051-5898-5 (alk. paper)
1. Surgery–Case studies. I. Watson, Christopher J. E. (Christopher John Edward) II. Title.
[DNLM: 1. Surgical Procedures, Operative–methods–Case Reports. 2. Surgical Procedures, Operative–methods–Problems and Exercises. WO 18.2 2008]
RD34.E45 2008
617–dc22

2008016695

ISBN: 978-1-4051-5898-5

A catalogue record for this book is available from the British Library.

Set in 9 on 12 pt Minion by SNP Best-set Typesetter Ltd., Hong Kong
Printed and bound in Malaysia by KHL Printing Co Sdn Bhd

3 2010

Contents

Preface

Sir William Osler, that great clinical teacher, wrote 'To study the phenomena of disease without books is to sail on uncharted seas – while to study books without patients is not to go to sea at all'.

Your surgical teachers will tell you that the best way to learn surgical diagnosis and management is to see as many patients as you can – in the accident and emergency department, the out-patients clinics and the wards – to see them at operation and then to study the pathological tissues removed from them. Your text books are there, first and foremost, to help you study your patients.

Nothing can substitute for 'the real thing'. However, when you come to revise for your examinations, there is a distinct need for well-illustrated and well-written books that present a series of clinical problems and discuss their investigation and management.

We hope that this series of our own patients, carefully chosen over the years, will help you. Their problems range over the wide field of 'general surgery'. Further details on each are given in our '*Lecture Notes in General Surgery*', 11th edition.

Harold Ellis
Chris Watson
2008

Acknowledgements

The authors are grateful to all the patients whose photographs are included in this book. In addition we are indebted to Dr Aileen Patterson for the histology photographs, and Dr Kathryn Nash and Dr Mark Gurnell for their advice.

The copyright for the following figures belongs to Cambridge University Hospitals NHS Foundation Trust: 1 (a), 3.2, 14.2, 15.3, 20.2 (a, b, c, d), 21.5, 23.1, 30.1, 31.3 (a, b), 46.4, 47.1, 49.2 (a, b, c, d), 51.1 (a, b), 63.3, 66.2, 79.1, 89.1, 92.1, 93.3, 95.3 (a, b), 97.1, 98.1, 101.2, 106.2, 108.3, 111.1, 111.3, 123.1, 123.2.

Some figures in this book are taken from:

Ellis, H. & Watson, C. (2001) *Pocket Diagnosis in General Surgery*, 3rd edition. Blackwell Science, Oxford.

Ellis, H. (2006) *Clinical Anatomy*, 11th edition. Blackwell Publishing, Oxford.

Ellis, H., Feldman, S. & Harrop-Griffiths, W. (2004) *Anatomy for Anaesthetists*, 8th edition. Blackwell Publishing, Oxford.

Ellis, H., Calne, R. & Watson, C. (2006) *Lecture Notes: General Surgery*, 11th edition. Blackwell Publishing, Oxford.

How to use this book

Clinical Cases Uncovered (CCU) books are carefully designed to help supplement your clinical experience and assist with refreshing your memory when revising. Each book is divided into three sections: Part 1, Basics; Part 2, Cases; and Part 3, Self-assessment.

Part 1 gives a quick reminder of the principles of surgical history and examination, and operating theatre etiquette. Part 2 contains many of the clinical presentations you would expect to see on the wards or crop up in exams, with questions and answers leading you through each case. Part 3 allows you to test your learning with several question styles (MCQs, EMQs and SAQs), each with a strong clinical focus.

Whether reading individually or working as part of a group, we hope you will enjoy using your CCU book. If you have any recommendations on how we could improve the series, please do let us know by contacting us at: medstudentuk@oxon.blackwellpublishing.com.

Disclaimer

CCU patients are designed to reflect real life, with their own reports of symptoms and concerns. Please note that all names used are entirely fictitious and any similarity to patients, alive or dead, is coincidental.

Approach to the patient

As with all medical specialties, the important elements in the assessment of the surgical patient are a thorough history and examination. The diagnosis is usually apparent from the history, and confirmed by clinical examination. In the acute situation a rapid appraisal of the patient's condition is necessary, and initiation of treatment for haemorrhage or septic shock may take priority over completion of a detailed history.

History

Document what the patient said, rather than your interpretation of what was said. Open questions are more helpful, and will direct you to what the patient wants to bring to your attention rather than what you perceive the patient's complaint to be. Hence questions like 'When were you last completely well?', and 'What happened next?' are more useful. When the history reveals a positive finding, such as pain, rectal bleeding or vomiting for instance, do not leave the subject until you know all that there is to know, for instance: when did the pain start; how did it start (sudden versus gradual); what made it better/worse; what associated features were there? Examples of such questions are given in Table 1.

Patients rarely share your knowledge of anatomy, so be sure to know what they mean, for instance, by stomach – it is usually taken to mean the peritoneal cavity rather than the J-shaped muscular tube in the epigastrium.

Remember the anatomical derivation of the abdominal organs when thinking about abdominal pain, and distinguish between visceral and parietal pain. Visceral pain relates to the organ itself, and is referred according to its embryological derivation. Hence gastritis is epigastric pain, because the stomach is a foregut structure and foregut pain is experienced in the epigastrium. Similarly the pancreatic ducts and bile ducts derive from the foregut, so pancreatitis, cholangitis and biliary colic give pain in the epigastrium. The midgut, from the mid-duodenum to the proximal two-thirds of the transverse colon, produces visceral pain, which is experienced in the umbilical region. Hence the pain of appendicitis, a midgut structure, is initially experienced in the epigastrium. Hindgut pain, arising from the distal colon and bladder, is experienced suprapubically. Parietal pain is derived from the parietal peritoneum, and localizes to the overlying dermatome. Hence in appendicitis, as the inflammatory process progresses, the inflammation involves the overlying parietal peritoneum, producing a pain that starts off centrally and migrates to the right iliac fossa.

Referred pain can cause difficulties with diagnosis. There are two circumstances that commonly cause problems, one is testicular pain, such as that of torsion, which radiates to the periumbilical region, the other is the pain of diaphragmatic irritation, which manifests as shoulder tip pain.

Past history is important, particularly details of any previous surgery. However, a patient's understanding of what occurred is often at odds with what actually occurred, or lacks sufficient detail so it is important that, wherever possible, you try to obtain copies of previous operation notes. Also enquire of any operative or anaesthetic difficulties that were encountered, since these may alter any future surgical or anaesthetic approach.

Examination

Examination follows the standard quartet of inspection, palpation, percussion and auscultation. Careful inspection is important, and may reveal signs that eager fingers miss. Note the general appearance of the patient: is he resting comfortably or in pain and restless or still; are there features of recent weight loss (clothes too big, gaunt face); is he tachypnoeic, or just breathing shallowly because deep inspiration hurts? After a general inspection, start the next phase by examination of the hands, then face, head and neck, chest and abdomen. Where appropriate examine the breasts in women and men (for example, where there is axillary lymphadenopathy).

Table 1 Example of features to determine in the history of patients presenting with pain or rectal bleeding.

Pain	Rectal bleeding
Time of onset	Estimation of amount of blood loss
Rate of onset	Colour of blood
Length of history	Timing of blood loss
Exact site	Relationship to passage of stool: Mixed in Following defaecation Not related to defaecation Present on paper only Present in pan, separate from stool
Radiation	Colour – bright red, dark red, black
Periodicity	Accompanying features – vomiting, haematemesis, pain
Nature – colicky or constant	Presence of shock/fainting
Severity	
Relieving and exacerbating factors	
Additional features, e.g. jaundice, vomiting, haematuria	

Examine the abdomen with the patient lying flat and comfortable. Complete exposure is important – failure to expose the upper abdomen may miss an abdominal aortic aneurysm, and failure to expose the groins will certainly render the diagnosis of an inguinal hernia impossible. Testicular cancer or torsion cannot be detected without examination of the scrotal contents. Any embarrassment you may feel in exposing the patient properly will be much less than the embarrassment of missing a life-threatening diagnosis.

Ask the patient to cough – not only will this demonstrate a hernia but it will also indicate whether there is any peritoneal irritation. In the presence of peritonitis, coughing causes severe pain as the peritoneal surfaces move. Following inspection, palpation should determine the presence and extent of any masses, cutaneous and subcutaneous lumps, and areas of tenderness. Percussion is important to confirm organomegaly, and elicit rebound tenderness. Auscultation should be used to listen for vascular bruits, the diagnosis of arteriovenous fistulae, and determining the presence and nature of bowel sounds. Finally, a rectal examination should be performed on any patient with gastrointestinal symptoms or an acute abdomen.

Introduction to the operating theatre

One of the more exciting, and intimidating, events in medicine is the visit to the operating theatre. Exciting, because it is a true theatre, with performances of art and skill in an atmosphere at one moment calm and at another tense and fraught. Anatomy is displayed, pathology demonstrated and treatments effected, with the surgeons reacting to the responsibility somewhere on a spectrum between calmness and anxiety. Nevertheless there is a code of conduct without which a trip to theatre will be a series of requests not to touch this, and exhortations not to go near to that.

At the centre of the theatre is the patient (Fig. 1). For most surgical procedures the anaesthetist stands at the head of the table next to the anaesthetic machine, a combination of ventilator and monitoring aids including electrocardiogram and oximeter. The patient is first anaesthetized, and then placed in the appropriate position for surgery. For an open nephrectomy or thoracotomy this would be lying in the lateral position; for laparotomies or other operations on the abdomen, the heart, breasts or head and neck, the patient is placed supine, facing up. The area to be operated on is prepared with an antiseptic such as iodine, and the prepared area then surrounded by sterile drapes. These are traditionally green in colour, but are now more commonly blue. Since they are sterile they should not be touched by anyone who is not 'sterile' (has scrubbed their hands and is gowned in an operating gown). A scrub nurse usually stands opposite the surgeon, and next to a trolley containing instruments that are appropriate for the operation to be performed. As an observer it is important not to desterilize personnel or instruments by touching

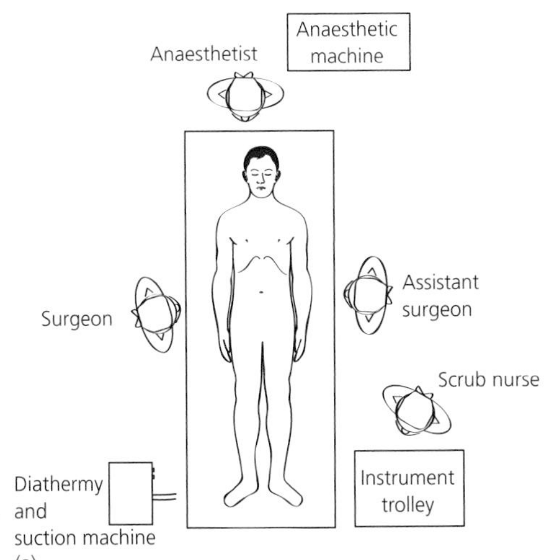

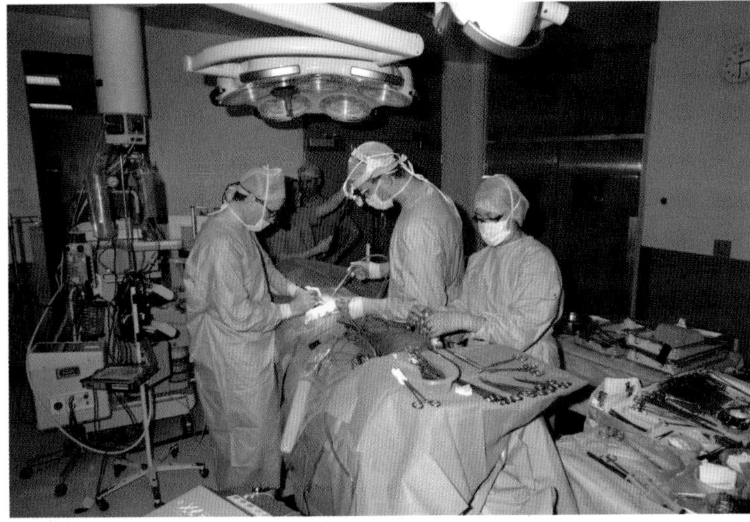

Figure 1 (a) Typical operating theatre layout. (b) Photo of operating theatre.

anything sterile, or crowding in on the operating personnel such that they inadvertently touch you.

Communication between surgeon, scrub nurse and anaesthetist is vital for a successful outcome. While they may talk between themselves about unrelated subjects, there will be times when they are silent when the procedure is taxing, or difficulties are encountered. It is distracting for the surgical team to hear unrelated conversations occurring in the background during such times of tension, so the observer is advised to keep quiet unless it is relevant to the case in question. This is particularly important when the patient is awake and having surgery under a local anaesthetic.

Case 1 Postoperative dyspnoea

A man aged 75 years, a heavy smoker, with a degree of chronic bronchitis, was admitted as an emergency. He had noticed a right-sided groin hernia some years before, which had gradually enlarged and descended into the scrotum when he coughed. Eight hours before admission, during the night, he had had a bad coughing spell. During this, the hernia became larger than usual, was painful for the first time and he could not reduce it. He vomited green fluid.

On admission he was found to have a strangulated, indirect, right inguino-scrotal hernia. He had a productive cough with mucopurulent sputum. He was operated upon 2 h later. The hernial sac contained a loop of strangulated but perfectly viable small intestine. This was reduced and the hernia repaired.

Figure 1.1 demonstrates the patient's temperature chart. After a rather stormy convalescence, he made a good recovery.

What is the most likely cause of his postoperative pyrexia, tachycardia and dyspnoea?

Postoperative pulmonary collapse. This is extremely common following thoracic, abdominal or groin surgery, especially in a patient with pre-existing pulmonary disease. Pyrexia so soon after surgery is unlikely to be due to wound infection or pulmonary embolism.

What causes this complication?

Retention of plugs of mucus in the bronchial tree.

What factors were likely to be responsible in this patient?

In any complication following surgery, consider preoperative, operative and postoperative factors.

- *Preoperative*: Heavy smokers often have chronic bronchitis, with excess of mucus in the bronchial tree.
- *Operative*: The anaesthetic drugs may irritate the respiratory mucosa and produce an excess of mucus secretion from the lining goblet cells; so does irritation of the endotracheal tube.
- *Postoperative*: The pain of the groin incision inhibits the expectoration of the accumulated bronchial secretions.

What physical signs would you have expected to find when you examined this patient on the first postoperative day?

As shown on the chart (Fig. 1.1), the patient would be tachypnoeic, pyrexial and have a tachycardia. There may have been cyanosis. He would have a 'fruity' cough, which he would try to suppress because of the pain this would cause in the wound. Chest expansion would be greatly reduced and percussion might reveal dullness also at the bases of the lungs. Auscultation might reveal diminished air entry and the presence of crackling adventitial sounds, especially at the lung bases, heard posteriorly.

What was the treatment?

Vigorous breathing exercises, with encouragement to cough in the upright position. The pain in the wound on coughing, which would inhibit this, was managed by repeated doses of morphine given by a patient-controlled delivery system (patient controlled analgesia, PCA). In his case, as the sputum was already mucopurulent, ampicillin was also prescribed.

As can be seen on the chart, there was a good response to this management regimen.

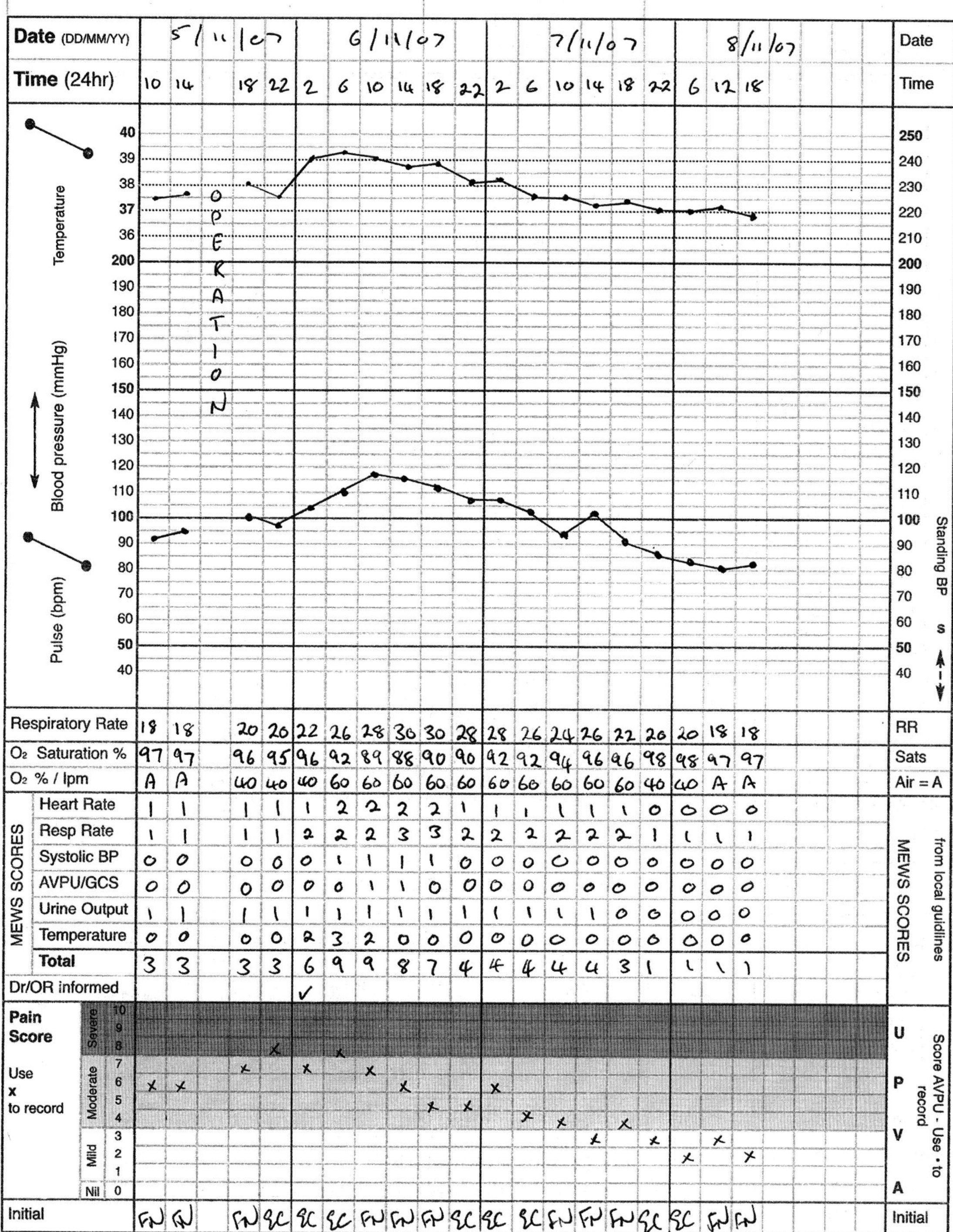

Addenbrooke's Hospital
Adult Observation Chart

Ward: C 12

Weight: 72 kg   Height: 1.62 m   Consultant: A. SURGEON

BOLSOVER
JASPER
DoB 13-1-1932

Freq. of obs (date and initial changes)

Date (DD/MM/YY)	5/11/07					6/11/07						7/11/07						8/11/07		
Time (24hr)	10	14		18	22	2	6	10	14	18	22	2	6	10	14	18	22	6	12	18
Respiratory Rate	18	18		20	20	22	26	28	30	30	28	28	26	24	26	22	20	20	18	18
O_2 Saturation %	97	97		96	95	96	92	89	88	90	90	92	92	94	96	96	98	98	97	97
O_2 % / lpm	A	A		40	40	40	60	60	60	60	60	60	60	60	60	60	40	40	A	A
MEWS SCORES: Heart Rate	1	1		1	1	1	2	2	2	2	1	1	1	1	1	1	0	0	0	0
Resp Rate	1	1		1	1	2	2	2	3	3	2	2	2	2	2	2	1	1	1	1
Systolic BP	0	0		0	0	0	1	1	1	1	0	0	0	0	0	0	0	0	0	0
AVPU/GCS	0	0		0	0	0	0	1	1	0	0	0	0	0	0	0	0	0	0	0
Urine Output	1	1		1	1	1	1	1	1	1	1	1	1	1	1	0	0	0	0	0
Temperature	0	0		0	0	2	3	2	0	0	0	0	0	0	0	0	0	0	0	0
Total	3	3		3	3	6	9	9	8	7	4	4	4	4	4	3	1	1	1	1
Dr/OR informed						✓														
Initial	FN	FN		FN	SC	SC	SC	FN	FN	FN	SC	SC	SC	FN	FN	FN	SC	SC	FN	FN

Figure 1.1 Sample temperature chart.

PART 2: CASES

Case 2 Inside out

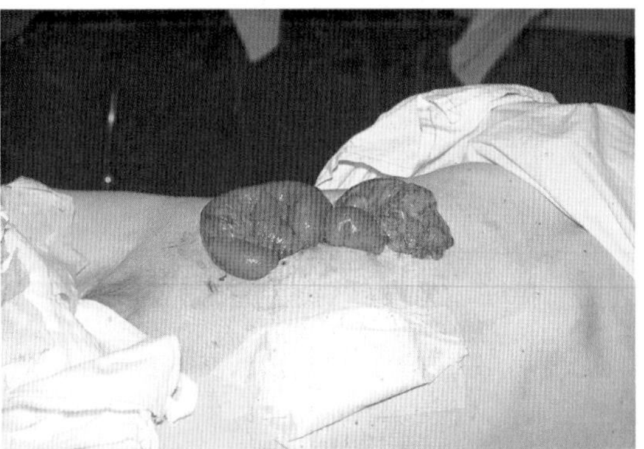

Figure 2.1

A civil engineer aged 58 years had a right hemicolectomy performed through a right paramedian incision for a carcinoma of the caecum. Postoperatively he developed quite a severe pulmonary collapse at both lung bases, which responded to vigorous chest physiotherapy. He also had a prolonged period of paralytic ileus and required nasogastric suction and intravenous fluids until flatus was passed on the seventh postoperative morning. During this time he was troubled with considerable abdominal distension. On the tenth postoperative day he had a spell of coughing and called the nurses because of the unpleasant sight shown in Fig. 2.1. The patient was, not surprisingly, very frightened, but was in no more than moderate discomfort.

What is this condition called?

The common term applied to this is burst abdomen. The rather more mellifluous expression is abdominal wall dehiscence.

What may be a warning sign of this before the abdominal wound completely ruptures?

The 'pink fluid sign'. This is produced by serous peritoneal exudate, tinged with blood and hence pink in colour, which oozes through the breaking down abdominal wound, sometimes for several days before complete dehiscence occurs.

The only other cause of such a discharge, which should be quite obvious, is the discharge of a large subcutaneous haematoma. The final disruption of all layers of the wound occurs either as a result of the patient coughing or straining, or when the skin sutures – the last things holding the edges of the wound together – are removed, usually around the tenth postoperative day.

If this sign is detected, the patient should be returned to the theatre and the wound explored under a general anaesthetic before complete rupture takes place.

How would you classify the factors that may be responsible for this emergency?

As in Case 1 (p. 4), the classification is into preoperative, operative and postoperative factors.

- *Preoperative factors*: These include factors that impair normal wound healing. These are numerous and include, most importantly, vitamin C deficiency, protein deficiency, jaundice, uraemia and anaemia, several of which may occur in the same patient, for example, one with advanced malignant disease. Preoperative factors that are likely to place undue strain on the surgical wound include chronic cough and abdominal distension.
- *Operative factors*: These are due to faulty technique – the sutures may have been poorly placed too near the wound edge, poorly tied or knotted, or the ends cut off too near the knot. The suture material to repair the abdominal wound should be non-absorbable (e.g. nylon) or only slowly absorbable (e.g. polydioxanone, PDS) material, and should not be too fine, and therefore readily breakable. Size 1 is commonly used.

Numerous controlled randomized and prospective studies have shown the value of the 'mass closure' technique of suturing the abdominal wound. All the layers of the abdominal wall apart from the skin and subcutaneous fascia are picked up a minimum of 1 cm from the

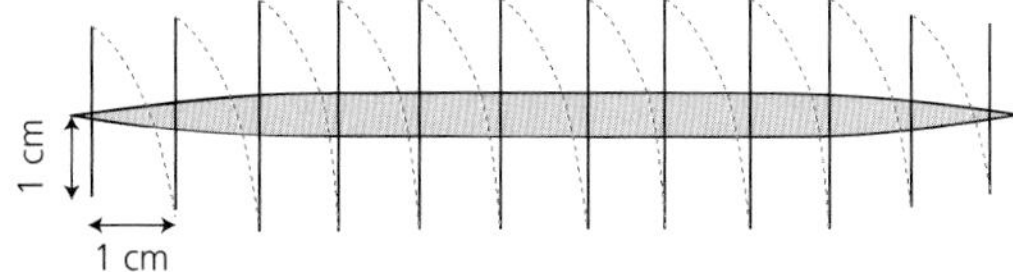

Figure 2.2 Jenkin's rule – the amount of the suture should be at least four times the length of the wound.

wound edge on either side and the sutures inserted 1 cm or less apart. The skin is closed as a separate layer. The formula is that, for a continuous suture, the length of suture used should be at least four times the length of the wound (T.P.N. Jenkins' rule), with sutures 1 cm apart and with 1 cm bites of the wound edge (Fig. 2.2).

- *Postoperative factors*: These are factors that either place undue strain on the abdominal wound (for example, postoperative cough or abdominal distension) or that weaken the tissues on either side of the incision – wound sepsis is important in this context.

How would you manage this situation?

- In every emergency, provided that your patient is conscious, remember that the first thing to do is to reassure the patient; in this particular instance he will certainly be terrified. (This rule is somewhat altered if the emergency patient is unconscious – in such an instance reassure the relatives!)
- Next give intravenous morphine, both as a sedation and pre-anaesthetic medication, together with an anti-emetic to prevent opiate-induced retching that might result in more bowel leaving the abdomen.
- The intestines cannot be reduced due to the rigidity of the abdominal wall; do not even attempt to do so. Cover the exposed viscera with a sterile towel or large dressing, soaked in warmed normal saline, and keep this in place with an abdominal binder or bandage. Arrange immediate transfer to the operating theatre. A general anaesthetic is required to relax the abdominal wall muscles and to allow reposition of the prolapsed viscera.
- Repair is carried out using interrupted nylon sutures, which are passed through all layers of the abdominal wall, including the skin (Fig. 2.3). The sutures are held open until all are inserted and then tied seriatim, great care being taken not to damage the underlying viscera.

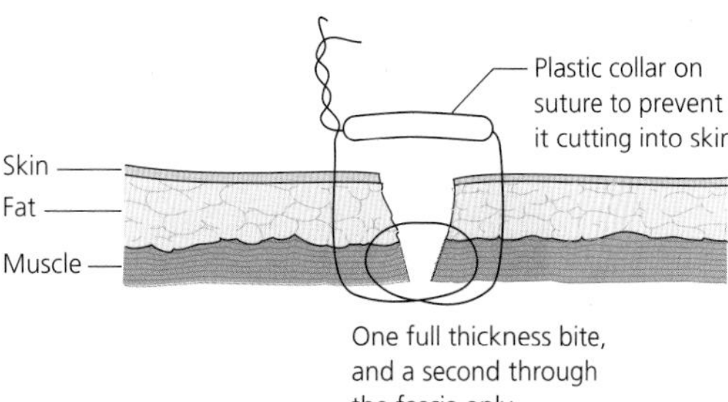

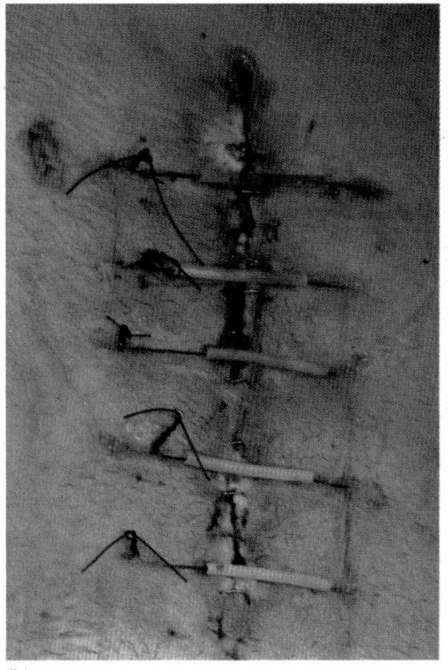

(b)

Figure 2.3 (a) Deep tension sutures pass through all layers of the abdominal wall with double bites of the musculo-facial layer. The plastic collar (b) prevents the suture cutting into the skin while the suture is in place, typically six weeks.

If the deep layers of the abdominal wound give way but the skin sutures hold, what will result?

An incisional hernia.

Case 3 A wound leak

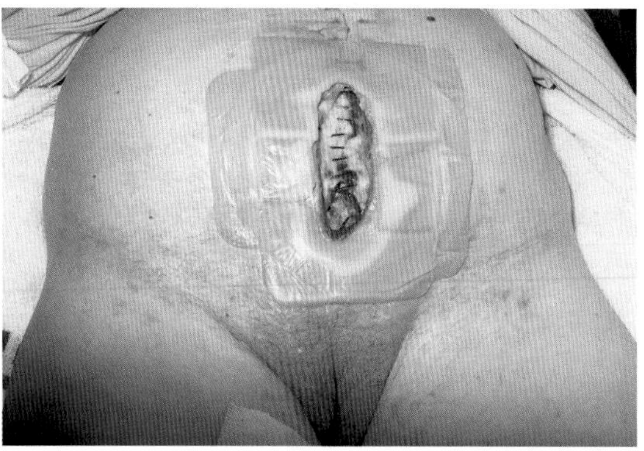

Figure 3.1

A housewife aged 68 years had a left hemicolectomy performed for severe diverticular disease complicated by a pericolic abscess. Her postoperative course was a stormy one. She developed a severe pulmonary collapse (she had been a heavy smoker), had a marked paralytic ileus, with severe abdominal distension and ran a persistent pyrexia. After a week, the abdominal scar was noted to be considerably inflamed and 3 days later faecal fluid and flatus began to discharge through its lower end, as shown in Fig. 3.1.

What is this condition called?

Postoperative faecal fistula, which has resulted from an – at least partial – break down of the large bowel anastomosis.

What is the definition of the term 'fistula'?

A fistula is a pathological communication between two epithelial surfaces – in this case, colon and skin. We have to add the word 'pathological' to this definition otherwise some purist would be able to call the alimentary tract a 'fistula between the mouth and the anal verge'!

What is the sheet of material that has been affixed around the fistula called and what is its importance?

This is a sheet of Stomahesive. A central hole has been cut out of it, which corresponds to the opening of the fistula. This material is invaluable. Unlike other dressings, it adheres to the skin even when this is wet and soggy. A collecting ileostomy pouch is attached to the Stomahesive. This prevents the enzyme-containing effluent intestinal contents from reaching, and digesting, the skin around the fistulous opening.

Before this material was available, gross excoriation of the skin was a distressing complication of bowel fistulae, especially of the upper alimentary tract, where the trypsin from escaping pancreatic juice is particularly harmful in this respect.

How can the track of the fistula be visualized radiologically?

By the injection of radio-opaque contrast fluid, for example Gastrografin, through a fine catheter into the fistula – a fistulogram. In Fig. 3.2 contrast is introduced into a midline wound fistula and rapidly fills a loop of small bowel and then moves on into the colon. There is contrast already in the rectum from a previous contrast enema.

In general terms, what conditions will prevent any fistula from healing spontaneously?

- If the two ends of the intestine are not in apposition to each other (Fig. 3.3a).
- If the mucocutaneous junction of the fistula has epithelialized (Fig. 3.3b). This is why a surgically established colostomy or ileostomy will not close – the surgeon sutures the mucosal edge of the bowel to

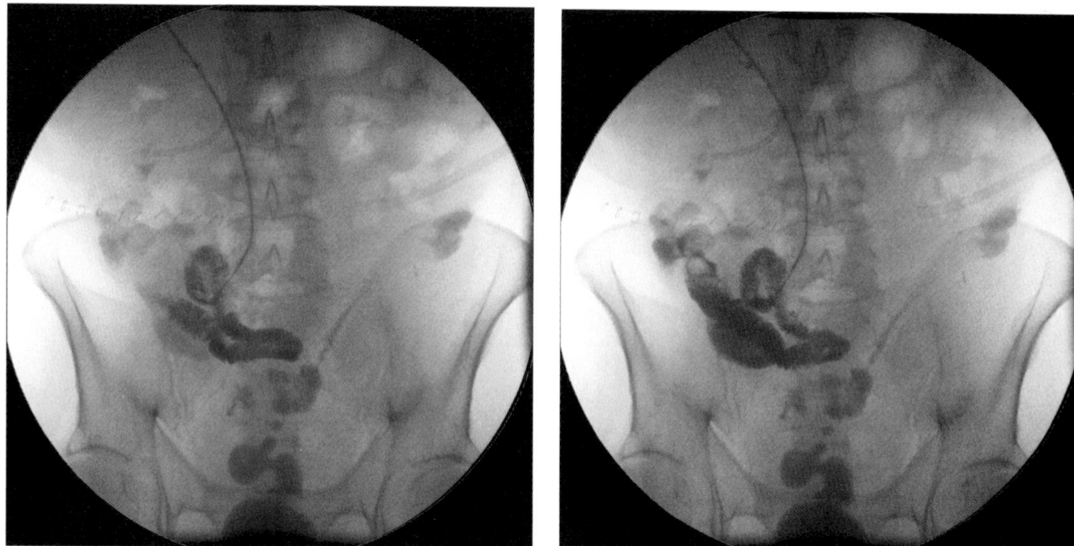

Figure 3.2 X-ray of a fistulogram.

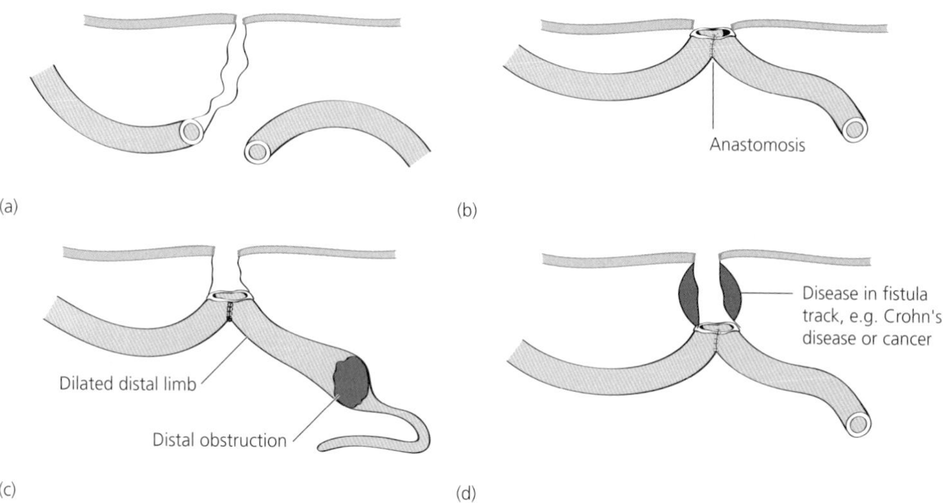

Figure 3.3 Causes of persistent fistulae: (a) bowel ends not in apposition, (b) mucocutaneous junction of the fistula has epithelialized, (c) distal obstruction to flow, and (d) disease in the fistula track.

the adjacent skin margin. The first step in closure of a stoma is to detach the mucosa from the skin edge.

• If there is distal obstruction (Fig. 3.3c); for example, a suprapubic cystostomy will close within a few days of removal of the cystostomy tube in the normal subject, but if there is distal obstruction, from an enlarged prostate or a urethral stricture, for example, the fistula goes on draining urine.

• If there is disease in the fistula track; for example, if the bowel fistula leads down to an area of Crohn's disease (Fig. 3.3d).

What are the principles in the treatment of a bowel fistula?

• Protect the skin around the fistula from excoriation by means of Stomahesive and a stoma pouch to collect the effluent.

• Replace the patient's fluid and electrolytes, ensure adequate nourishment and restore the haemoglobin level if necessary. (Note that in a high intestinal fistula this will require intravenous nutrition by means of an intravenous central line.)

• Investigate the anatomy of the fistula by means of a fistulogram and drain any pus collection. If any factors are found to be present that will prevent spontaneous healing of the fistula (see question above), proceed to appropriate surgery when the patient's general condition has been returned to as near normal as possible.

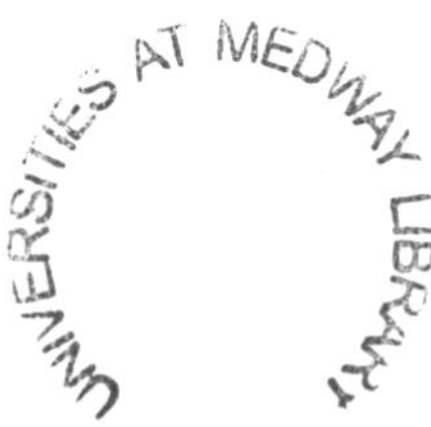

Case 4 An inflamed neck

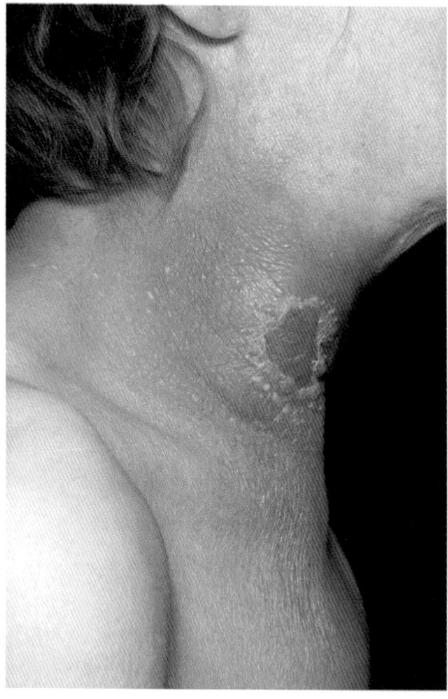

Figure 4.1

This 55-year-old woman developed this painful and tender lesion (Fig. 4.1) 2 days after a scratch on the neck.

What is this condition called?

Cellulitis.

What is the meaning of this term?

A spreading infection of cellular tissues – in this case the superficial fascia of the neck and the overlying skin. It may involve other cellular tissues, for example orbital cellulitis, which affects the connective tissues of the eye socket.

What are the characteristic clinical features of cellulitis?

- Those of any acute superficial infection – classically 'calor, dolor, rubor, turgor', that is heat, pain, redness and swelling. The heat and redness result from vasodilatation, the pain from the stimulation of the pain receptors in the skin and superficial tissues, and the swelling results from tissue oedema. There may be blistering of the overlying skin and occasionally skin necrosis (gangrene).
- The cellulitis may progress to the formation of an abscess (defined as a local collection of pus). Associated features may be lymphangitis (inflammation involving the draining lymphatic channels), which manifests as visible red streaks in the skin along the course of the lymphatics, and lymphadenitis where the draining lymph nodes become swollen and tender.
- Systemic features may often accompany a severe cellulitis. There is usually pyrexia, the patient feels ill and may have rigors.

How is this condition treated?

- If possible, the part is put to rest. A septic hand, for example, is splinted and elevated in a sling. In this case, a cervical collar would make the patient much more comfortable.
- The area is swabbed and blood cultures taken. Antibiotic therapy is then commenced. The initial choice of antibiotic would be intravenous benzyl penicillin to cover the group A (β-haemolytic) streptococci (e.g. *Streptococcus pyogenes*) and flucloxacillin to cover *Staphylococcus aureus* (most community-acquired staphylococci are flucloxacillin-sensitive). Erythromycin is the antibiotic of choice in patients who are allergic to penicillins. Metronidazole is added if there is ischaemic tissue or the subject is diabetic to cover anaerobes.
- If pus formation occurs, the abscess is drained (see Case 5, p. 12).

Case 5 Postoperative infection

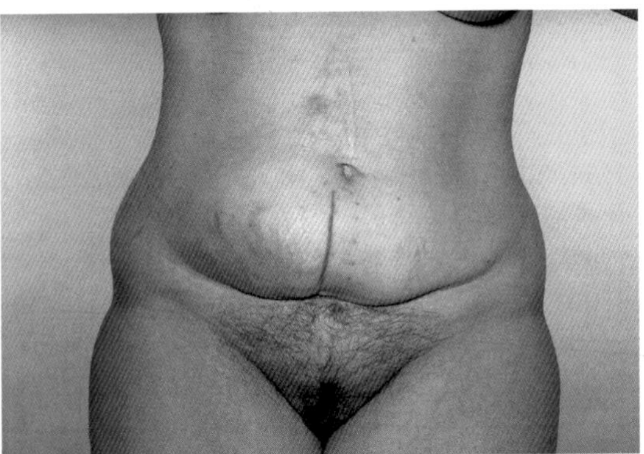

Figure 5.1

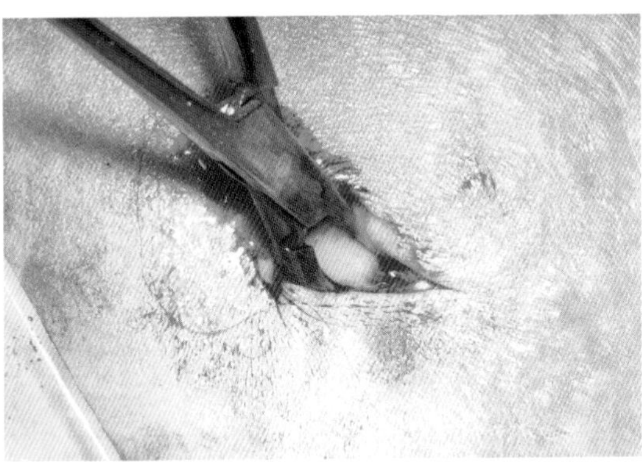

Figure 5.2

A housewife aged 42 years was admitted to hospital with a 48 h history of acute abdominal pain, having previously been entirely well. On examination she had the typical clinical features of a general peritonitis. She had a temperature of 38°C, she was toxic, tachycardic and had a coated tongue. Examination of the abdomen revealed generalized guarding and tenderness, especially over the right iliac fossa, where there was marked muscular rigidity. On rectal examination, there was pain on pressing anteriorly in the pouch of Douglas.

She underwent emergency laparotomy later that day through a midline lower abdominal incision and a perforated gangrenous appendix was removed. Metronidazole, penicillin and gentamicin had been started preoperatively, and the course was completed.

Nasogastric suction and intravenous fluids were used and she made a smooth recovery. However, 3 weeks after surgery, having been at home for nearly a fortnight, she presented with a large abscess in the superficial tissues of the lower right abdomen (Fig. 5.1). She was readmitted to hospital and the surgical procedure that she underwent is shown in Fig. 5.2.

What is the definition of an abscess?

An abscess is a localized collection of pus. Pus itself is defined as living and dead phagocytes, usually containing living and dead bacteria.

What general manifestations often accompany an abscess?

A swinging pyrexia, tachycardia, malaise, anorexia and sweating. There is usually a polymorph leucocytosis.

What is the likely cause of the abscess in this case?

Contamination of the tissues of the abdominal incision by pus that escaped at the time of the initial operation. Even if copious lavage is carried out at the time of surgery and prompt antibiotic treatment is initiated, contaminated wounds such as this have a 15–20% risk of the development of postoperative infection.

The fact that the wound infection did not become manifest until 3 weeks after surgery is explained by bacterial inhibition produced by the antibiotic regimen. It is not at all rare to see postoperative infections such as this to be delayed for many weeks – even months – after the initial episode of contamination. Often the pus will be seen to have formed around a piece of suture – a 'stitch abscess'.

What procedure is being performed in Fig. 5.2?

The abscess is being drained. A small skin incision is made immediately over the centre of the abscess – often this site is through the old incision itself. The track is explored bluntly by forceps, since a scalpel might injure deep structures. This technique is termed Hilton's method.*

When pus is reached, a swab is taken for bacteriological examination. The report on this, by the way, often comes back as 'sterile on culture', again as a result of the previous antibiotic treatment. A drain is then inserted. This can be a gauze wick or a piece of plastic tubing or a corrugated sheet according to the surgeon's preference. The drain is shortened daily to allow the track to heal from below upwards.

The abscess would have eventually discharged spontaneously, probably through the old incision itself. However, during this time the abscess would have continued to act as a source of toxaemia, the patient would have continued to be febrile and ill and there would be the risk of necrosis of the overlying skin.

*John Hilton (1805–1878), surgeon at Guy's Hospital, London.

Case 6 A sore neck

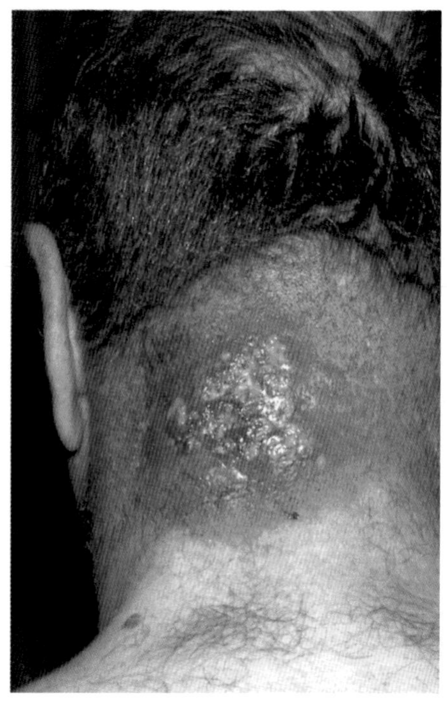

Figure 6.1

This man, a lorry driver aged 60 years, reported to the accident and emergency department with this unpleasant-looking and painful lesion on the neck (Fig. 6.1). He had first been aware of 'something there' 5 days before. It became progressively more swollen and sore, and was now discharging.

What is this lesion called and how is it defined?

A carbuncle. The definition of this is an area of subcutaneous necrosis that discharges onto the surface through multiple sinuses. (A sinus itself is defined as a track leading to an epithelial surface.) It is these multiple openings that give a carbuncle its characteristic appearance. The neck is the commonest site for this lesion, and it is often produced by excoriation of the skin from the edge of a collar.

What is the usual causative organism?

Staphylococcus aureus. This can be established by bacteriological examination of a smear of the pus and its subsequent culture. Its antibiotic sensitivities are checked.

What are the bacteriological features of this organism?

Staphylococcus aureus is a Gram-positive coccus, which grows readily on culture to form typical golden yellow clumps (*aureus* is Latin for golden). Under the microscope the cocci clump together like bunches of grapes (*staphyle* is Greek for bunch of grapes, as opposed to *streptos*, which means chain, hence *Streptococcus*).

What simple laboratory investigation should be carried out on this patient in A&E?

This condition is particularly likely to occur in diabetics. Therefore the urine should always be tested for glucose and, if this is positive, a confirmatory blood glucose estimation performed. Always think of the possibility of diabetes mellitus in a patient with an unusual septic condition, of which this is an example. Other instances are gangrene of the foot, necrotizing fasciitis and severe urinary infection.

In this patient, there was no evidence of diabetes, but the average A&E department is likely to pick up several examples of previously unrecognized diabetes each year.

How should this patient be treated?

• A bacteriological swab of the pus is taken for a Gram stain and culture to determine the organism's antibiotic sensitivities.

• The area is kept clean and is protected with sterile dressings.
• A cervical collar prevents undue movement of the neck and relieves a good deal of discomfort.
• Antibiotic treatment is commenced, usually with flucloxacillin (or erythromycin if the patient states that he is penicillin-sensitive). The antibiotic sensitivity of the organism will be checked in the microbiology department and the antibiotic changed, if necessary, as a result of this. If the patient is known to be a carrier of methicillin-resistant *Staphylococcus aureus* (MRSA), vancomycin is used instead since these organisms are also resistant to flucloxacillin.

Case 7 Hidden infection

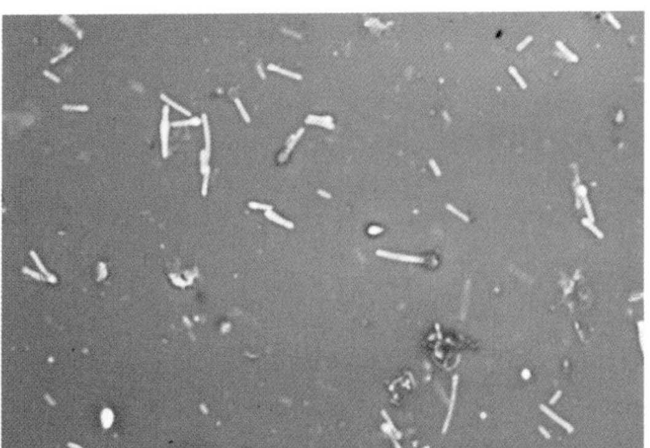

Figure 7.1

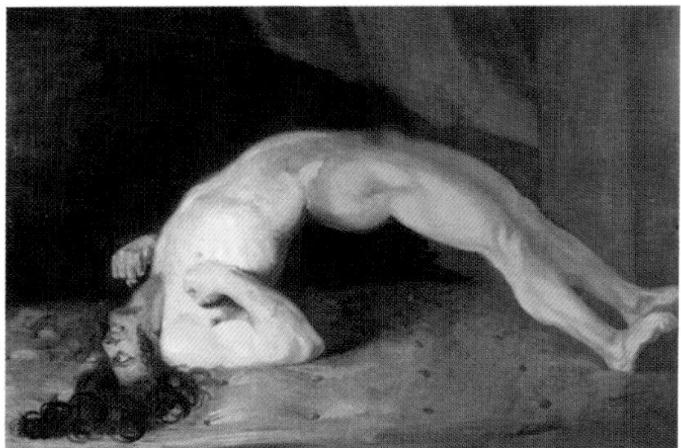

Figure 7.2 A soldier dying of tetanus from wounds received at the battle of Corunna in northern Spain, during the Napoleonic wars, 1809. Note the dramatic opisthotonus. Painting by Sir Charles Bell (1774–1842) hung in the Royal College Surgeons of Edinburgh.

Figure 7.1 shows a smear of a bacterial culture of a swab taken from an infected puncture wound on the hand of a farm labourer admitted to hospital with the clinical diagnosis of tetanus. He admitted that he had never had tetanus prophylaxis.

What does the smear show?

The characteristic Gram-positive bacilli with terminal spores ('drumstick' spores) typical of *Clostridium tetani.*

What is the normal habitat of this organism?

It is a normal inhabitant of faeces and of well manured soil – characteristically of farms and gardens.

What are its bacteriological features?

It is a Gram-positive, capsulated, terminal spore-bearing, exotoxin-producing rod, which can only grow in strictly anaerobic conditions. Because of this last important feature, tetanus can only occur when the organism contaminates devitalized tissues where anaerobic conditions exist – for example, when a gardener puts a garden fork through his foot, or when a compound fracture is produced by a high velocity missile with considerable soft tissue destruction.

What are the effects of the tetanus exotoxin?

The exotoxin, tetanospasmin, is produced at the site of inoculation into ischaemic tissue and tracks along peripheral nerve axons to the central nervous system, where it becomes fixed in the anterior horn cells of the spinal cord and the motor nuclei of the cranial nerves. There it blocks the release of inhibitory neurotransmitters such as γ-aminobutyric acid (GABA) thus permitting unopposed excitatory activity from motor and autonomic neurons. This results in widespread spasm of the muscles in response to minimal sensory stimulation. Typically, the facial muscles become fixed in a 'smile' – the risus sardonicus – and spasm of the spinal muscles produces the extraordinary appearance of opisthotonus (Figs 7.2 and 7.3).

List the effective prophylactic measures against this condition.

• Active immunization with tetanus toxoid (formalin-treated exotoxin) with booster doses at intervals of 10 years or at the time of injury.

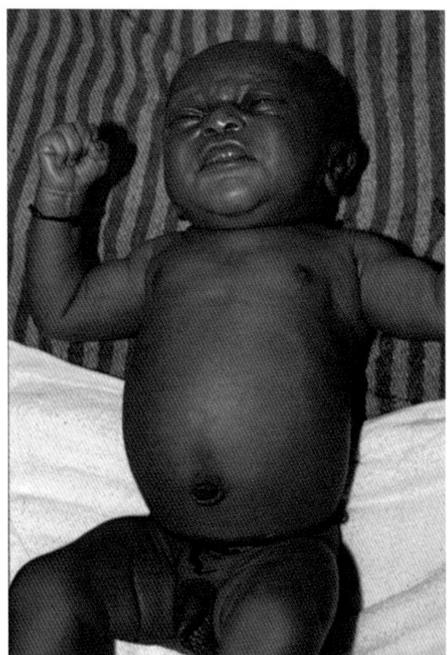

Figure 7.3 Neonatal tetanus following umbilical infection in Sierra Leone; note the risus sardonicus. (Photograph taken by one of us (CW) on our student elective.)

• Wound toilet comprises adequate excision of contaminated or potentially contaminated wounds to remove all dead tissue, combined with a course of prophylactic penicillin.

• Passive immunization is required where the patient has not been previously immunized (i.e. toxoid has not been given previously). This comprises human tetanus immunoglobulin, prepared from fully immunized subjects and should be given if the wound is heavily contaminated or is a puncture wound. A course of toxoid should also be given.

Case 8 Burnt thorax

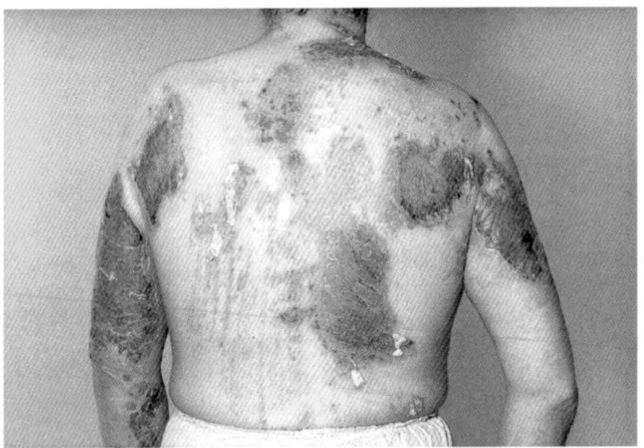

Figure 8.1

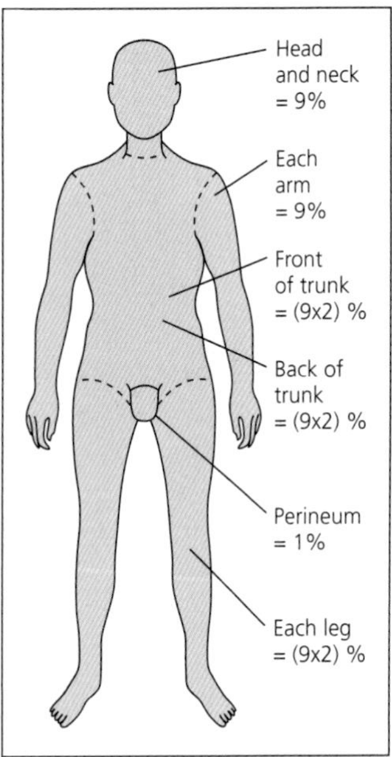

Figure 8.2 The 'rule of nines' – a useful guide to the estimation of the area of a burned surface. (Note also that a patient's hand represents 1% of the body surface area.)

The patient was an industrial worker in his fifties who sustained burns to the back of his chest and upper arms in a factory accident. Figure 8.1 was taken 10 days after the accident.

Can you estimate approximately the area of his body surface that has been affected?

Approximately 14%. The 'rule of nines' states that the

area of the front of the trunk is $2 \times 9\%$ of the body's surface area, the back of the trunk $2 \times 9\%$, each upper limb 9%, each lower limb $2 \times 9\%$, the head and neck 9%, and the perineum 1% (Figure 8.2). Using this, we can see that about half the back of the trunk that has been burned, about 9%. Using the patient's hand as representing 1% of the total body area, the scattered burns on the arms can be estimated to make up another 5%, total 14%. An alternative to the rule of nines would be the Lund and Browder chart (Fig. 8.3), which is particularly useful in children.

Why is it important to estimate the area of the burn in planning treatment?

In this patient, the 14% burn area is borderline for intravenous fluid replacement. The standard teaching is that intravenous fluid resuscitation is indicated if the area of burn is more than 15% of the body surface in adults (10% in a child). The amount of fluid replacement in the first 24 h is based on the Parkland formula:

$$\text{Fluid replacement in first 24 h (in ml)} = 4 \times \text{weight of patient (in kg)} \times \%\text{ area of burn}$$

Half this volume is given in the first 8 h following the burn, and the second half over the ensuing 16 h. This is in addition to the patient's normal daily fluid requirements (3 L of crystalloids in adults under temperate conditions). The fluid of choice is Ringer's lactate (Hartmann's) solution.

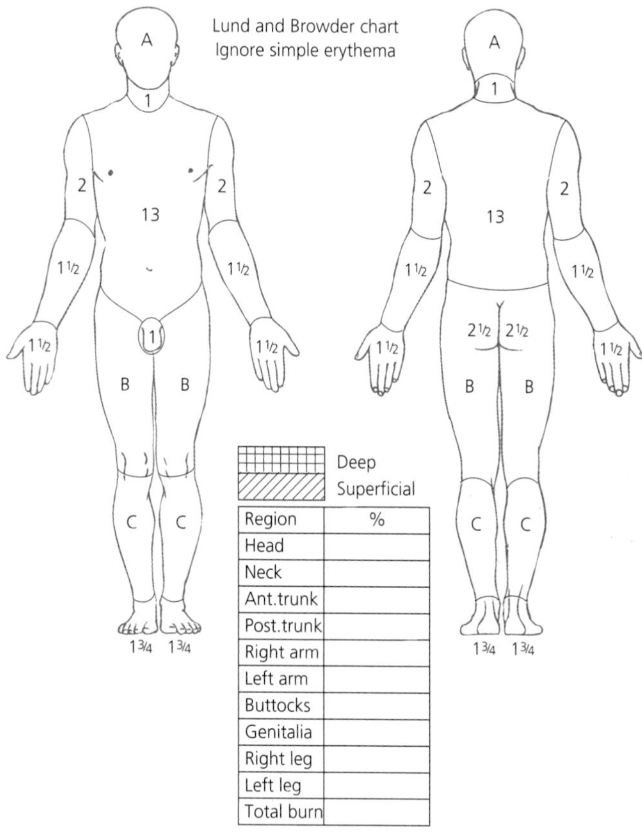

Relative percentage of body surface area affected by growth surface

Area	Age 0	1	5	10	15	Adult
A = 1/2 of head	9.5	8.5	6.5	5.5	4.5	3.5
B = 1/2 of one thigh	2.75	3.25	4.0	4.5	4.5	4.75
C = 1/2 of one leg	2.5	2.5	.2.75	3.25	3.25	3.5

Figure 8.3 The Lund and Browder chart allows more accurate estimation of burn surface area and is particularly useful in children. The extent of the burn is marked on the chart. The areas of burns on the head, thighs and lower legs (A, B and C on the chart) are calculated and multiplied by the age factor in the table.

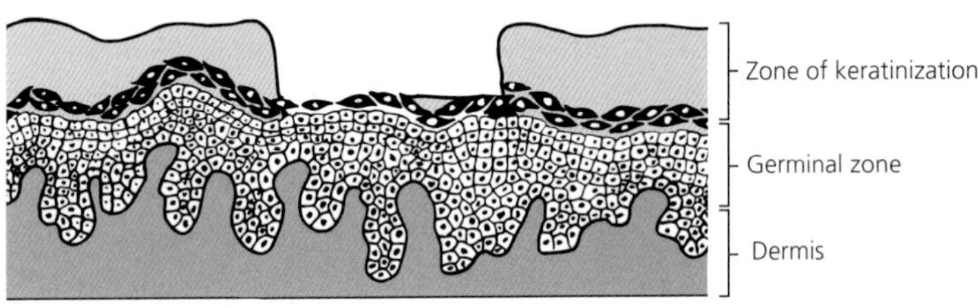

(a) Partial thickness burn

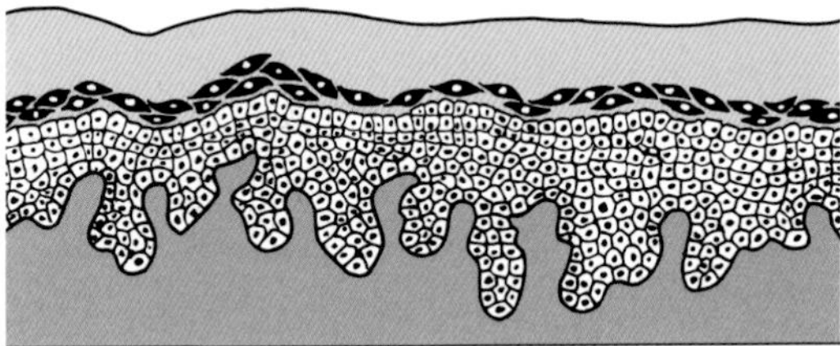

(b) Healed partial thickness burn

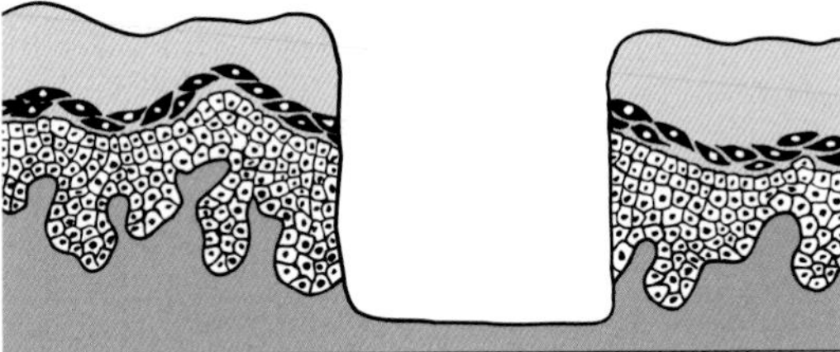

(c) Full thickness burn

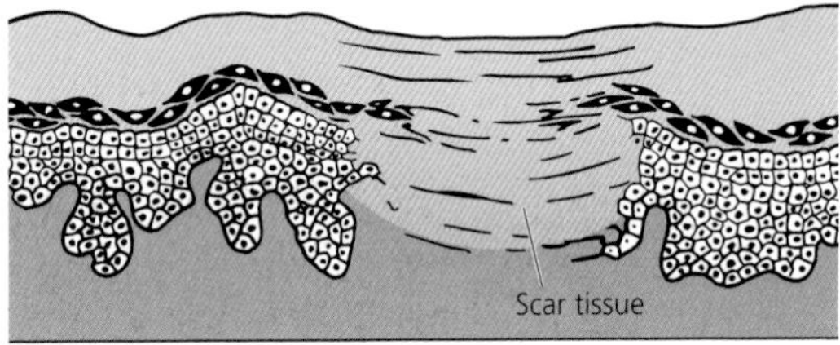

(d) Healed full thickness burn

Figure 8.4 A partial-thickness burn (a) leaves part or the whole of the germinal epithelium intact, so complete healing takes place (b). A full-thickness burn (c) destroys the germinal layer and, unless very small, can only heal by dense scar tissue (d).

How deep are these burns?

The burns over most of the back are partial thickness. The underlying germinal layer of the skin has remained unharmed, has proliferated, and healing can be seen to be taking place. As the scabs of superficial layers of the epidermis flake off, healthy new pink epithelium can be seen. The burns over the arms and the area over the right scapula, however, are full thickness. Here the germinal layer has been involved and the overlying coagulum of dead epithelium is adherent to the underlying granulation tissue (Fig. 8.4).

What further treatment will be necessary for these areas of full thickness burns?

These areas were excised the following day and covered with split-skin grafts taken from the thigh (see Case 9, p. 22).

What local treatment should be given to these burns immediately, as a first aid measure, and then on admission to hospital?

• First aid comprises stopping the burn process at once. The patient must immediately be removed from danger – the source of the burn – his clothes removed (they retain heat), and the burns cooled with cold running water.

• In hospital the burns can be treated by the closed technique, using silver sulphadiazine (flamazine), covered by thick layers of sterile dressings. Alternatively, if only the anterior or, as in this case, the posterior aspect of the body, or the face, are involved, the open technique (or exposure method) may be used. Here the area is left open and a dry scab rapidly forms.

Case 9 Burn treatment

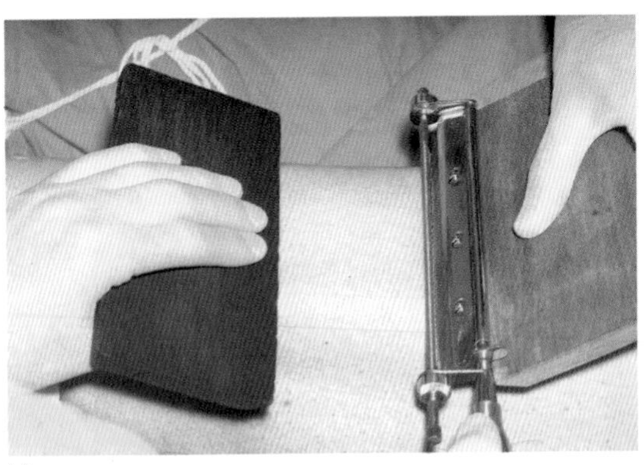

(a)

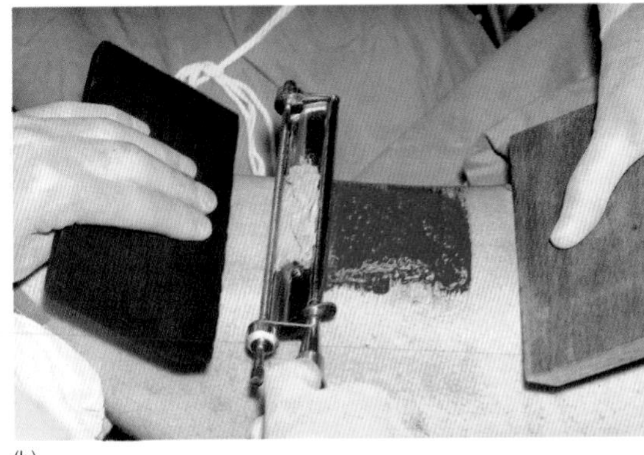

(b)

Figure 9.1

Figure 9.1 shows the stages of the operation performed on the thigh of the patient discussed in Case 8 (p. 18) on the next day.

What operation is being performed?

Skin is being taken in order to perform a skin graft.

What layer of skin is being removed by the surgeon?

This is a split-skin graft, being taken through the germinal layer of the epithelium (see Fig. 8.3), and leaving islands of the layer on the donor site. The surgeon can tell that he is in the right plane because the sheet of skin he is taking is translucent, while on the donor site there is punctuate bleeding of the areas of dermis between the islands of residual epithelium.

What will happen to the raw area left behind on the patient's thigh?

This is dressed with paraffin gauze covered with a thick sterile gauze dressing. The remaining islands of germinal epithelium at the donor site will proliferate, so that the raw area will become re-epithelialized in about 10 days. In very extensive full thickness burns, the donor sites can be re-utilized over and over again.

What are the areas of priority for grafting in patients with extensive full thickness burns?

The eyelids have top priority, followed by the face, hands and flexor aspects of the joints. These are the areas where scarring contractures would produce considerable deformity and disability.

Case 10 Lumps on the scalp

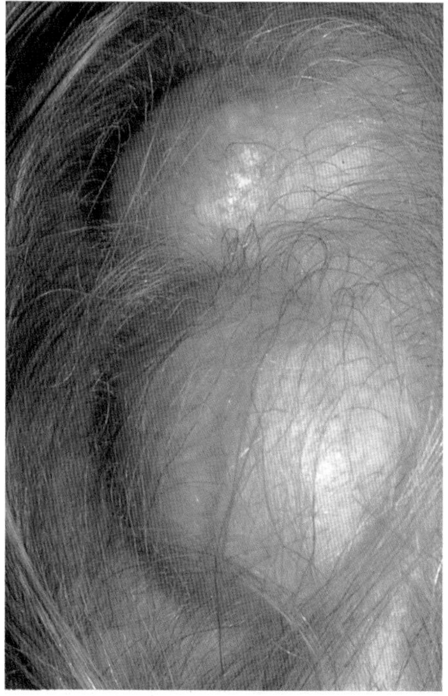

Figure 10.1

Figure 10.1 is a close-up of the scalp of a female hospital cleaner in her late sixties. She presented to the surgical outpatient clinic stating that she had first noted these lumps a couple of years before. They are quite painless, but they are slowly enlarging and bare patches are showing over them. She is worried that they might be some sort of a growth.

On examination, these lumps were found to be smooth, attached to the skin, but mobile on the underlying skull. They demonstrated the sign of fluctuation between two fingers (performed in two directions), and transilluminated when a torch was applied to them in the darkened examination cubicle.

What is the likely diagnosis?

This has all the features of sebaceous cysts of the scalp – a very common lesion.

Describe the physical signs of a cystic swelling

- *Fluctuation*: The tip of the index finger of one hand is placed at the side of the lump, which is pressed upon by the tip of the opposite index finger – the 'watching' finger is felt to elevate. The test is repeated with the fingers moved at right angles to their previous position; again fluctuation is elicited.
- *Transillumination*: In addition, the lump can be shown to transilluminate when a bright torch is help against it, but this must usually be done in a darkened room. Transillumination is especially well seen in the examination of a ganglion, hydrocele or cyst of the epididymis (see Case 121, p. 249).

Why bother to do the test for fluctuation in two directions at right angles to each other?

Try the experiment on yourself: 'fluctuate' transversally across the quadriceps muscle of your thigh – you can even do this experiment through your trousers or skirt – your watching finger will be elevated as you push the muscle mass transversally. Now try again with the fingers now at right angles, placed one above the other – now no movement is detected. You have not got cystic degeneration of your quadriceps!

Are there any other lumps that may occur on the scalp and which would therefore be a differential diagnosis to sebaceous cyst?

- An ivory osteoma of the skull vault is uncommon. It will not fluctuate, nor will it be moveable.

• Secondary deposits in the skull will give similar signs to an osteoma and there might well be clinical evidence of a primary tumour – breast in the female, prostate in the male and bronchus in both sexes are the headlines. Invasion of the skull by an underlying meningioma is a rarity.

Where else are sebaceous cysts found and where do they never occur?

Apart from the scalp, which is the commonest site, they are often found on the face, lobule of the ear, scrotum and vulva. They cannot occur on the sebaceous gland-free palms of the hands and soles of the feet.

What do these cysts look like when they are excised and cut open?

There is a white lining membrane (of squamous epithelium). The contents are white and cheesy, with an unpleasant smell.

What complications may they undergo?

Infection (the commonest), ulceration ('Cock's peculiar tumour'*), calcification, horn formation and malignant change (rare).

What treatment would you advise this woman to have?

Because of the common risk of infection, patients should always be advised to have their sebaceous cysts excised. This can be done quite simply under local anaesthetic. If acutely inflamed, surgical drainage is required, followed later by excision of the capsule wall to prevent further flare-ups of infection. However, the inflammatory scar tissue now makes excision of the cyst a more difficult operation.

*Edward Cock (1805–1892), surgeon, Guy's Hospital, London.

Case 11 A lump on the wrist

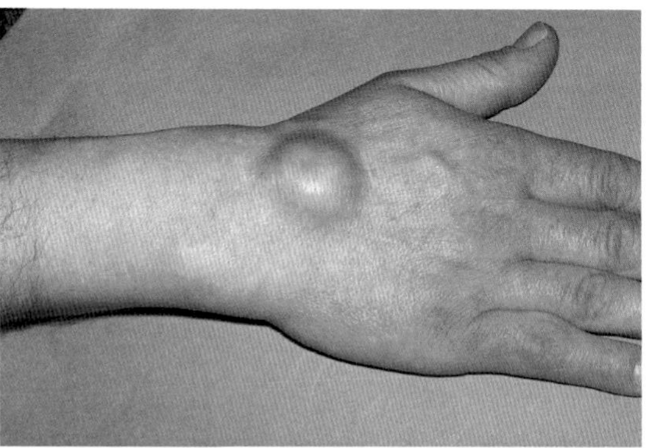

Figure 11.1

This 28-year-old civil servant presented to his family doctor with a painless swelling on the dorsum of his wrist, which he noticed first about a year before. If anything, it was rather larger now and he had recently experienced some aching of the wrist after long sessions on the word processor. He was otherwise perfectly well but was quite worried by this lump and asked to have something done about it.

Just looking at Fig. 11.1, what would be your 'spot' diagnosis?

A ganglion on the wrist.

What physical signs would you elicit to confirm the diagnosis?

The skin can be moved freely over the lump, as can the overlying extensor tendons, but it is tethered to the underlying capsule of the wrist joint. Confirm that the lump is cystic by fluctuation in two directions (see Case 10, p. 23). These ganglia transilluminate brilliantly when a torch is applied to them – even in broad daylight.

Where else are these cysts commonly found?

The dorsum of the foot (arising from the joint capsule), on the flexor tendon sheaths of the fingers and on the peroneal tendon sheaths.

What is their cause?

Although they are so common, their aetiology is still something of a mystery, they may represent a benign myxoma of a joint capsule or tendon sheath, a hamartoma or myxomatous degeneration of the joint capsule or tendon sheath as a result of minor trauma.

What material does the cyst contain?

Mucoid fluid having the appearance of Wharton's jelly* of the umbilical cord. This is contained within the compressed collagen capsule.

What is the prognosis after surgical excision?

Recurrence is unfortunately quite common after surgical excision, and the patient must be warned of this. It is quite a tricky operation, which is performed under general or regional anaesthetic and in a bloodless field produced by a tourniquet to avoid leaving a fragment of the capsule of the cyst behind. Ganglia on the dorsum of the wrist, such as the one shown in Fig. 11.1, commonly lead right down to the ligament between the scaphoid and the lunate.

*Thomas Wharton (1614–1673), physician, St Thomas's Hospital, London.

Case 12 Recurrent abscesses over the sacrum

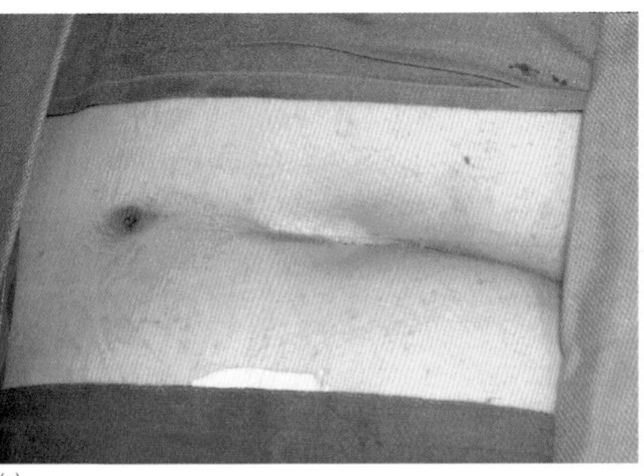
(a)

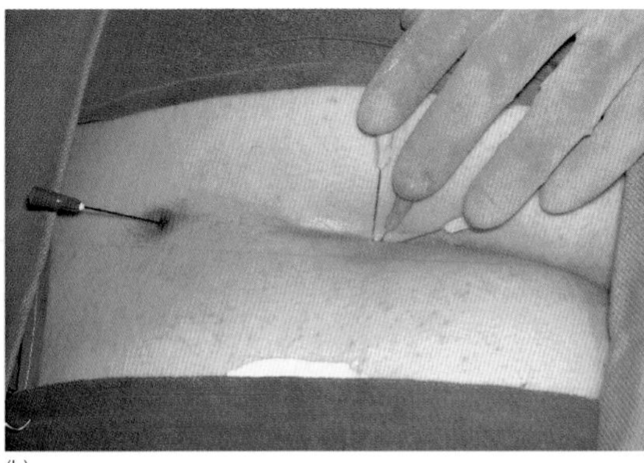
(b)

Figure 12.1

A 25-year-old, rather overweight, male office worker was referred to the surgical outpatient clinic with a history of recurrent abscesses 'at the lower end of the spine'. He was admitted for surgery. Figure 12.1a shows the appearance of his sacral region as he lay anaesthetized on the operating table with his buttocks strapped apart. In Fig. 12.1b, probes have been placed into three small orifices just above the anal verge and into a larger, higher opening, which is at the site of the previous recurrent abscesses.

What is the diagnosis?

This can only be a group of pilonidal sinuses with an associated recurrent abscess.

What does the term pilonidal mean?

It comes from the Latin *pilus* meaning hair and *nidus* meaning a nest – a nest of hair.

Define the term sinus

A sinus is a blind track that leads to an epithelial surface.

What is the aetiology of this condition?

It is believed that hairs shed from the head and trunk collect in the natal cleft (which is deeper in obese subjects). Movement of the buttocks against each other, especially in the sitting position, produce a negative pressure that allows these hairs to implant into the hair follicles. Here they set up a foreign body reaction, which leads to abscess formation. The pus tracks either proximally, as in this case, or to one or other side of the natal cleft. The abscess discharges spontaneously or is drained surgically, but repeated episodes of infection will occur unless the underlying cause is removed.

This aetiology explains how pilonidal sinuses can occur at other sites. Barbers commonly develop them in the interdigital clefts of the fingers, as demonstrated in Fig. 12.2. In these cases the hair comes from the customer and not from the patient! Similarly they have been described between the toes of abattoir workers; here animal hair is implicated. They also occur in the axilla, umbilicus and in the folds of amputation stumps that have redundant skin.

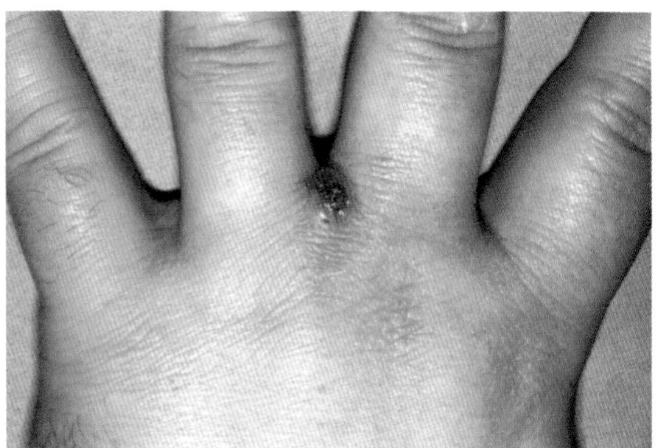

Figure 12.2 Pilonidal sinus between the fingers of a men's barber.

What are the principles of treating this condition?

- If there is an abscess, this must first be drained.
- Once this is resolved, surgery is performed to remove the underlying sinus tracks.
- Subsequently the patient is advised to keep the natal area meticulously free of hair.

Case 13 A septic great toe

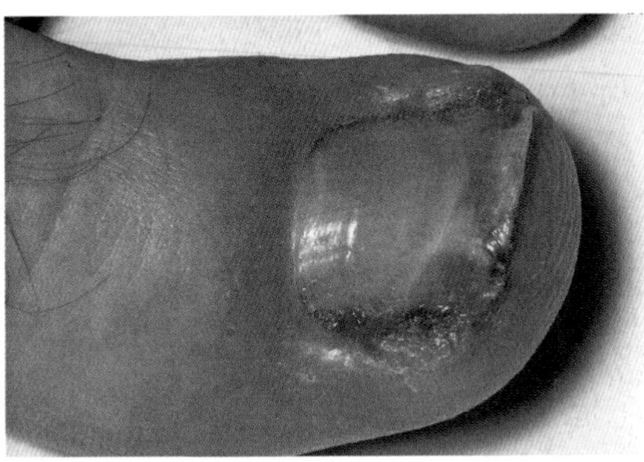

Figure 13.1

Figure 13.1 shows the left hallux of a keen young amateur footballer. He limps into the accident and emergency department of his local hospital complaining of a very painful, swollen great toe.

There are two pathological processes here; what are they and how do they inter-relate?

- The primary condition is ingrowing of the toenail. In this case, both sides of the nail are involved.
- The secondary condition, on the medial side, is paronychia – infection of the soft tissues at the side of the nail, with all the classical features of acute infection – pain, swelling, heat and redness. This has resulted from trauma to the soft tissues by the ingrowth of the nail, which has allowed ingress of bacteria.

How could the primary condition, the ingrowing toenail, have been treated and this complication avoided?

The patient is advised as follows: Avoid cutting the nail downwards into the nail fold – cut the nail transversely. Avoid tight shoes. Tuck a pledget of cotton wool daily into the side of the nail bed to enable the nail to grow out of the fold. Once this has been achieved, there is no risk of further trouble.

How should the infection be treated in the acute phase?

- Drainage of the pus by removal of the side of the nail under general anaesthetic or a ring block with local anaesthetic.
- If the condition affects both sides of the nail, avulsion of the whole nail is necessary.
- Antibiotics are not usually required and resolution is rapid.

What treatment may be necessary in recurrent cases?

The toenail is avulsed and regrowth is prevented either by excision of the nail root (Zadek's operation*) or by treating it with undiluted phenol.

*Frank Raphael Zadek (1914–1995), orthopaedic surgeon, Wigan.

Case 14 A skin tumour

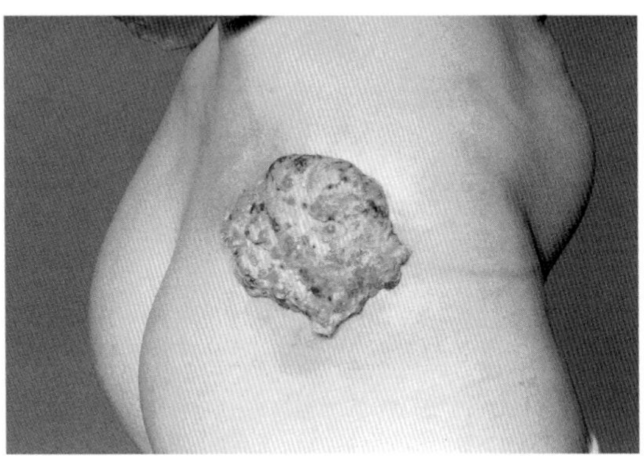

Figure 14.1

This 58-year-old woman actually worked in the kitchen of our hospital canteen. She stated that she had noticed a little lump above her right buttock some 10 years previously. This had slowly but surely enlarged over the years but did not hurt and never bled (Fig. 14.1). She had carefully hidden the lump from her family, including her husband, all this time. Eventually she plucked up her courage and showed her lump to a junior female doctor, who brought her round at once to the surgical outpatient clinic.

What would be your 'spot' diagnosis on looking at this lesion?

It certainly looks like a large squamous carcinoma of the skin.

What would you expect to find on further examination, and where would you examine for evidence of possible metastatic disease?

Sure enough, palpation revealed that the lump was rubbery-hard in consistency, with raised, everted edges. The groins were carefully palpated and enlarged, rubbery-hard nodes were felt on the right side. The rest of the clinical examination found an otherwise perfectly healthy – but very anxious – woman.

This is a relatively unusual site for this tumour. Where is it more often found?

Squamous carcinoma of the skin usually occurs at sites exposed to sunlight – the face and the backs of the hands.

What are the predisposing factors for the development of this tumour?

Predisposing factors to the development of squamous carcinoma of the skin include, as already mentioned, exposure of white skin to sunshine or to irradiation, exposure to carcinogens (e.g. pitch, tar and soot, malignant change in senile keratosis, lupus vulgaris and chronic ulcers (Marjolin's ulcer*), malignant change in Bowen's disease† (carcinoma in situ) and in patients on long-term immunosuppressive drugs.

Left untreated, what causes death in these patients?

Blood-borne metastases are unusual in this condition. Death occurs from repeated haemorrhages and infection of the mass, when it eventually and inevitably ulcerates, or haemorrhage from ulceration of the involved lymph nodes infiltrating the groin vessels.

How was this patient treated?

The diagnosis was first confirmed by taking a biopsy under local anaesthetic from the tumour edge. This revealed the typical appearances of a moderately well differentiated squamous carcinoma of the skin

*Jean Nicholas Marjolin (1780–1850), surgeon, Hôpital St Eugénie, Paris.

†John Templeton Bowen (1857–1941), dermatologist, Harvard Medical School, Boston.

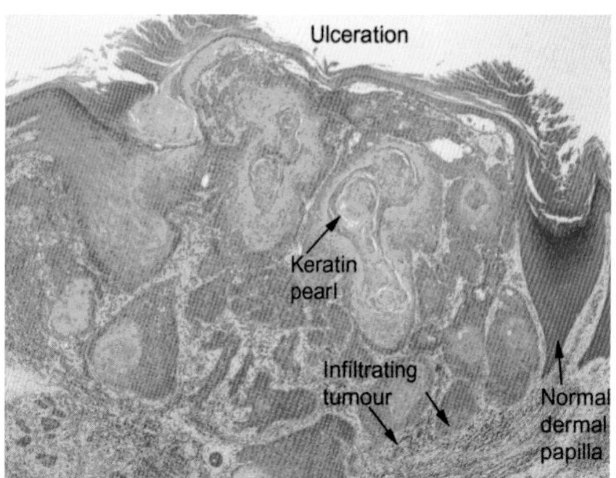

Figure 14.2 Histology of a squamous carcinoma of the skin (magnification × 10, haematoxylin and eosin stain).

(Fig. 14.2). There is ulceration, and tumour is seen infiltrating into the normal adjacent dermis; note the 'keratin pearls' typical of squamous carcinomas.

Wide excision of the primary tumour was performed, with split-skin grafts to the resulting defect, followed by block dissection of the nodes in the groin. She achieved long-term survival!

Case 15 Two old gentlemen with facial ulceration

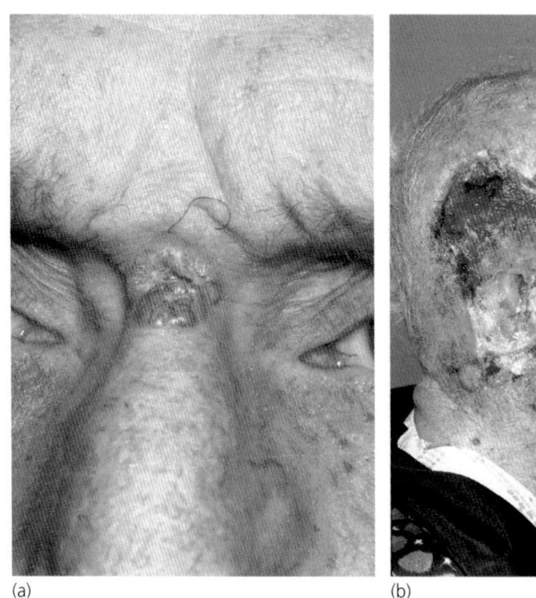

Figure 15.1 (a) (b)

These two patients presented in consecutive weeks in surgical outpatients. Figure 15.1a shows the nose of a 78-year-old retired merchant-seaman, now living in London. He had noticed a little lump on the bridge of his nose about 3 years before, which had slowly grown to its present size. It was painless and had never bled.

On examination, it was firm to touch, not tender, and showed some classical features – pearly nodules, with small blood vessels coursing over its surface and with rolled, rather than everted, edges. These are shown in the sketch made in the patient's clinic notes (Fig. 15.2).

Figure 15.1b shows the extraordinary appearance of the second patient, a retired building worker aged 83. At first he would not tell us how long this lesion had been there, but then admitted that it had started as a 'little pimple' just above the pinna of his right ear 'about 10 or so years ago'. Slowly the lump got bigger, his ear disappeared and the lesion bled from time to time; it also became very smelly but only gave him mild discomfort. He lived by himself and hid the lesion from the neighbours under a scarf.

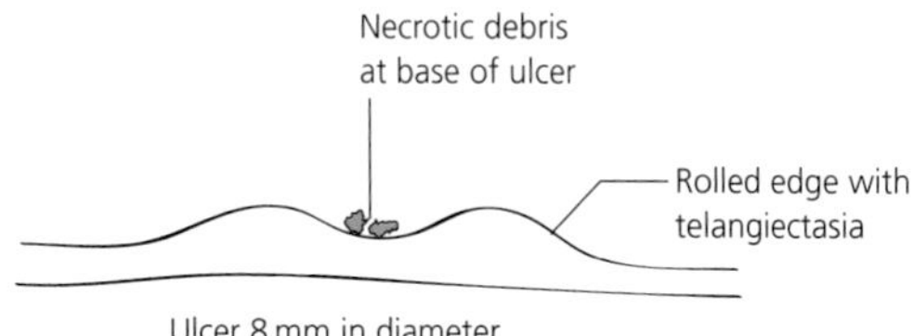

Figure 15.2 Diagram illustrating a rodent ulcer.

Examination revealed not only the ulcer, which exposed the skull and the cartilage of the external auditory meatus, but also numerous maggots. These were killed with surgical spirit before this photograph was taken, but not before a (male) medical student in the clinic had fainted. The regional lymph nodes were impalpable.

What are the scientific and 'popular' names for this lesion?

Basal cell carcinoma and rodent ulcer, respectively.

What is the typical cutaneous distribution of this tumour?

Over 90% are found on the face above a line that joins the angle of the mouth to the external auditory meatus. It is particularly common around the eye, in the nasolabial fold and along the hairline of the scalp.

What is its typical microscopical appearance?

Under the microscope, solid sheets of uniform, darkly staining cells are seen, which arise from the basal layer of the epidermis (basal cell tumour). Prickle cells and epithelial pearls, typical of squamous cell carcinoma of the skin, are absent. Note the central ulceration and islands of basaloid cells in the deep dermis (Fig. 15.3).

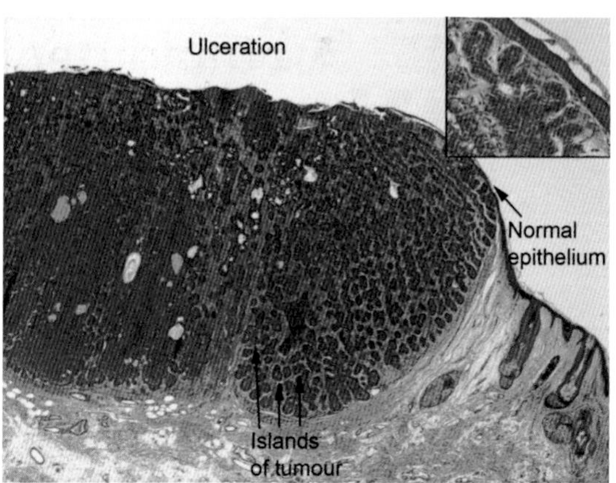

Figure 15.3 Histology of a rodent ulcer (magnification × 2 (inset × 10), haematoxylin and eosin stain).

How does this tumour spread?

Spread is by slow but steady infiltration of the surrounding tissues, which may include the underlying skull and meninges, face, nose and eye (hence the term 'rodent'). Lymphatic spread and blood-borne metastases are extremely rare, and have not been seen by either of the authors.

How are these lesions treated?

A small basal cell tumour can be treated by surgical excision, where this can be done with an adequate margin and without cosmetic deformity. Surgery may also be indicated in late cases, where the tumour has recurred after radiotherapy or where it has invaded underlying bone or cartilage. In these cases, major plastic surgery reconstruction is usually necessary. In most cases, such as in the first patient, the lesion is treated by radiotherapy after biopsy confirmation of the diagnosis.

Case 16 A pigmented spot on the face

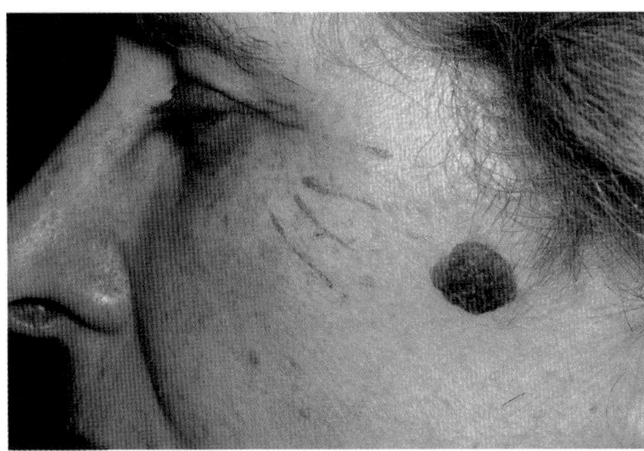

Figure 16.1

This 34-year-old housewife has had this pigmented lesion on her face 'ever since she was a girl' (Fig. 16.1). She does not think it has changed in size but she would now like it removed for cosmetic reasons and because she is worried about what she has read in the papers about malignant melanomas.

How frequent are benign melanomas in the white population?

Nearly everyone with pale skin will have one or more benign melanomas, or 'moles'; often hundreds are present.

What is their cutaneous distribution?

The intradermal melanoma may be found anywhere on the skin apart from the palms of the hands, soles of the feet, the scrotum or the labia. Junctional melanomas may occur on any part of the skin surface.

This lesion was excised and the histology report came back as an intradermal melanoma. What does that term mean?

An intradermal melanoma is situated entirely in the dermis, where melanocytes form non-encapsulated masses (Fig. 16.2b).

What is meant by a junctional melanoma?

In contrast, the junctional melanoma shows melanocytes clumping together in the basal layer of the epidermis, at the junction between the epidermis and dermis (Fig. 16.2c). It is the junctional melanoma that may, in a small percentage of cases, undergo malignant change (Fig. 16.2c).

When should a pigmented lesion of the skin be removed?

Excision of a pigmented lesion of the skin should be carried out under the following circumstances:

- If the patient is worried about it – and this applies disproportionately among doctors, nurses and medical students – or if it is cosmetically unpleasant.
- If it is situated on the hand, sole, nail bed or genitalia – where it is likely to be a junctional melanoma.
- If the lesion shows any of the features that suggest malignant change might have taken place. This will be considered with Case 17 (p. 35).

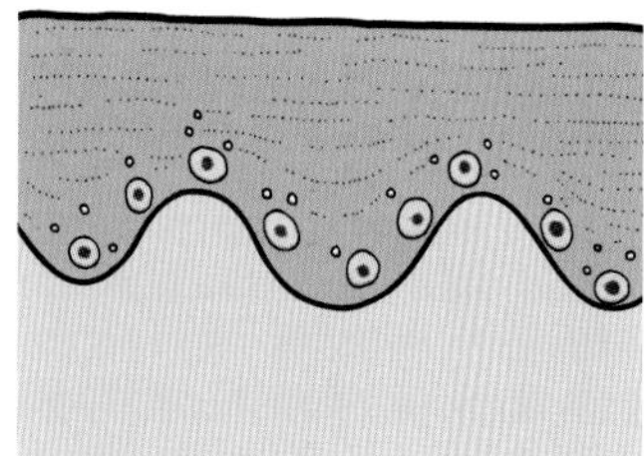

(a) Normal

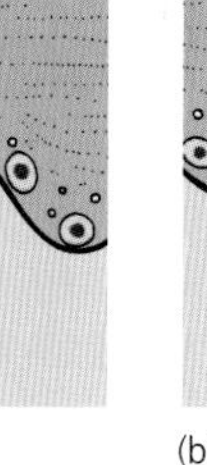

(b) Intradermal melanoma

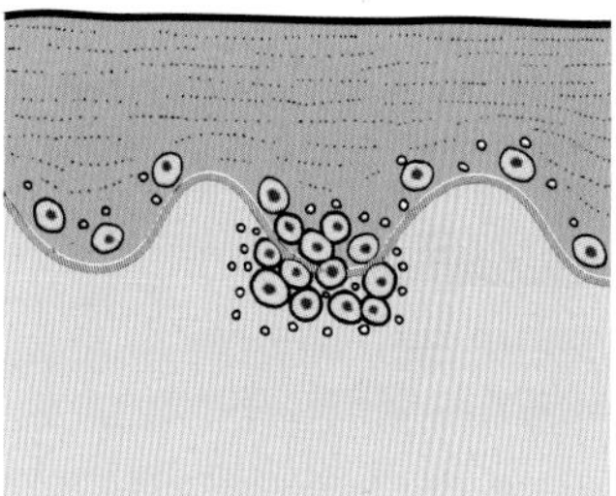

(c) Junctional melanoma

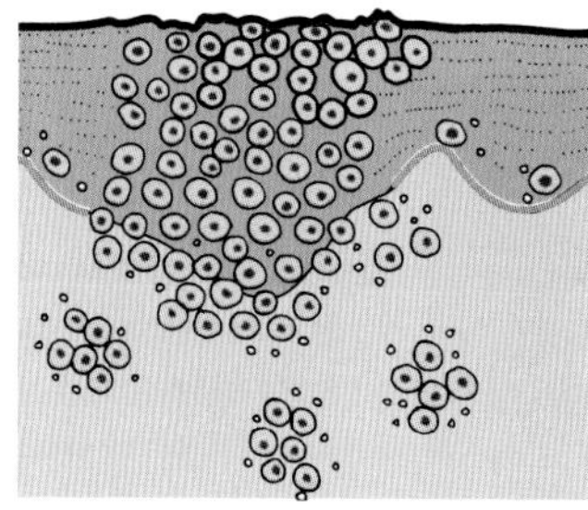

(d) Malignant melanoma

Figure 16.2 (a) Normal skin contains melanocytes (shown as cells) and melanin pigment (shown as dots). The pigment increases in sunburn and freckles. (b) A benign intradermal naevus; the melanocytes are clumped together in the dermis to form a localized benign tumour. (c) A junctional naevus with melanocytes clumping together in the basal layer of the epidermis. These are usually benign but may occasionally give rise to an invasive malignant melanoma (d).

Case 17 A pigmented skin lesion that has got bigger

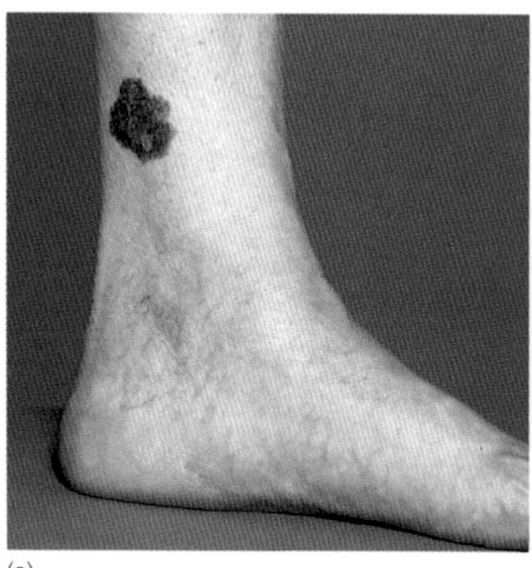

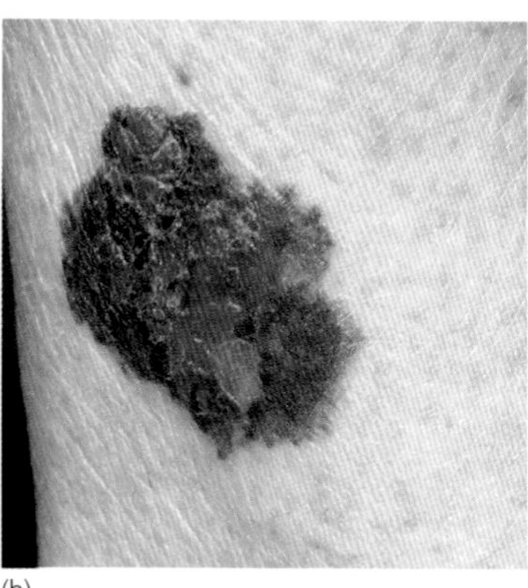

Figure 17.1 (a) (b)

Figure 17.1a shows a pigmented lesion above the left ankle of a schoolmistress aged 40 years. She had noticed a brownish spot there for many years but over the past few months she was aware that it had begun to enlarge quite rapidly. Naturally, she was extremely anxious about this. Figure 17.1b is a close-up view of the lesion.

What features suggest that this is a malignant melanoma?

The story of recent enlargement is important. Careful inspection shows irregularity in its outline, its surface and its pigmentation – all highly suspicious.

What other features, not present in this patient, indicate malignant change?

Other features are bleeding, ulceration, spread of pigment beyond the edge of the tumour and surrounding daughter nodules. A history of itching or pain is also suspicious.

Where would you examine the patient next for evidence of metastatic spread?

Examine all the way along the lower limb for the presence of satellite nodules deposited along the lymphatics. Carefully examine the groin for inguinal lymphadenopathy.

Where else, apart from the skin, may malignant melanomas occur?

Malignant melanomas may occur on the mucosa of the nose, mouth, anal canal and intestine. In the eye, malignant melanomas may be found in the conjunctiva, choroid and pigmented layer of the retina.

What factors determine the prognosis in patients with cutaneous malignant melanomas?

The prognosis in a case of cutaneous malignant melanoma depends on the following:

- The thickness of the primary tumour (the Breslow depth*). If this is less than 0.75 mm, the outlook is excellent. The deeper the lesion, the worse becomes the survival rate; this is associated with the greater danger of lymphatic spread as the invading tumour reaches the lymphatic vessels, which lie in the dermis (Table 17.1).
- A superficial spreading lesion has a better prognosis than a penetrating and ulcerating melanoma – for exactly the same reason.

*Alexander Breslow (1928–1980), pathologist, George Washington University Hospital, Washington DC.

Table 17.1 Survival according to Breslow depth.

Depth (mm)	Five-year survival
<0.75	>95%
0.75–1.5	90%
1.5–4.0	70%
>4.0	<50%

• Melanomas on the limbs have a better prognosis than those of the trunk, the eye and the viscera.

• The presence of cutaneous or lymphatic deposits greatly increases the gravity of the prognosis, while blood-borne metastases, for example to the liver, make the prognosis virtually hopeless.

This patient was treated along standard lines. What are these?

• The lesion was excised and the diagnosis confirmed histologically by frozen section. A wider local excision was then performed with a clearance of 1 cm for every millimetre of Breslow depth of the lesion and the defect repaired by means of a split-skin graft taken from the other thigh (see Case 9, p. 22).

• The sentinel lymph node† in the groin was identified by injection of blue dye around the melanoma preoperatively and was excised – in this case it was free of tumour.

• At follow-up a careful check was performed at each visit on the local area, the skin along the line of the lymphatics of the lower limb and the groin lymph nodes.

• Should inguinal node metastases develop, a block dissection of the groin would be performed.

†A sentinel lymph node is the first lymph node to receive the lymphatic drainage from a tumour. If it is free of tumour on histological examination, lymphatic metastasis has not occurred. If it is positive (tumour is identified), the lymphatic field is excised (block dissection).

Case 18 Lump on the chest wall

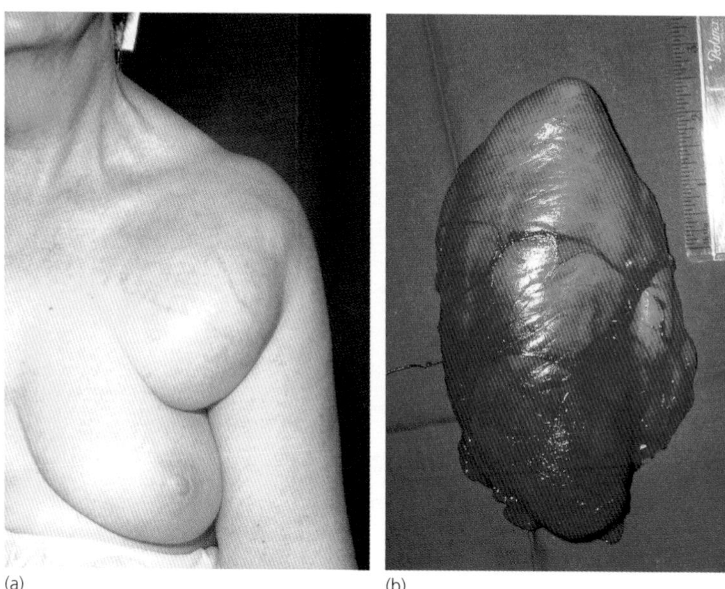

Figure 18.1 (a) (b)

Figure 18.1a shows the appearance of a lump on the chest wall of a housewife aged 58 years. She presented to the surgical outpatient clinic with a history that she had noticed the lump many years before – perhaps 20. It had slowly but surely enlarged over this time, but had never hurt her. Now it was beginning to show through her clothes and both she and her husband were getting embarrassed by this.

She was operated upon in the day surgery unit. Under local anaesthetic infiltration, a transverse skin crease incision was made over the mass. The lump enucleated easily and almost bloodlessly from the subcutaneous tissues. The appearance of the excised specimen is shown in Fig. 18.1b.

On the information given to you at this stage, what is the most likely diagnosis?

A large, benign, subcutaneous lipoma.

What physical signs would you have expected to find on examination of the lump?

The lump would have been soft, lobulated and subcutaneous, with the skin moving over it. It would have been freely moveable on the underlying pectoralis major muscle when this was tensed by getting the patient to put her hand on her side and to press firmly. Fluctuation in two directions at right angles to each other and trans-illumination with a torch in a darkened room would be positive.

Why do subcutaneous lipomas fluctuate?

Fluctuation occurs because lipomas are made up of aggregates of fat cells, each cell containing a microscopic globule of liquid fat. Note that students often reply to this question by saying that fat is liquid at body temperature – yet subcutaneous fat does not come pouring out of a wound when the surgeon makes an incision through the skin!

Lipomas are widely distributed over the surface of the body, but there are three areas of skin where they never occur – name them and give the reason for this

The palm of the hand, the sole of the foot and the scalp. In these areas fat occurs, but lies within dense fibrous septa.

Very rarely these tumours are malignant. What clinical features would suggest this?

A history of recent, rapid enlargement, possibly accompanied by pain. On examination, the mass feels firmer than a benign lipoma, may be less mobile and appears more vascular. Malignant change is so uncommon that removal of a lipoma that is not bothering the patient is not necessary.

Case 19 A patient with a chest drain

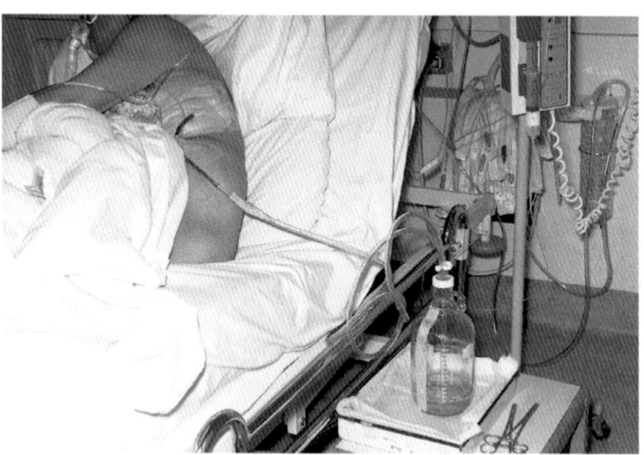

Figure 19.1

This patient underwent a left thoracotomy the day before through the seventh intercostal space. He is now back on the ward breathing spontaneously and is receiving oxygen by means of a face mask. He has a drip of dextrose saline via the cephalic vein at his left wrist and is also on oral fluids.

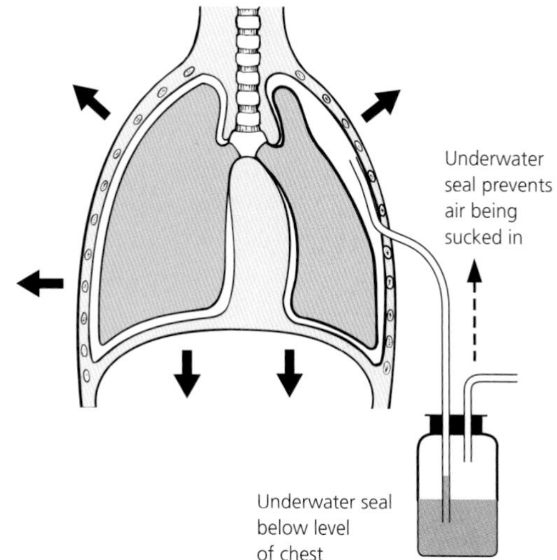

Figure 19.2 Underwater seal chest drain in the treatment of a pneumothroax. Air escapes from the pleural cavity on expiration but cannot be sucked back through the water seal on inspiration (as shown here). The water bottle is placed below level of chest to ensure fluid does not reflux into the thoracic cavity.

What type of drainage system is shown in Fig. 19.1?

An underwater chest drain (details of this are shown in Fig. 19.2). Air escapes from the pleural cavity on expiration but cannot be sucked back when the intrapleural pressure falls in inspiration, as shown here. The water bottle is placed well below the level of the chest to ensure that fluid does not reflux into the chest.

Note the two large drain clamps placed alongside the drainage bottle; if the bottle has to be lifted for any reason – for example, if the bed has to be shifted – the tubing is double clamped to prevent the risk of this reflux from occurring.

What is a pneumothorax?

A pneumothorax means a collection of air in the pleural cavity. It can occur on one or occasionally both sides. A tension pneumothorax results if the pleural tear is valvular, either after trauma, where a bony spicule has lacerated the lung, as shown in Fig. 19.3, or spontaneously, as a result of rupture of an emphysematous bulla of the lung. A tension pneumothorax is an urgent indication for the insertion of a chest drain.

What other pleural injury commonly accompanies chest trauma?

A haemothorax. This may also have an associated pneumothorax; the two together constitute a pneumohaemothorax. This may complicate a closed injury, where the fractured rib may have lacerated an intercostal artery or vein, or arise as a consequence of an underlying contused

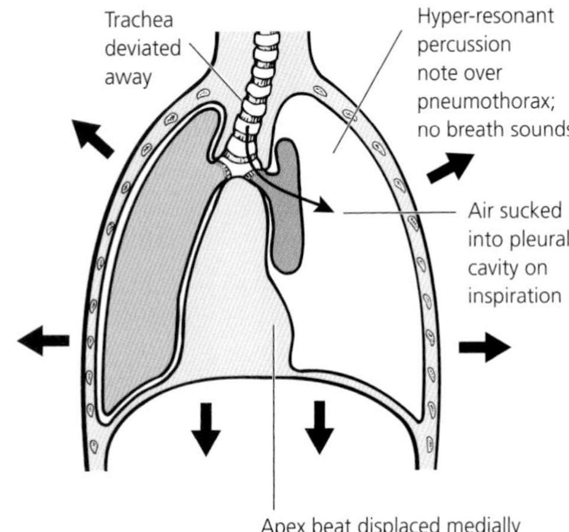

Figure 19.3 Tension pneumothorax produced by a valvular tear in the lung. Air is sucked into the pleural cavity on inspiration and cannot escape on expiration.

lung. It may also result from a penetrating wound of the chest from a stab wound or gun shot injury. On occasions, it may complicate trauma to the heart or great vessels.

How is a traumatic haemothorax treated?

An under water pleural drain is inserted. The fifth intercostal space in the mid-axillary line is recommended as the site for this. The bleeding usually ceases, but continued haemorrhage is an indication for urgent thoracotomy.

Case 20 A fatal lung disease

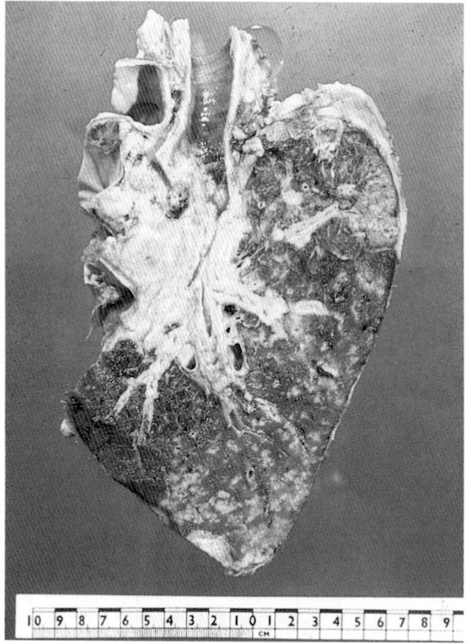

Figure 20.1

Figure 20.1 is the postmortem specimen of the lung of a man aged 68 years.

What is the obvious pathology?

An extensive carcinoma of the lung, which is invading the left main bronchus and with involvement of the hilar lymph nodes.

About how many deaths are attributed to this disease annually in the UK?

About 33 500 deaths in 2005 – making it far and away the leading cause of deaths from malignant disease in the UK, accounting for over one-fifth of all cancer deaths. It is commoner in men than women, but this disparity is lessening year by year. Survival is dismal, with 1- and 5-year survivals of 25% and 6%, respectively.

What are the known predisposing factors in this disease?

The main predisposing factor is cigarette smoking, although the condition occasionally occurs in lifetime non-smokers. Other factors include air pollution with diesel, petrol and other fumes. The incidence is higher in urban than in rural populations. Radioactive carcinogens in certain mines are associated with lung carcinoma.

List the main histological types of this disease

- Twenty per cent are small cell (oat cell) carcinoma (Fig. 20.2a).
- Eighty per cent are non-small cell lung cancer (NSCLC). Of these, 20–25% are squamous cell (Fig. 20.2b), 50–60% are adenocarcinoma (Fig. 20.1c) and the remainder are undifferentiated large cell carcinoma (Fig. 20.2d).

List the pathways of spread of this tumour

There are four potential pathways of spread of a malignant tumour, and carcinoma of the lung may manifest all four of these in its advanced stage.

- *Local*: Invasion of the lung parenchyma, eventually reaching the pleural surface and chest wall; spread along the bronchus.
- *Lymphatic*: To the hilar, mediastinal and cervical lymph nodes.
- *Blood*: Especially to the liver, bone and brain.
- *Transcoelomic*: Seeding over the pleura, with resulting pleural effusion.

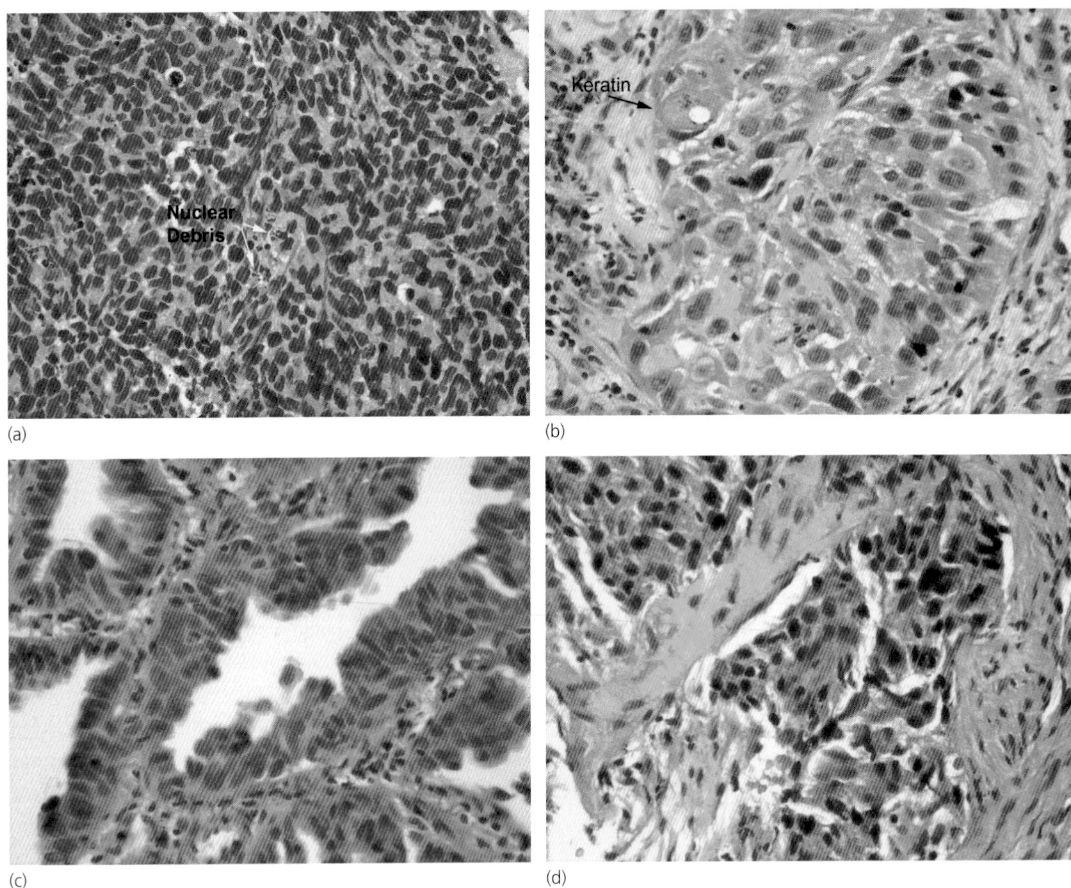

Figure 20.2 The different types of lung cancer. (a) Small cell carcinoma. There are numerous infiltrating small cells with prominent nuclei and little cytoplasm. The cells are fragile and prone to 'smear' artefact, and typical nuclear (karyorrhectic) debris. (b) Squamous cell carcinoma. Note the large eosinophilic cells and keratin in the tumour (arrowed). (c) Adenocarcinoma showing a typical glandular architecture with tall columnar cells. (d) Large cell carcinoma with large pleomorphic cells. (Magnification × 40, haematoxylin and eosin stain.)

Case 21 A pulsating abdominal mass

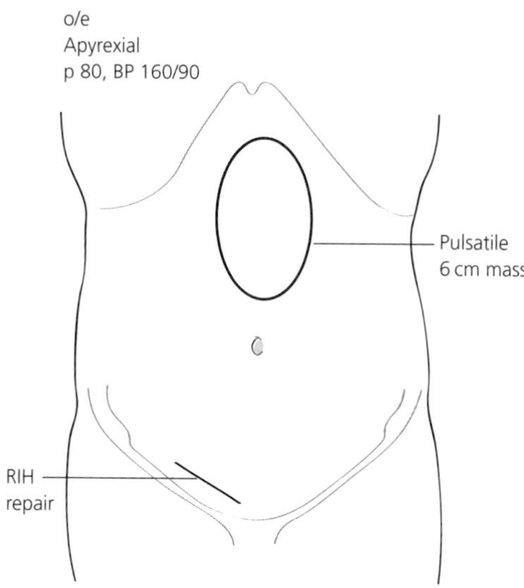

Figure 21.1

A solicitor, still very fit and fully employed at the age of 70 years, had a particularly conscientious family practitioner, who was keen on giving the septuagenarians in his practice a full medical check-up. To the doctor's surprise, he detected an obvious pulsating mass in the abdomen; his sketch of his findings, recorded in his notes, is shown in Fig. 21.1. Apart from a mild degree of hypertension the examination was otherwise negative.

What was the doctor's (correct) clinical diagnosis, and why?

An abdominal aortic aneurysm. The abdominal aorta is palpable in the normal subject. Its pulse is felt by downward pressure in the midline. This pulsation ceases where the aorta bifurcates into the common iliac arteries in front of the fourth lumbar vertebra. This is located at the level of the supracristal line that joins the iliac crests on each side (Fig. 21.2). A pulsating mass below this line

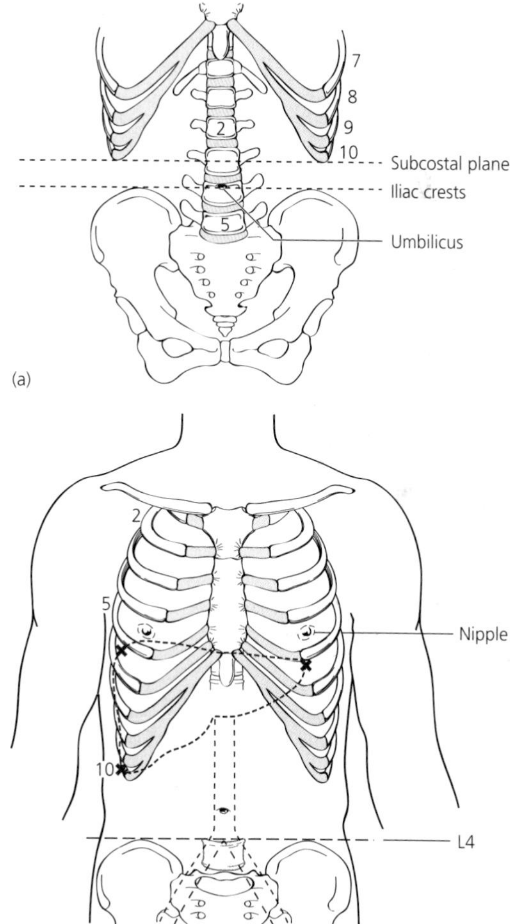

(b) X's mark the outline of the liver which reaches from the 5th intercostal space R to the 5th intercostal space L in mid clavicular line, and lower margin 10th rib

The aorta bifurcates at L4 which is in line with the iliac crests

Figure 21.2 Boundaries, bony landmarks and vertebral levels of the abdomen.

cannot therefore be an aortic aneurysm. It is either an iliac aneurysm or a pelvic mass with transmitted pulsation from the iliac arteries.

Whereas the normal aortic pulse gives a forward and backwards impulse to the examining fingers, an aneurysm gives an expansile sensation detected by a finger placed on either side of the mass. Auscultation of an aortic aneurysm is usually negative since turbulent flow is not usually a feature of an aneurysm in this situation. However, in the acute situation a machinery murmur suggests an aorto-caval fistula.

His doctor arranged an urgent plain abdominal X-ray to be carried out at the local hospital. What does this demonstrate?

The abdominal X-ray (Fig. 21.3) demonstrates the calcified wall of the aneurysm (arrowed). Note that this bulges over to the left side – a very typical appearance – away from the inferior vena cava, which runs along its right border.

What is the usual proximal extent of the aneurysm?

Interestingly, the great majority of abdominal aortic aneurysms are infrarenal, that is to say, they lie distal to the origins of the renal arteries and therefore distal to where the left renal vein crosses over the front of the aorta, below the origin of the superior mesenteric artery (Fig. 21.4).

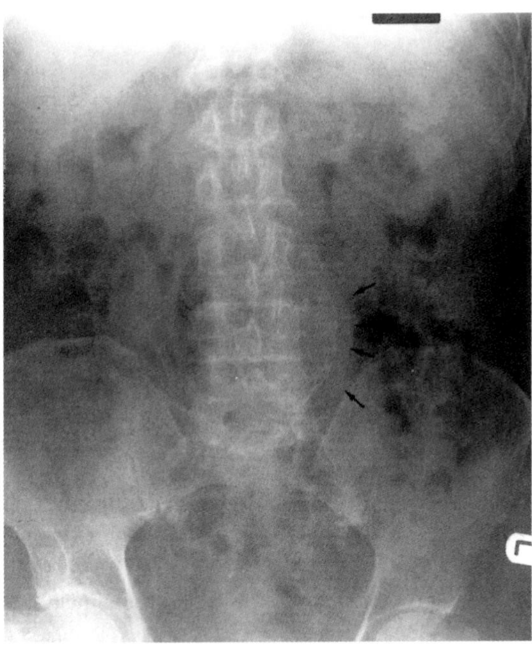

Figure 21.3 Abdominal X-ray showing the aneurysm (arrowed).

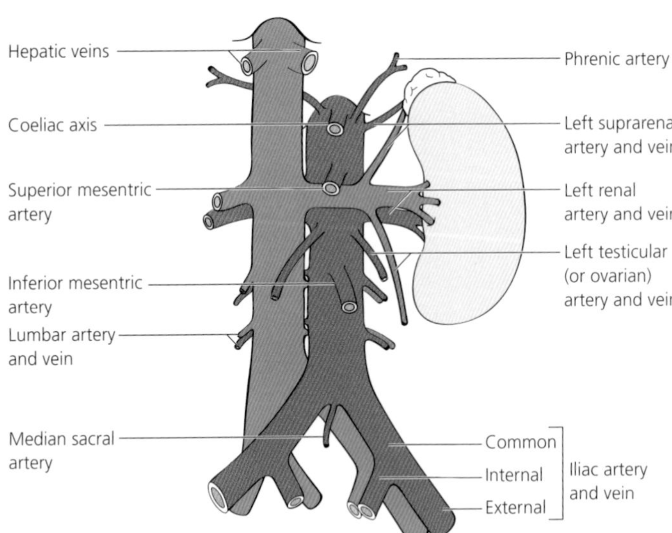

Figure 21.4 The abdominal aorta and inferior vena cava and their main branches.

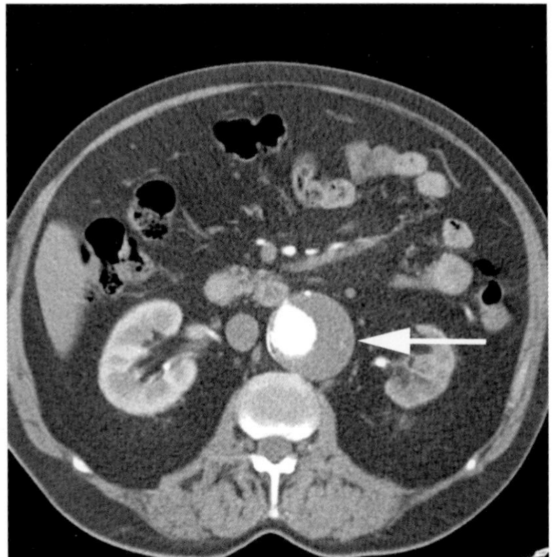

Figure 21.5 A CT scan showing a transverse section through the abdomen with a large abdominal aortic aneurysm (AAA, arrowed). The white area within the AAA is contrast material in the lumen of the aorta injected intravenously a few seconds prior to scanning. Lateral to the contrast-containing lumen is a clot within the aneurysm sac.

The occasional suprarenal aortic aneurysm presents a technically difficult problem, since, to deal with it, the aorta needs to be controlled above the origins of the superior mesenteric, coeliac and renal arteries. This requires a thoraco-abdominal approach and all these arteries are reimplanted into the graft.

What further imaging methods are used to delineate the aneurysm?

Abdominal ultrasound is a useful and accessible imaging method and is used in population screening and in the measurement of the anteroposterior diameter of the aneurysm. Computed tomography (CT), with intravenous contrast enhancement, gives very accurate delineation of the aneurysm (Fig. 21.5) and detects associated aneurysms of the common and internal iliac arteries, which are not uncommon.

What is the principal complication of this condition and what is its mortality?

- Rupture, first retroperitoneally and then into the peritoneal cavity.
- The mortality is in the region of 80%.

What is the management of this patient?

Elective repair of the aneurysm is advised in patients when the risk of death from rupture is greater than the operative mortality. This corresponds to an aortic aneurysm anteroposterior diameter over 5.5 cm on ultrasound scanning; the operative mortality is around 4%. Repair can be performed by the open method, replacing the aneurysm with a tube of Dacron, or by the closed method. In the latter, a graft is passed endoluminally from the femoral artery across the aneurysm sac where it is anchored proximally and distally with intraluminal stents.

Case 22 Abdominal bruising

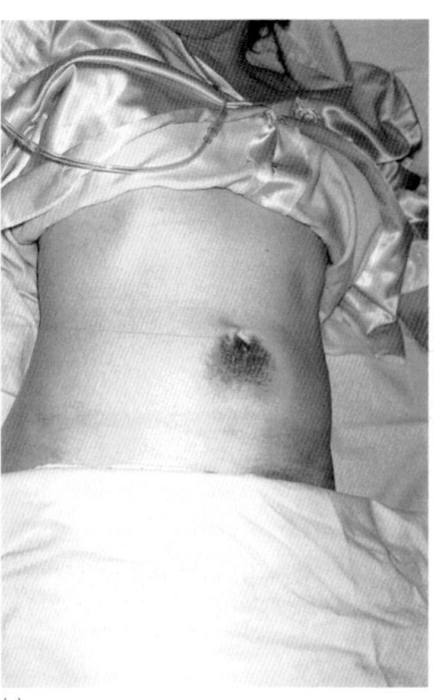

(a)

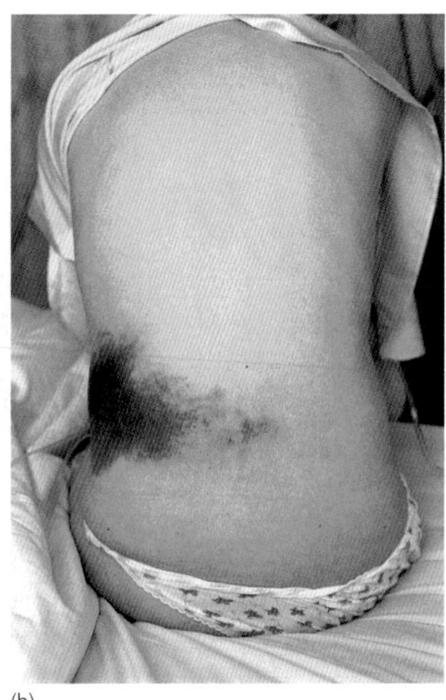

(b)

Figure 22.1

A fit 72-year-old woman presented with a 12 h history of sudden onset severe abdominal pain radiating to her back. With the onset of the pain she collapsed, and on recovering could not stand without feeling faint. On presentation the following day she had developed bruising of the abdominal wall (Fig. 22.1). She underwent a CT scan.

What are the two eponymous signs and what do they signify?

Cullen's sign and Grey Turner's sign. Thomas Cullen (1868–1953), a gynaecologist at Johns Hopkins, Baltimore, described a periumbilical bluish discolouration in a case of ruptured ectopic pregnancy in 1922. George Grey Turner (1877–1951), a surgeon from Newcastle upon Tyne and later the Royal Postgraduate Medical School, Hammersmith Hospital, London, described lumbar discolouration as a feature of acute pancreatitis in 1920.

What conditions are they associated with?

They are associated with causes of retroperitoneal haemorrhage, such as acute haemorrhagic pancreatitis, ruptured abdominal aortic or iliac aneurysm and ruptured ectopic pregnancy.

This patient underwent a plain X-ray and CT scan. What do they show and what is the diagnosis?

The abdominal X-ray shows absence of the left psoas shadow and the descending colon stretched laterally (Fig. 22.2a). The CT scan shows a 6 cm abdominal aortic

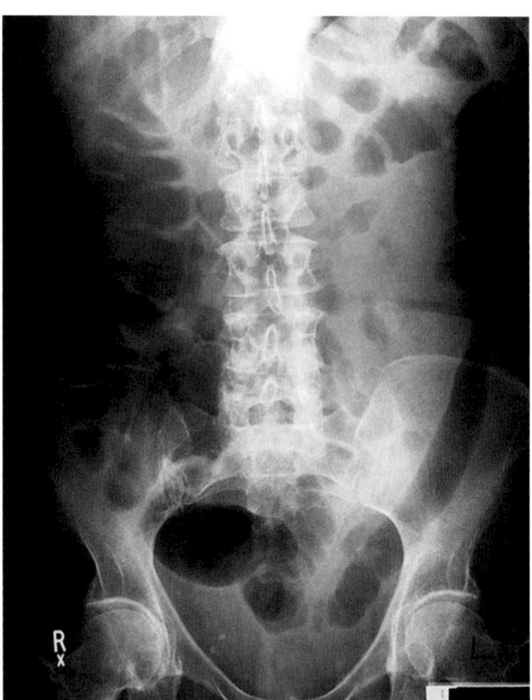

(a)

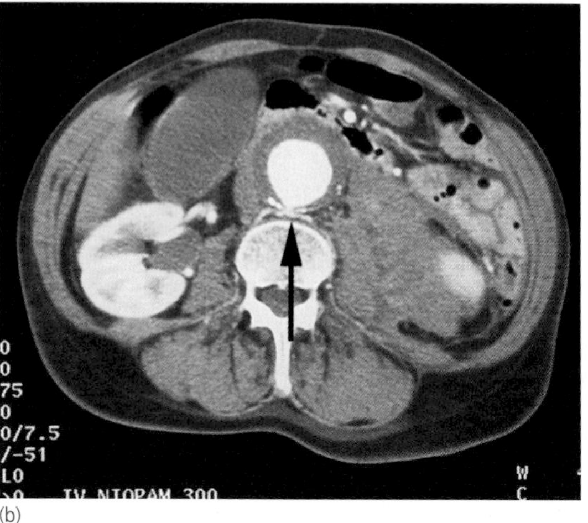

(b)

Figure 22.2 (a) Plain X-ray, (b) CT scan of the patient.

aneurysm with a rind of thrombus (called mural thrombus) around the lumen, which is white due to the administration of contrast medium (Fig. 22.2b). The rind is deficient posteriorly, the site of a rupture (arrowed). There is extensive haemorrhage around the lower pole of the left kidney and the descending colon is seen displaced posterolaterally around the haematoma. She has suffered a ruptured abdominal aneurysm with a contained retroperitoneal haematoma.

Case 23 A painful calf

A building construction worker aged 48 years is referred by his family practitioner to the vascular clinic of a university hospital. His excellent referral note reads as follows:

> The patient has been a heavy smoker since his teens. He has attended the surgery for the past year or so with pain in the left calf on walking. I have tried, without any success at all, to cut down his 30 cigarettes a day habit. Recently the pain has got much worse, so that he can now only hobble a few yards, and I have had to sign him off work. On examination the left foot is cold and pale. Although I can feel all the pulses in his right leg, I can only find his left femoral pulse. His BP is 150/80 and there is no glycosuria.

What is your provisional diagnosis on reading this letter?

He has severe claudication pain affecting the calf muscles of the left leg as a result of occlusion of the arterial supply to his lower limb. The block is somewhere between the femoral artery at the groin, whose pulse can be felt, and the popliteal artery, whose pulse is impalpable.

Are there any further details you would want to elicit in your history and examination of this patient?

Yes indeed. You would want to find out if there is clinical evidence of other areas involved in this occlusive arterial disease. Enquire carefully for any history of angina pectoris or transient ischaemic attacks (TIAs), and any story that might suggest a previous myocardial infarct or cerebral vascular accident. Carefully examine the heart and central nervous system, and examine the blood vessels of the retina through an ophthalmoscope.

Locally, is the skin of the foot cold, does it look pale or cyanotic, does it blanche on elevation and become cyanosed when hanging dependent (Buerger's sign*), and do the superficial veins of the leg 'gutter' when the leg is elevated? Is the return of capillary circulation to the toes delayed when the skin is blanched by firm pressure?

A useful measurement is to take the brachial blood pressure and then the lower limb pressure using a special long blood pressure cuff. Normally, the brachial and ankle pressures are about the same. 'Critical ischaemia' is defined as when the ankle pressure is less than 50% of the brachial pressure (the ankle–brachial pressure index, ABPI). It will almost inevitably be so in this case, but the test provides useful objective documentation.

At the peripheral vascular clinic, an urgent arteriogram was ordered, and is shown here. What does it demonstrate?

There is a short block at the bifurcation of the left common femoral artery (Fig. 23.1, arrowed); the main vessels show irregularities due to arteriosclerosis. Collateral vessels can be seen around this occlusion.

What is the condition of the artery distal to the obstruction on the left side, and why is this important?

The distal superficial femoral artery and the popliteal artery are patent. This means that there is a 'good run-off' and, other things being equal, the patient is suitable for some sort of reconstructive procedure.

How can the patient's disabling symptoms be treated?

Smoking must be prohibited. There is little point in carrying out any reconstructive procedure unless the patient gives up the habit because of the very high risk of re-occlusion. This short section of occlusion is best treated by angioplasty using a balloon catheter under X-ray control, with or without insertion of a stent.

---

*Leo Buerger (1879–1943), born in Vienna, surgeon, Mount Sinai Hospital, New York.

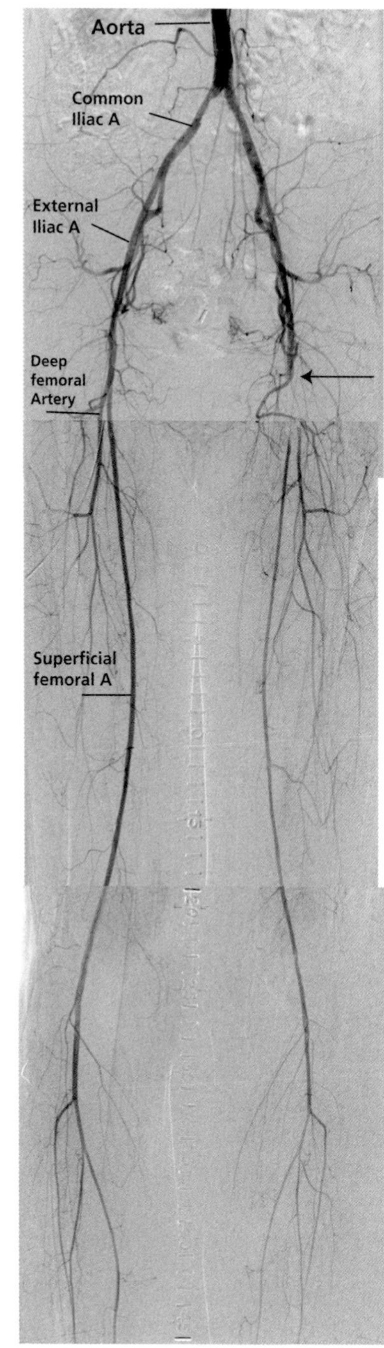

Figure 23.1 Arteriogram of the patient showing the arteries from aortic bifurcation to calf. The block in the left superficial femoral artery is arrowed. A, artery.

Case 24 Black toes

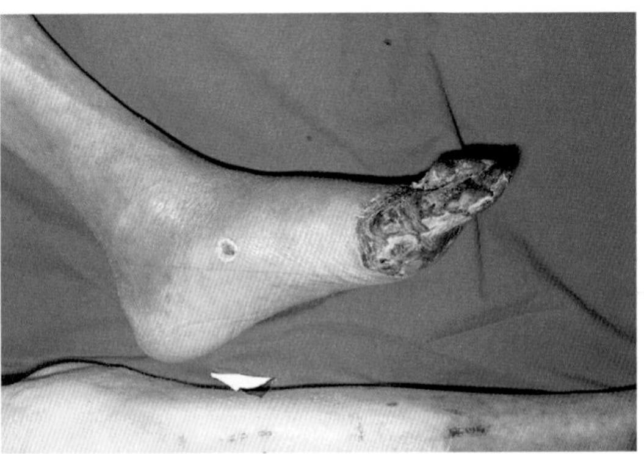

Figure 24.1

A 40-year-old, unemployed labourer presented to the accident and emergency department with these black, but not especially painful, toes on his left foot (Fig. 24.1). He was a known diabetic, on insulin, but confessed to being very bad about taking it and was rather confused about his correct dosage. He admitted that he often neglected the advice given to him in the diabetic clinic concerning his diet and care of his feet and, all too frequently, indulged in drinking bouts with his mates. He smoked 'as many cigarettes as he could get' – probably about 20 a day.

On examination, the left hallux and the second and third toes were obviously gangrenous and infected. There was some pitting oedema over the dorsum of the foot. All the pulses in the right lower limb were present. On the left side, the femoral and popliteal pulses were easily felt but not the ankle pulses. However, these could be picked up using the Doppler probe. There was diminution of sensation to both vibration and fine touch (10 g nylon monofilament) over both feet. Clinical examination was otherwise normal and this included fundoscopy, with no evidence of diabetic retinopathy. The urine tested strongly positive for sugar in the A&E department.

What is the, pretty obvious, diagnosis?

Diabetic gangrene of the left foot with clinical evidence of diabetic neuropathy.

What factors in his diabetes contributed towards development of the gangrene?

- *Diabetic microangiopathy*: This affects the blood vessels at arteriolar level with subintimal hyperplasia. The same pathology leads to the characteristic changes of diabetic retinopathy.
- The poorly controlled diabetes also predisposes to infection of the poorly vascularized tissues.
- *Diabetic neuropathy* (typically glove and stocking distribution of diminished sensation): This increases the risk of minor, unnoticed trauma to the skin of the foot, allowing ingress of bacteria into the ischaemic soft tissues.

What factors in smoking contribute to this condition?

- Nicotine produces vasospasm at an arteriolar level.
- Inhaled carbon monoxide in the smoke is taken up by haemoglobin to form carboxyhaemoglobin, which reduces the oxygen-carrying capacity of the blood. It is slowly dissociated, so this phenomenon persists long after the cigarette is stubbed out.
- Smoking increases platelet adhesiveness and so encourages thrombosis.

How should the patient be treated initially?

He requires emergency hospital admission. The diabetes is brought under control with insulin and diet adjustment. Broad spectrum antibiotic treatment is commenced after a bacteriological swab has been taken, the organisms identified and their sensitivities determined. Smoking is vetoed.

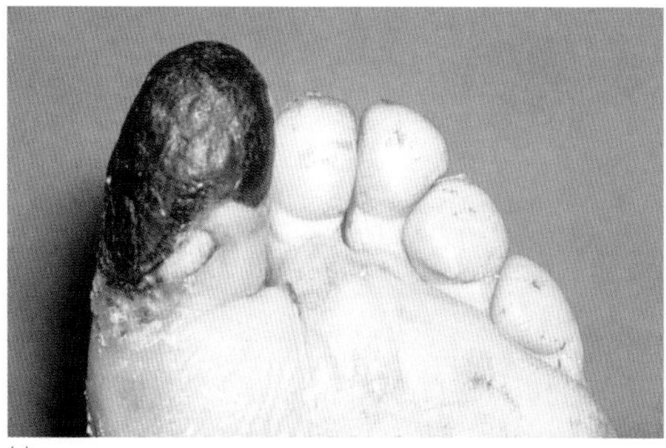

(a)

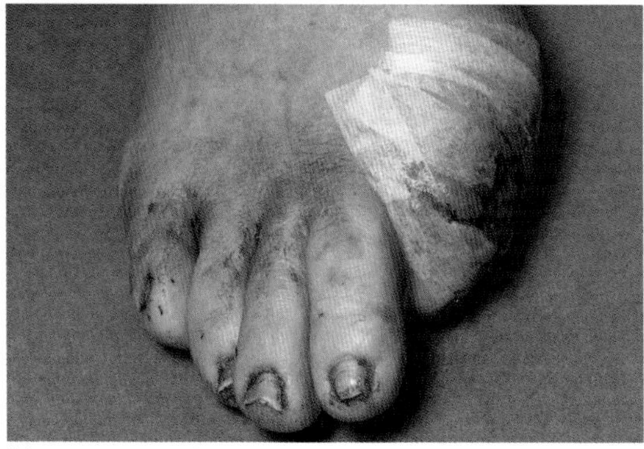

(b)

Figure 24.2 (a) Before and (b) after surgery in a diabetic patient with diabetic gangrene.

Is major amputation likely to be necessary in this patient?

This is unlikely in the first instance. The peripheral pulses are present, so this is a local phenomenon due to the factors already described. Under a general anaesthetic, all the necrotic tissues are excised as a forefoot amputation, resulting in a deformed but useful foot. Such local amputation is demonstrated in these 'before and after' photographs of a similar patient with diabetic gangrene (Fig. 24.2). If the patient persists in smoking and continues ignoring his diabetes he will inevitably develop further diabetic complications necessitating a more proximal amputation.

Case 25 A useful instrument in vascular surgery

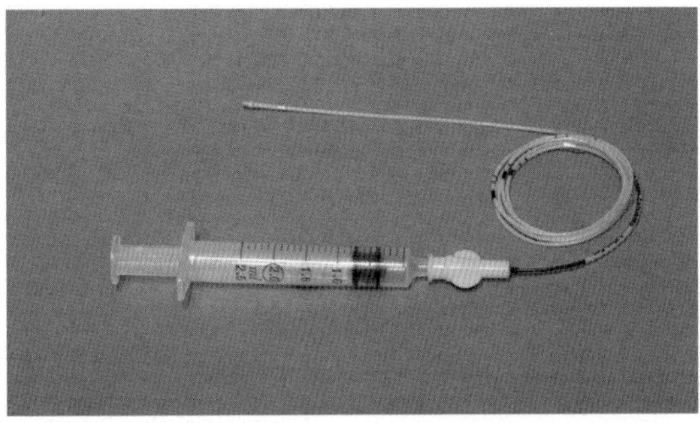

(a)

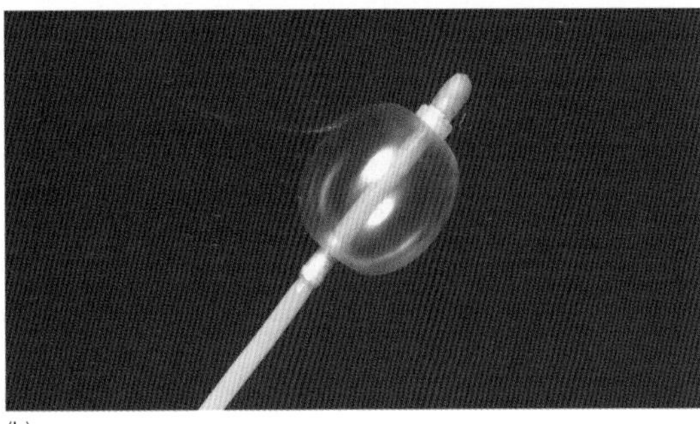

(b)

Figure 25.1

Figure 25.1a shows a valuable instrument used in arterial surgery. Figure 25.1b is a close-up of its tip when inflated.

What is it called?

A Fogarty balloon catheter.

What was the status of the inventor when he designed it?

Thomas Fogarty* thought of this while he was a medical student, and his reputation was made by the time he became a surgical resident.

*Thomas Fogarty (b. 1934), surgeon, Portland, Oregon.

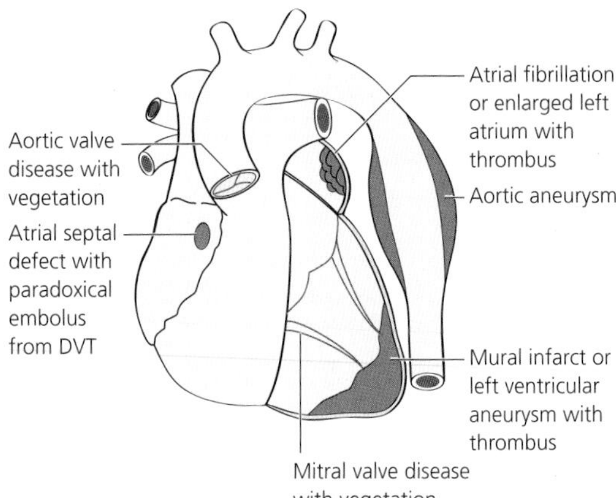

Figure 25.2 Sources of peripheral emboli. DVT, deep vein thrombosis.

What vascular emergency is it used for?

Its principal use is to remove an occluding embolus and propagated clot from a blocked peripheral artery. It is slid down the artery through a proximal arteriotomy, the balloon is then inflated and the catheter withdrawn, allowing the embolus and distal clot to be withdrawn. The procedure is repeated till all the occluding material has been removed, as shown by free back-bleeding.

What drug should be commenced at once by the intravenous route in this condition?

Intravenous heparin should be commenced at once to prevent further propagation of clot.

What is the most important prognostic factor in deciding the fate of the limb in a case of peripheral embolism?

The likelihood of success of embolectomy is inversely proportional to the time interval from the onset of the block to the embolectomy. After 24 h have elapsed, successful disobliteration becomes unlikely. A limb that is unlikely to be viable even after disobliteration of the artery is characterized by the development of purpuric skin staining that does not blanche on pressure ('fixed staining').

What is the definition of an embolus?

An embolus is abnormal, undissolved material carried in the blood stream from one part of the vascular system to impact in a distant part. While the embolus may comprise air, fat or tumour, it is usually thrombus which becomes detached from its source, usually in the heart or the major vessels. The common sources of embolism are shown in Fig. 25.2.

Case 26 A young woman with cold hands

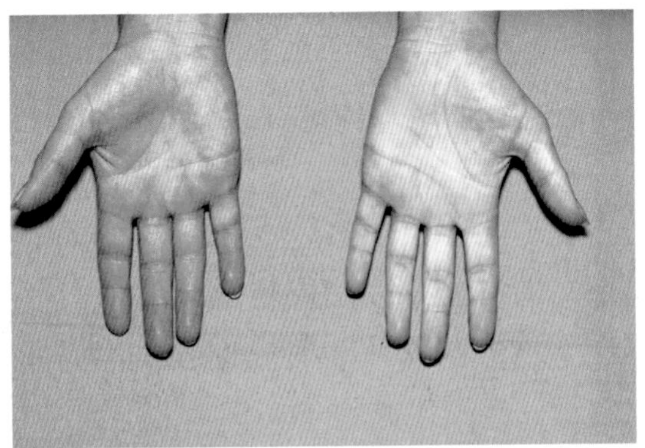

Figure 26.1

Figure 26.1 shows the hands of a secretary aged 20 years, which was taken on a warm, sunny day, when she is usually free of symptoms. However, the left hand has just been immersed in a bowl of water with ice cubes floating in it for a period of 5 min.

What do you notice about the appearance of the left hand?

The left hand has become bluish-white compared with the normal appearance on the right side. The patient also says that the left hand has now become painful, tingling and numb. This exactly mimics what her hands and feet feel like in the cold weather.

What disease do you suspect she has?

Raynaud's disease, named after Maurice Raynaud,* a 19th century Parisian physician who gave a good clinical description of this condition.

*Maurice Raynaud (1834–1881), physician, Paris.

What are the clinical features of this condition?

It nearly always affects females. Cold, painful, numb hands (and often feet) dating back to childhood and occurring in cold weather. Symptoms are absent or much milder in warm weather. The extremities become bluish-white when exposed to cold. Gangrene of the tips of the digits may occur, but is very rare. As the hand is warmed and the circulation improves, the affected areas turn red and throb.

What is the assumed pathology of this condition?

Idiopathic spasm of the digital arterioles. The peripheral pulses are perfectly normal in this condition.

What other conditions produce arterial impairment in the upper limb?

A whole variety of vascular diseases can produce ischaemic symptoms and signs in the upper limb. These are grouped together under the term Raynaud's phenomenon, in contrast to Raynaud's disease. These include arterial trauma, embolism (Fig. 26.2a), arteriosclerosis, cervical rib, scleroderma, other collagen diseases (Fig. 26.2b), and cryoglobinaemia; it also occurs in workers using vibrating tools. In contrast to patients with Raynaud's disease, gangrene of the fingers may occur in these patients.

What treatment can be advised for this patient?

Some patients emigrate to a hot, sunny climate. For those less fortunate, the use of fur-lined or heated gloves and boots is advised during cold weather. Smoking should be stopped, as should β-blockers. A trial should be made of vasodilator drugs such as calcium channel antagonists like diltiazem and nifedipine. Sympathectomy produces dramatic improvement but, unfortunately, this is often not long-lasting.

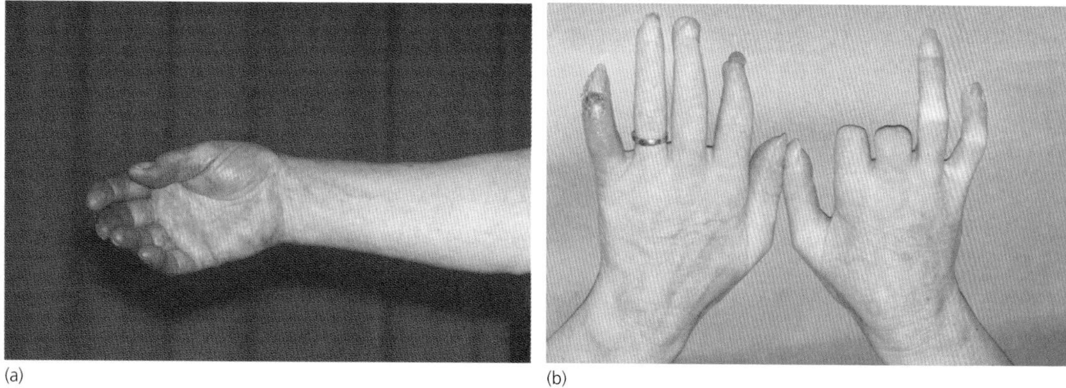

(a) (b)

Figure 26.2 (a) A hand following digital emboli. (b) Hands of a patient with scleroderma.

Case 27 A complication of varicose veins

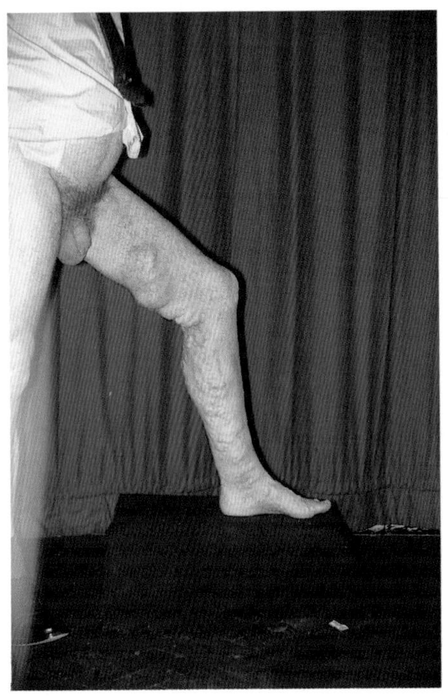

Figure 27.1

This patient is a brick-layer aged 55 years. He has had varicose veins on both his legs, left worse than right, for many years. They have gradually become more noticeable, but as they did not interfere with his heavy work, he never bothered about them. However, in the past few days the veins in his left thigh have become hard and painful and he noticed that the overlying skin had become very red (Fig. 27.1).

What complication of his varicose veins has taken place in his left thigh?

Acute phlebitis. The stagnant column of blood in the varices has clotted and set up a sterile inflammatory reaction.

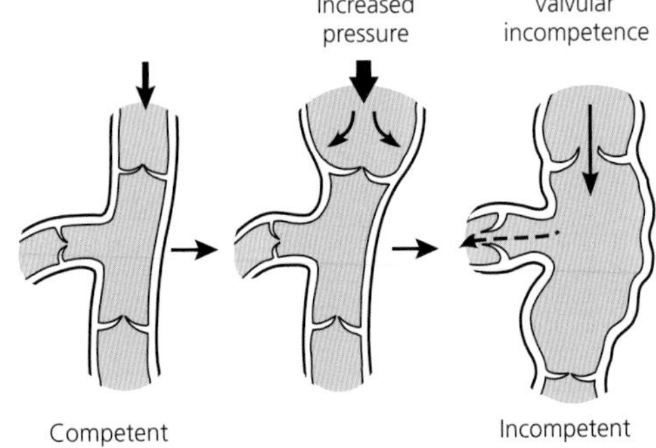

Figure 27.2 Normal veins and incompetent varicose veins. Note the vein dilates under pressure and the valve becomes incompetent.

How should this complication be treated?

Bed rest and elevation of the leg – the foot higher than the knee, the knee higher than the thigh. Antibiotics are rarely indicated as this is a sterile inflammatory process in the great majority of cases.

If you see a teenager with varicose veins, what would you usually find in the family history?

There is usually a story that one or both parents and often siblings and other family members are also affected. This presumably means that there is a congenital predilection for some defect in the valves, the basis of the development of varices (Fig. 27.2).

This patient has a particularly large bulge at the saphenous termination at his groin. What is this called, and how would you confirm the diagnosis?

A saphena varix. This swelling is often misdiagnosed as a femoral hernia, but there should be no difficulty in making the correct diagnosis. With the patient standing, the lump gives a characteristic thrill to the examining finger on coughing, as a column of blood refluxes into the varix. The tap test is performed by having the patient stand, placing your finger over the varix and tapping over distally placed varices – a transmitted thrill will be detected. Finally, the varix disappears immediately when the patient lies down.

If traumatized, large varicose veins like these can bleed furiously if the patient is standing up. In this position, the veins are at high pressure, with a column of blood, unsupported by valves, extending up to the right atrium! How would you treat this dangerous emergency?

Lie the patient flat, raise the leg vertically in the air and apply a firm dressing to the bleeding point. When he was a house surgeon, one of the authors treated a woman with this emergency who had nearly died of blood loss.

Case 28 A chronic leg ulcer

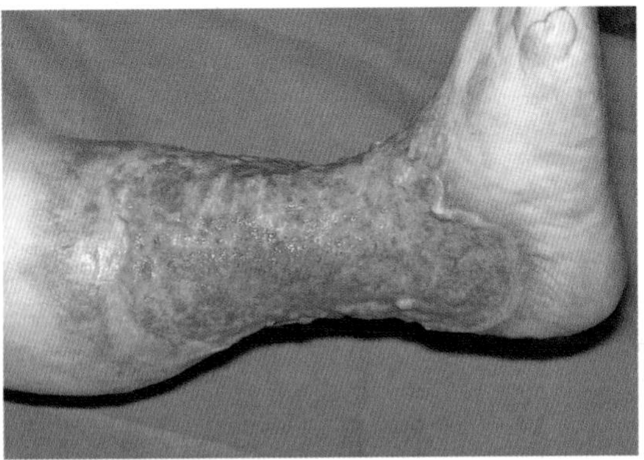

Figure 28.1

This patient, a housewife aged 72 years, had had this ulcer on her leg for many years (Fig. 28.1). She thought it had followed a 'swollen leg' that she had during her last (fourth) pregnancy when she was 38 years old. She had treated her leg with various balms and ointments from the chemist's shop, but had never sought medical advice. Apart from this lesion, general examination revealed an obese, but otherwise healthy, old woman. A routine blood count was normal and her blood sugar was within normal limits.

What names are given to this common condition?

The popular term is varicose ulcer, which is often a misnomer, as will be discussed below. Other names are venous ulcer or gravitational ulcer.

On examination, there was no evidence of varicose veins on either leg, so what is the likely aetiology of the ulcer in this patient?

A preceding deep vein thrombosis (presumably complicating her last pregnancy). This would have caused damage to the valves of the deep veins in her leg, which would have resulted in venous hypertension and, therefore, poor cutaneous blood supply to the skin and subcutaneous tissues of the lower leg.

What do you notice about the patient's foot and the skin surrounding the ulcer? Can you explain these changes?

The foot is oedematous as a result of the venous hypertension in the lower leg (remember Starling's law of fluid exchange in the tissues). The skin surrounding the ulcer shows the typical pigmentation, often called 'varicose eczema', which results from diapedesis of red cells through the capillaries. These break down and deposit haemosiderin in the soft tissues.

What is a dangerous, but fortunately uncommon, complication of longstanding cases of this disease?

Malignant change at the edge of the ulcer into a squamous carcinoma – an example of a Marjolin's ulcer* (malignant change in any chronic ulcer). Indeed, we were suspicious that this might have taken place at the lower edge of this woman's ulcer, but a tissue biopsy revealed no evidence of tumour. A clinical feature that suggests malignancy is a non-healing ulcer with a raised margin, particularly one that has shown a recent unexplained deterioration in appearance.

What are the other possible causes of a chronic ulcer of the leg?

Venous ulcers are by far the commonest cause of a chronic ulcer of the leg in the Western world, and account for about 90% of cases. However, it is important to remember that other causes occur, whose treatment and prognosis may be very different. These can be listed as follows:

• Venous ulcer: Complicating deep venous insufficiency.

---

*Marjolin – see Case 14, p. 29.

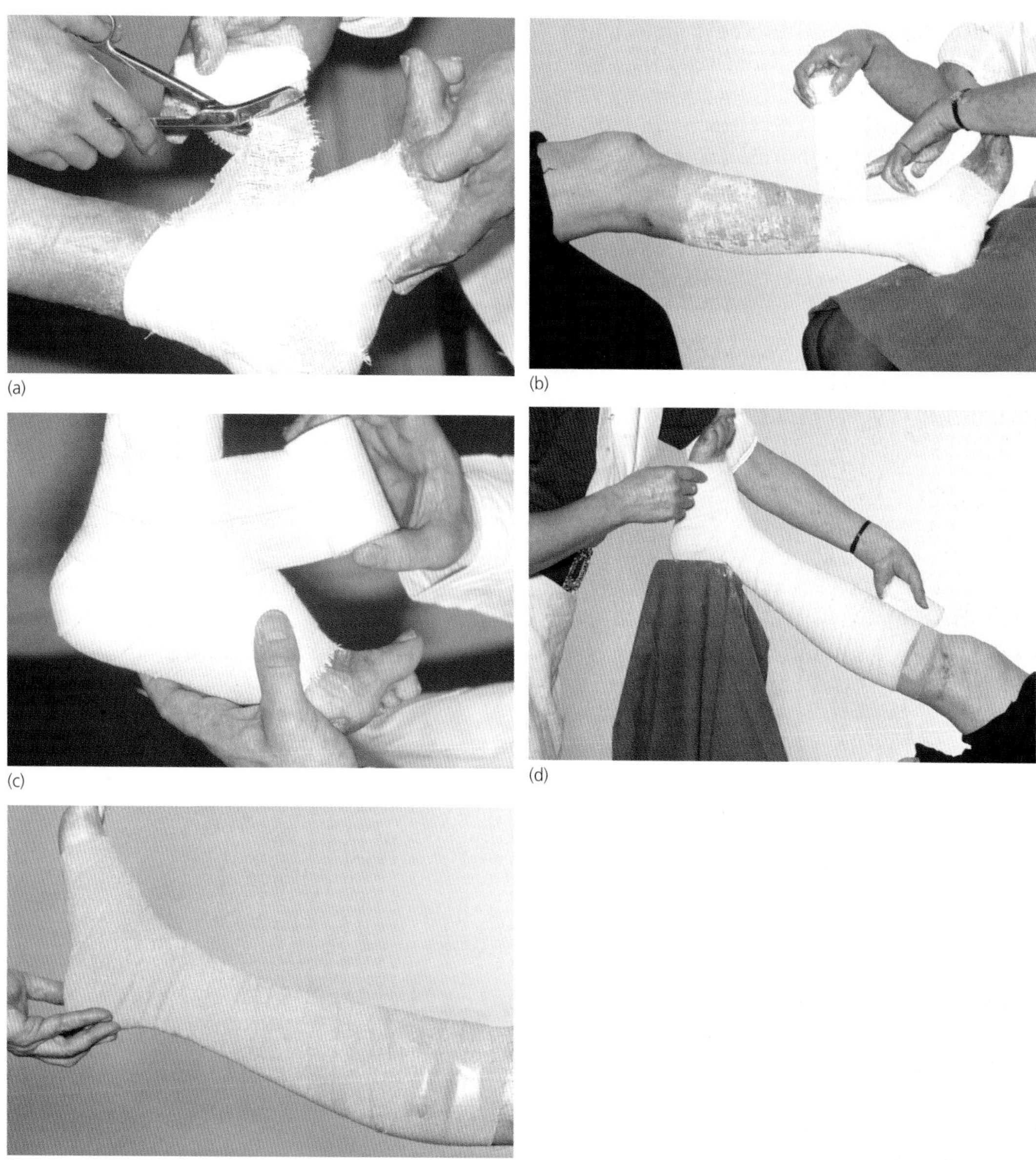

Figure 28.2 Steps in the application of bandages for the treatment of venous ulceration.

- Ischaemic ulcer: Due to impaired arterial blood supply; the peripheral pulses must always be examined and the ankle–brachial pressure index (ABPI) checked.
- Neuropathic ulcer: Particularly common in diabetics, where it is often compounded by ischaemia due to diabetic microangiopathy.
- Malignant ulcer: A squamous carcinoma, often arising in a pre-existing chronic ulcer or an ulcerated malignant melanoma.
- Ulcer complicating systemic disease, e.g. acholuric jaundice, ulcerative colitis and rheumatoid arthritis
- Arteriovenous fistula-associated ulcer.
- Repetitive self-inflicted injury.
- Gummatous ulcer of syphilis: Usually affects the upper one-third of the leg.

An example of the importance of remembering differential diagnoses will be discussed in Case 29 (p. 61).

How should this patient be treated?

A number of important steps are taken:

- She is advised to keep the leg elevated whenever possible – in bed at night and when sitting during the day. The foot should be higher than the knee, the knee higher than the hip. This eliminates the venous hypertension in the leg during the hours the leg is elevated and allows ingress of oxygenated blood.
- All ointments and medicaments should be thrown away.
- The ulcer is covered with a simple, non-adherent dry dressing, held in place by a paste bandage to the leg, and over this elastoplast bandaging is applied from the toes to below the knee (Fig. 28.2). Again, this counters the venous hypertension. The bandages are changed initially at weekly intervals, but as healing progresses and the amount of oozing is reduced the intervals between dressings can be increased.
- A split-skin graft can be applied if the ulcer remains indolent.
- Once the ulcer is healed, elastic stocking support is mandatory to prevent the very real risk of recurrence.

Case 29 Another leg ulcer

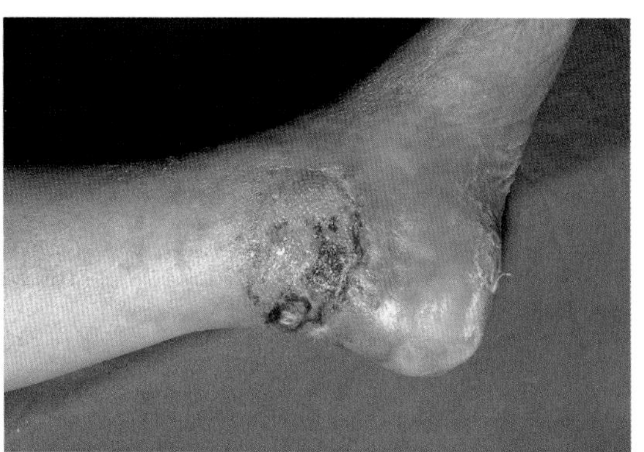

Figure 29.1

This 69-year-old lady has had her ulcer of the left leg treated for many months by the district nurse using conventional bandaging. As it showed no signs of healing – indeed, if anything it seemed to be getting worse – she was referred to the vascular clinic at her local hospital. Here she gave a history of left calf pain on walking. This had been present for about a year and she was now only able to limp about 50 yards before having to stop and rest because of the pain. However, she put this down to the presence of the ulcer. She had no problems with her right leg, gave no history of angina or of transient ischaemic attacks (TIAs), but did admit to being a 'life-long' cigarette smoker.

On examination, the ulcer had sloping edges and a necrotic base (as shown in Fig. 29.1). The left foot was colder than the right, the toes were blue and Buerger's test (see p. 48) was positive. There were no varicose veins on either leg. All the pulses could be detected in the right leg but only the femoral pulse was present on the left.

What is your clinical diagnosis?

An arterial ulcer due to arteriosclerotic disease with occlusion of the left superficial femoral artery.

Why the calf pain on walking?

This is classical calf claudication pain due to muscle ischaemia.

How can a Doppler ultrasonic probe be used to help confirm the diagnosis?

It is used in conjunction with a sphygmomanometer to compare the arm systolic blood pressure with that obtained in the leg. (A special long cuff must be used to take the blood pressure in the lower limb.) There will be a considerable lowering of the ankle blood pressure compared with the brachial pressure (the ankle–brachial pressure index, ABPI). Indeed, 'critical ischaemia' is defined as an ankle systolic pressure that is lower than 50% of the brachial pressure (ABPI < 0.5), although the presence of tissue loss (the ulcer) also signifies that the ischaemia is 'critical'. Sure enough, this was so in the present case.

What other investigation is required?

She requires further investigation by means of a femoral arteriogram to delineate the arterial tree in the left leg. We need to know if there is a stenosis or total occlusion and whether or not there is an adequate run-off (Fig. 29.2). This will allow reconstruction of the vascular tree, either by a balloon angioplasty, with or without a stent, or surgical reconstruction, using a saphenous vein graft. If there is a totally inadequate run-off, she may well come to amputation of the left leg.

Revise the differential diagnosis of the causes of leg ulcers

See the list on p. 58, Case 28.

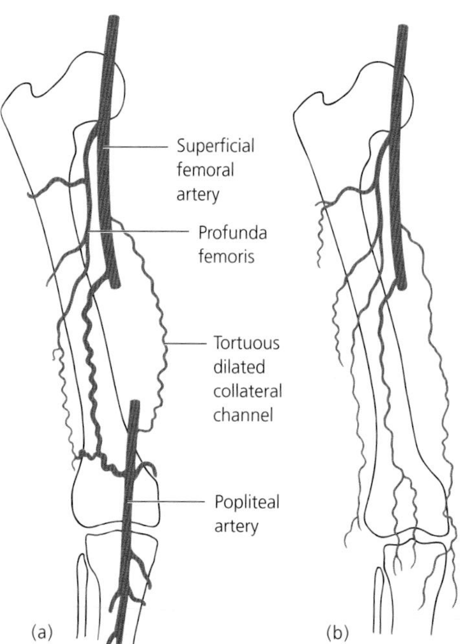

Figure 29.2 Tracings of arteriograms. (a) An example of a good run-off with a patent popliteal artery; this is suitable for reconstructive surgery. (b) The main arterial tree is obliterated and reconstruction cannot be carried out.

Case 30 A cerebral mass on magnetic resonance imaging

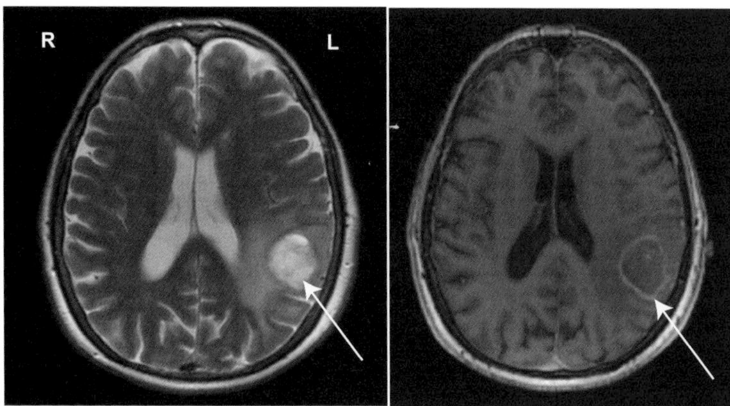

Axial T2 weighted image IV Contrast (gadopentetic acid) **Figure 30.1**

These are two images from a magnetic resonance (MR) imaging scan series of a 45-year-old man who had complained of increasingly severe headaches over a couple of months, particularly worse in the morning. More recently he had started to vomit for no apparent reason, and had developed mild dysphasia.

Clinical examination revealed marked papilloedema on fundal examination and a mild right hemiparesis. Because of this, an urgent MR scan had been ordered.

Describe the lesion (which has been arrowed)

There is an irregular heterogeneous enhancing mass in the left parietal region on the axial T2-weighted image with surrounding oedema. The wall of the mass has taken up contrast. The lesion is solitary; this is in favour of a primary tumour since metastases in the brain – the commonest pathology of tumours of the central nervous system (CNS) – are usually multiple.

What effect is this having on the ventricular system?

The lateral ventricle is being compressed on the left, and the midline is displaced slightly to the right.

A needle biopsy, performed through a burr hole, confirmed that this was a poorly differentiated astrocytoma. From which cells does this tumour arise, and what proportion of brain tumours does it comprise?

Gliomas arise from the glial supporting cells. In fact, there are no tumours that derive from neurons themselves. Gliomas account for about 45% of tumours encountered in neurosurgical units. They are graded according to their degree of differentiation, with low grade lesions being grades I and II; anaplastic astrocytomas are grade III, while the high grade glioblastoma multiforme is grade IV. Low grade tumours have a better prognosis than the high grade glioblastomas. Secondary deposits in the brain (often from lung, breast, renal or melanoma primaries), are the commonest tumours of the CNS overall, but these patients do not generally come under the care of the neurosurgeon.

Where do intracranial tumours typically occur in children?

In the cerebellum, where the commonest histological type is the medulloblastoma.

What treatment is available for this patient and what is his likely prognosis?

Overall, prognosis is extremely bad in these large and poorly differentiated tumours. Small growths, less than 3 cm in diameter, may be suitable for stereotactic radiosurgery, the so-called 'gamma knife'. Larger tumours, deemed operable, may be resected and this is usually followed by radiotherapy. In a large tumour, such as this, palliative radiotherapy is given which may be combined with surgical decompression. Cytotoxic drugs may confer additional benefit in some tumours, for example oligodendrogliomas.

Case 31 A cerebral vascular catastrophe

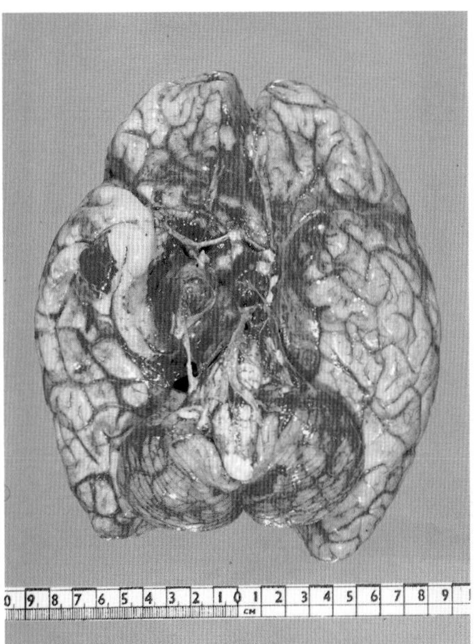

Figure 31.1

A previously healthy schoolmaster, aged 41 years, collapsed in his classroom. He was taken by ambulance to hospital, where he was found to be deeply unconscious, not responding to painful stimuli, breathing stertoriously, and with marked neck stiffness. Shortly after arrival, he had respiratory arrest and was intubated and put on a ventilator. Four days later his brainstem reflexes were found to be absent and he was pronounced dead; following his premortem wishes he became a multiorgan donor.

Figure 31.1 shows the appearance of the inferior aspect of his brain at autopsy.

Describe the pathological findings revealed in this specimen

There is a large right-sided aneurysm of the circle of Willis* which has ruptured. There is blood in the subarachnoid space.

Describe the circle of Willis; what is its importance?

The arterial circle of Willis is a rich anastomosis between the anterior, middle and posterior cerebral arteries on both sides. The posterior cerebral links to the middle via the posterior communicating artery, while the anterior cerebral links to its opposite via the anterior communicating artery. The middle and anterior cerebral arteries on each side are formed by the bifurcation of the internal carotid artery (Fig. 31.2).

Its importance is that it provides a highly effective anastomosis between the carotid system on either side. For example, in the healthy subject, ligation of the internal carotid artery can be performed without infarction of the brain on that side.

What is the commonest cause of this condition?

The great majority of circle of Willis aneurysms are congenital. About 20% are multiple and 85% occur on the anterior half of the circle. They may be associated with polycystic kidneys and with collagen diseases such as the Ehlers–Danlos syndrome.† Rarely, they result from arteriosclerosis, trauma or infection (mycotic aneurysm).

What is the natural history of the course of the untreated disease?

About a quarter of patients with haemorrhage from rupture of the aneurysm die without recovering consciousness, as in this case. Untreated, more than half will

---

*Thomas Willis (1621–1675), physician and anatomist, Oxford and then London.

†Edward Lauritz Ehlers (1863–1937), dermatologist, Copenhagen; Alexandre Danlos (1844–1912), dermatologist, Paris.

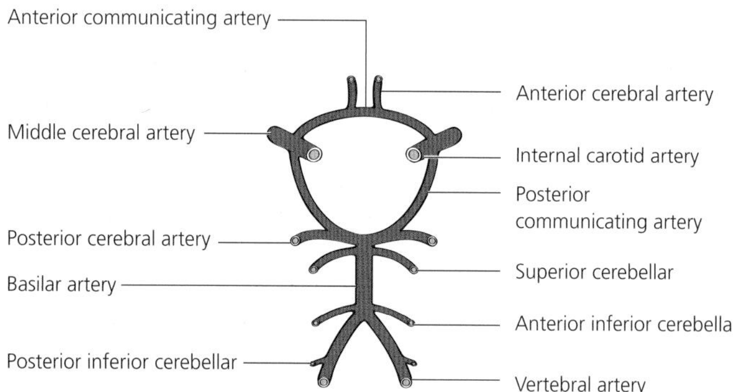

Figure 31.2 Anatomy of the circle of Willis.

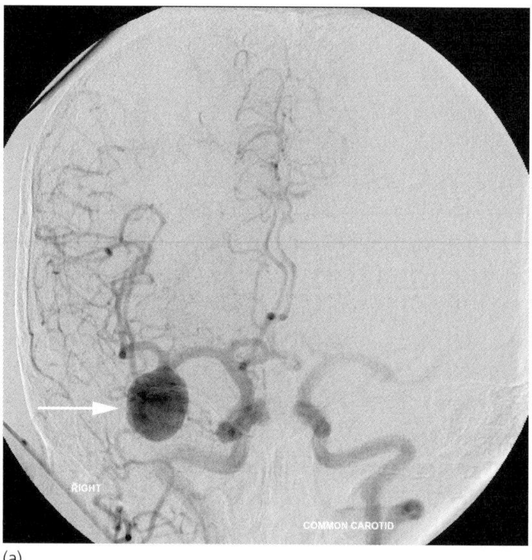

(a)

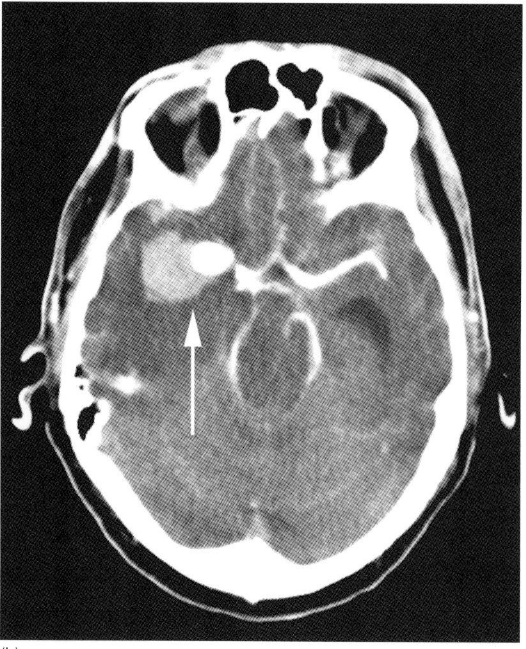

(b)

Figure 31.3 Middle cerebral artery (MCA) aneurysm. (a) An angiogram illustrating a large right MCA aneurysm (arrowed). (b) This is also visible on the contrast-enhanced CT, which also shows a recent haemorrhage (light grey, arrowed), with surrounding oedema, some midline shift to the left, and obliteration of the right lateral ventricle.

bleed again within 6 weeks of the initial bleed and the mortality of this is high. After 6 weeks, the risk of a further bleed becomes less, but is still present.

Outline the management of this condition

When the patient is in coma or has a dense hemiplegia, nursing care only is indicated. If the patient recovers from the initial bleed, CT, MR or cerebral angiography are performed to localize the aneurysm (Fig. 31.3). If an aneurysm is demonstrated, surgical treatment is indicated. This may be possible by percutaneous transarterial embolization or open operation with ligation or clipping of the neck of the aneurysm. About one-third of the angiograms are negative. These probably indicate that thrombosis has taken place in a small aneurysm. In such cases, the treatment is conservative and the prognosis is good.

Case 32 A baby with a large head

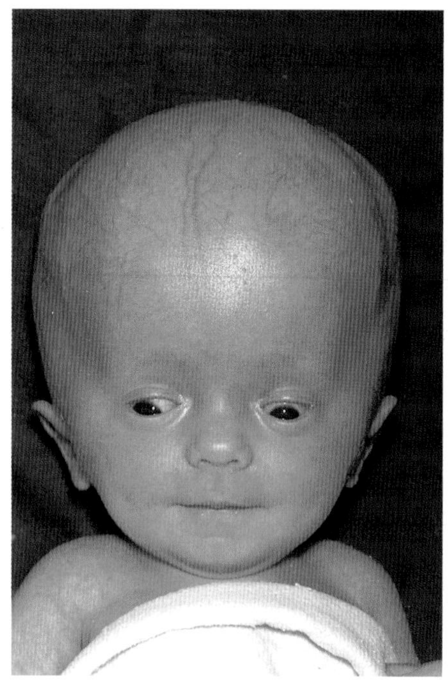

Figure 32.1

Figure 32.1 illustrates the head of a 3-week-old baby girl.

What is this condition called?

Congenital hydrocephalus.

What do you notice that is typical about the eyes in this child?

The eyes are deviated downwards due to compression of the upper brainstem. There may also be a squint and nystagmus in this condition.

Is papilloedema present on examining the fundi of these infants?

Characteristically, no.

What other physical signs might be commonly found on examining the enlarged head?

- The fontanelles bulge, the cranial sutures are widened (noticeably the sagittal suture) and dilated subcutaneous veins can be seen coursing over the cranial vault, as is shown in Fig. 32.1.
- X-rays of the skull in older children may show 'copper beating' of the bones of the vault and erosion of the pituitary fossa.

What other congenital anomaly is typically associated with this condition?

Spina bifida (see Case 36, p. 75).

What is the surgical treatment of this condition?

A shunt using a Spitz–Holter valve* between the lateral cerebral ventricle and the right atrium or peritoneal cavity (Fig. 32.2).

---

*John Holter (1916–2003), machinist at the Yale and Town lock company, Philadelphia; Eugene Bernard Spitz (1919–2006), paediatric neurosurgeon, Philadelphia. The Spitz–Holter valve is a one-way valve that releases controlled amounts of cerebrospinal fluid from the brain. John Holter had a son with hydrocephalus, and designed the valve in 1956 to treat the condition. His son lived for 5 years.

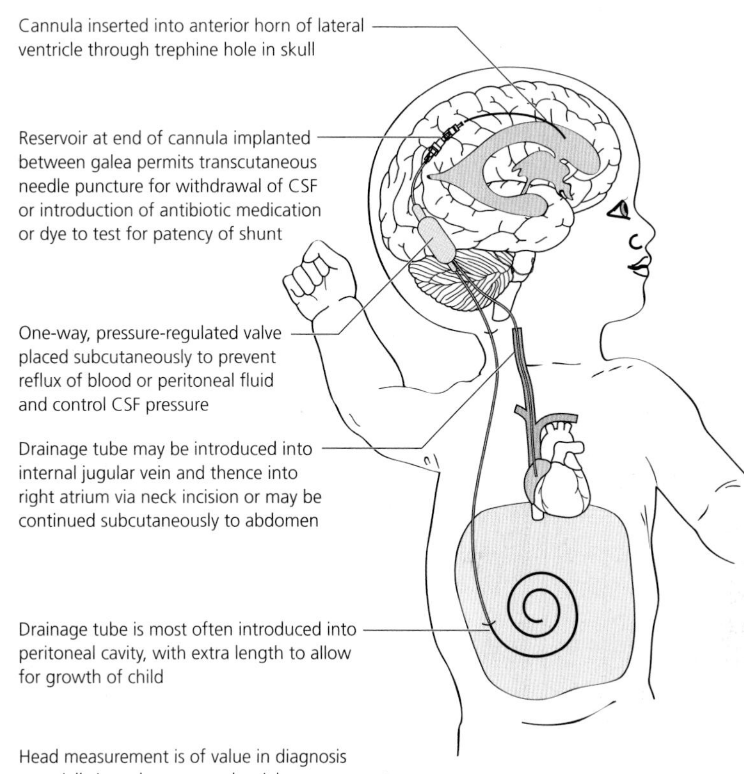

Figure 32.2 Shunt procedure for hydrocephalus using a Spitz–Holter valve. CSF, cerebrospimal fluid.

Case 33 A blow to the skull

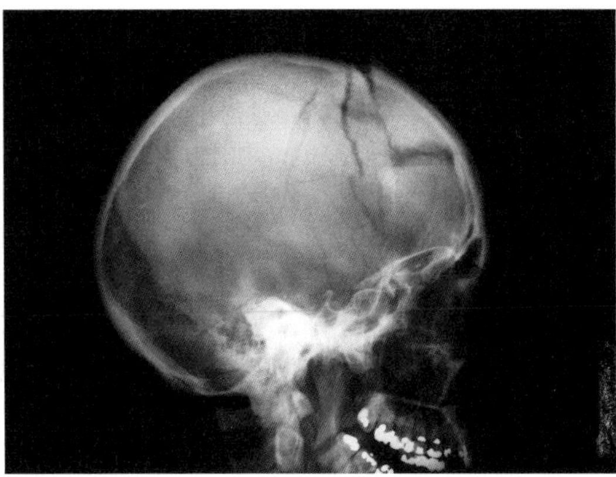

Figure 33.1

This is the lateral skull X-ray of a young man who came off his motorcycle at considerable speed and struck his forehead against the kerb. The force was so great that he split his helmet.

What abnormality can be seen on the X-ray?

Severe multiple linear fractures involving the frontal, parietal and temporal bones.

This was a closed fracture – the overlying scalp was intact. What sort of skull fracture is nearly always compound in the adult patient?

Depressed fractures of the skull vault, sufficient to depress the bone below the level of the rest of the skull outline, are nearly always compound injuries.

What type of skull fracture only occurs in children?

A 'pond' fracture. The soft, pliable bones of the child's skull can be indented, in the way you can indent a table-tennis ball.

What nasal discharge can occur if the fracture involves the frontal and/or ethmoid sinuses, and what is the danger of this?

Leakage of cerebrospinal fluid (CSF) from the nose (CSF rhinorrhoea). The danger of this is that the tear of the dura allows a pathway for infection from outside air via the nasal cavity to the meninges, i.e. meningitis.

How is this discharge distinguished from the discharge of blood-stained mucus that is so often seen in patients with facial injuries?

The fluid is collected and tested for sugar. CSF contains sugar, unlike mucus, where sugar is not found. Jugular compression may increase the flow of CSF from the nose.

Case 34 A severe head injury

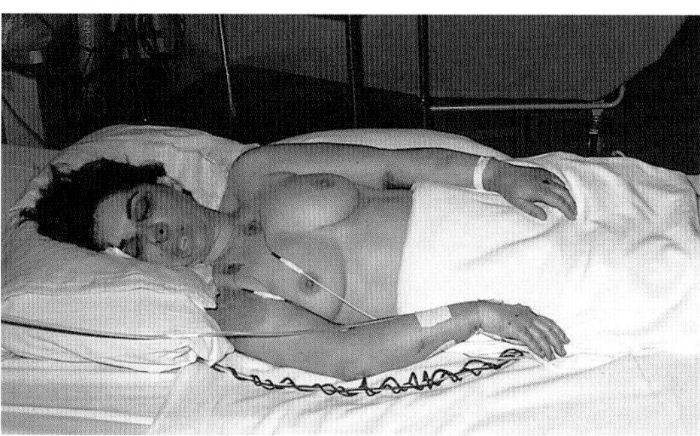

Figure 34.1

A 38-year-old overseas tourist, visiting London, stepped off the pavement looking to the left and not to the right and stepped straight in front of a bus. She was rapidly brought into hospital by ambulance, lying on her side and with a cervical collar in place.

When assessed by the casualty officer, she was deeply unconscious. There were bilateral periorbital haematomas, as can be seen in Fig. 34.1, with subconjunctival haemorrhage, but the pupils were normal, equal and responded to light. She withdrew her arm when her hand was pricked with a pin, and there was a similar response when her feet were pricked. When spoken to loudly, she made incomprehensible noises only. Using the Glasgow Coma Scale (Box 34.1), the doctor graded her as scale 7 (E1, V2, M4).

Apart from quite extensive bruises on her legs and right shoulder, there were no other obvious injuries on full examination.

What is the most important thing to ensure in the immediate management of an unconscious patient from whatever cause?

Maintenance of the airway. The patient in coma will die within a few minutes if the airway is blocked.

Box 34.1 The Glasgow Coma Scale (GCS)

Eye opening (E)
4 Spontaneously
3 To speech/command
2 To pain
1 None

Best verbal response (V)
5 Orientated – knows who he or she is and where he or she is
4 Confused conversation – disorientated; gives confused answers to questions
3 Inappropriate words – random words; no conversation
2 Incomprehensible sounds
1 None

Best motor response (M)
6 Obeys commands
5 Localizes pain
4 Flexes to pain – flexion withdrawal of limb to painful stimulus
3 Abnormal (decorticate) flexion – upper limb adducts, flexes and internally rotates so that it lies across chest; lower limbs extend
2 Extends to pain (decerebrate) – painful stimulus causes extension of all limbs
1 None

Figure 34.1 shows how this has been achieved in her case. What does it demonstrate?

The nasal and oral airways are in place. These were sufficient to maintain an adequate airway and endotracheal intubation was not necessary.

Why did the ambulance men transport her on her side?

She was transported in the 'tonsil position', so-called from the position children are placed in when recovering from the anaesthetic after tonsillectomy. The patient is turned on her side with the body tilted head-downward. This allows the tongue to drop forward so as not to occlude the oropharynx. With the patient tipped head-down, bronchial secretions, vomit or blood drain from the mouth rather than being inhaled into the respiratory passages. If necessary, the tongue is drawn forward by pushing the angle of the jaw forward on each side.

At present, she has an intravenous line with a drip of dextrose saline. What will be the simplest way of giving this comatose patient food and drink?

A fine nasogastric tube is passed (ensure it is in the stomach and not the trachea). This allows adequate hydration and nourishment to be given, even in prolonged periods of coma.

What are the standard imaging investigations carried out in patients with severe head injuries, such as in the present case?

- Skull X-rays.
- X-rays of the cervical spine (cervical vertebral fractures are common in head injuries and, of course, the unconscious patient cannot complain of neck pain or of symptoms of cord involvement).
- CT scan of the head (and cervical spine if plain films fail to show all seven cervical vertebrae and the C7/T1 junction).
- X-rays should be taken, also, of any other area where there is clinical evidence of injury.

> *Under careful nursing care and close monitoring, this woman made a steady recovery and was fit to leave hospital 3 weeks after her accident.*

Is there a clinical method of assessing the severity of the head injury after the patient has recovered?

Yes; determine the period of amnesia, both up to the time of the injury – the retrograde amnesia – and the amnesia following the accident – the post-traumatic amnesia. For some unknown reason, the former is always considerably shorter than the latter. If the period of amnesia is measured in minutes or a few hours, prognosis is excellent. If, however, the amnesia lasts for days or even weeks, this indicates a severe cerebral injury with poor prognosis for return of full mental function.

Case 35 Another severe head injury

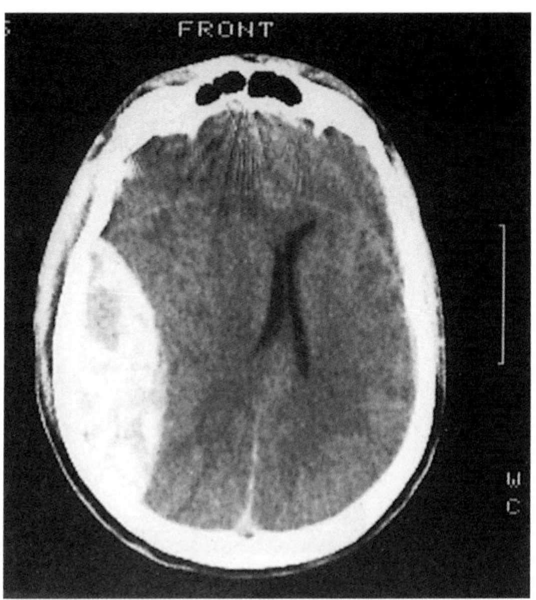

Figure 35.1

Figure 35.1 is one slice of a CT scan of the head of an amateur cricketer aged 19 years who was hit on the right side of the head by a cricket ball as he fielded in the slips. He immediately fell to the ground and could not be roused. However, within a few minutes, after he had been carried into the pavilion, he was beginning to wake up and was fully conscious a quarter of an hour after the accident.

He was taken by car to the district general hospital and, while in the A&E department, he started to become drowsy and within a couple of hours was in coma. He was intubated and an urgent CT scan performed.

What can you see on his CT scan?

There is a localized fluid collection in the right temporal region with displacement of the lateral ventricles to the left.

What is the period of regained consciousness called?

The 'lucid period'. Although very typical of an extradural bleed, it is by no means invariable in this condition. If the initial injury is sufficiently severe, the initial coma due to the cerebral concussion can merge imperceptibly into the coma produced by the cerebral compression due to the expanding haematoma.

What physical signs would you expect the patient to have shown when he relapsed into coma?

- A rising blood pressure, slowing of the pulse (Cushing's reflex* response to raised intracranial pressure) and possibly a hemiparesis or hemiplegia on the contralateral side.
- Dilatation of the pupil on the side of the compression due to pressure of the haematoma against the third (oculomotor) cranial nerve against the edge of the tentorium cerebelli. The oculomotor nerve transmits parasympathetic pupilloconstrictor fibres to the ciliary muscles of the eye; if these are knocked out, that leaves intact the pupillodilator sympathetic fibres. If compression continues, and this golden period for surgery missed, both pupils become fixed and dilated and prognosis for recovery drops sharply.

Should a lumbar puncture be performed at this stage?

No, you would almost certainly kill the patient. The intracranial pressure is high. If cerebrospinal fluid is drawn off at lumbar puncture, the raised pressure within the skull will force the cerebellar tonsils through the

*Harvey Cushing (1869–1939), Professor of surgery, Harvard Medical School, Boston.

foramen magnum, which will compress the medulla, with its vital cardiac and respiratory centres, and there is prompt cardiac arrest!

What urgent treatment is needed here to save the patient's life?

- Maintain the airway by means of endotracheal intubation.
- Transfer at once to theatre for a right-sided craniotomy, evacuation of the extradural haematoma (Fig. 35.2) and to control the source of the bleed. This is frequently due to a tear of the middle meningeal artery and/or vein, but may be from a tear of the sagittal sinus or of a diploeic vein in the skull bone marrow.

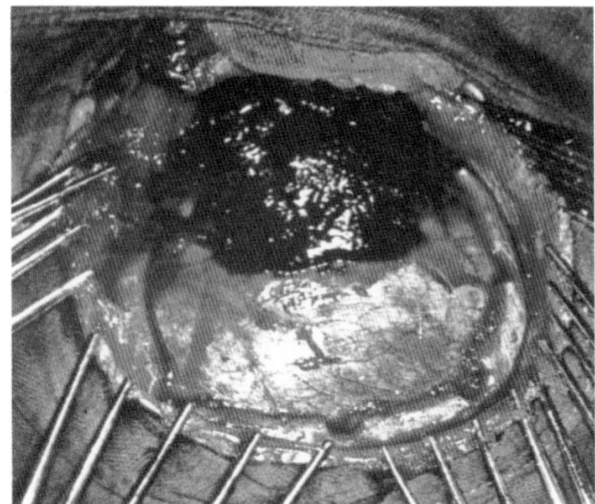

Figure 35.2 Extradural haematoma evacuation.

Case 36 A spinal abnormality in a newborn child

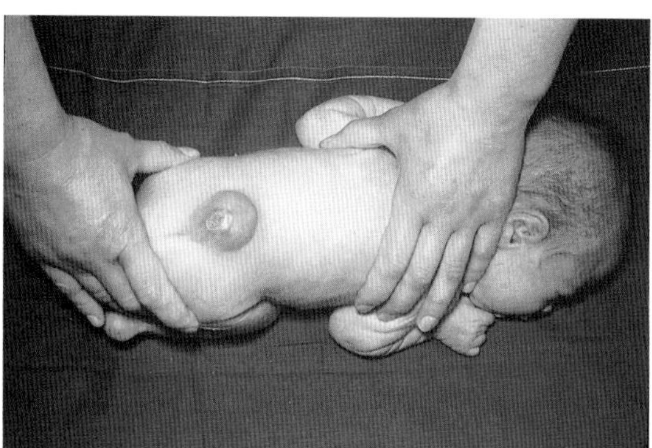

Figure 36.1

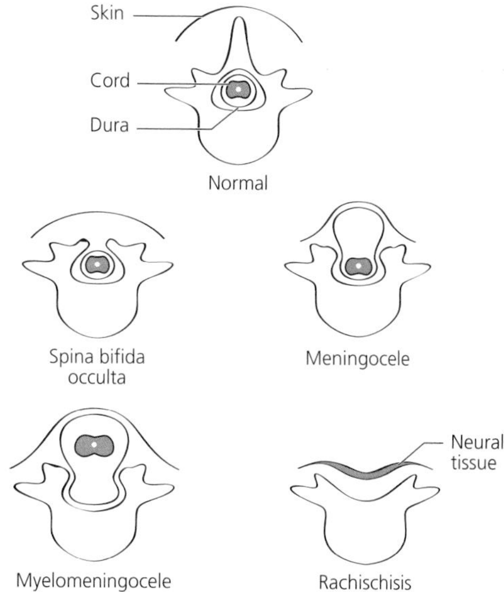

Figure 36.2 The different varieties of spina bifida.

Figure 36.1 demonstrates an obvious spinal abnormality in a newborn child. The parents were deeply upset, but at least they were expecting to see this condition.

What is this lesion called?

Spina bifida with meningocele – protrusion of the meninges through the vertebral defect without nervous tissue involvement.

How are the various types of this lesion classified?

The following range of anomalies may be found, in ascending order of severity (Fig. 36.2):

• *Spina bifida occulta*: Failure of vertebral arch fusion only. This is symptomless and is picked up incidentally on spinal X-ray. It may occur anywhere along the spinal column, but the great majority of defects involve L5 (6% of the population) or upper sacrum (11%). It may sometimes be associated with a tuft of hair, a lipoma or an overlying dimple in the skin.

• *Meningocele* (as in this case): Protrusion of the meninges without nervous tissue involvement.

• *Myelomeningocele*: Neural tissue (the spinal cord or roots) protrudes into and may adhere to the meningeal sac.

• *Myelocele* (or rachischisis): Failure of fusion of the neural tube, which results in an open spinal plate that occupies the defect as a red granular area weeping cerebrospinal fluid from its centre. This condition is incompatible with survival.

How did the parents know about this condition before the baby was born?

Prenatal screening by means of ultrasound, with confirmatory elevation of the α-fetoprotein level in the amniotic fluid, enables the defect to be diagnosed with a high degree of confidence. In severe degrees of this lesion, parents may elect for termination of the pregnancy.

What other congenital condition may typically coexist with this lesion?

Hydrocephalus occurs in 75% of cases of myelomeningocele (the Arnold–Chiari malformation, see Case 32, p. 68). Hydrocephalus is very rare in an uncomplicated meningocele, such as in this child.

How should this lesion be treated?

The sac is excised and the skin defect repaired.

Case 37 Back injury

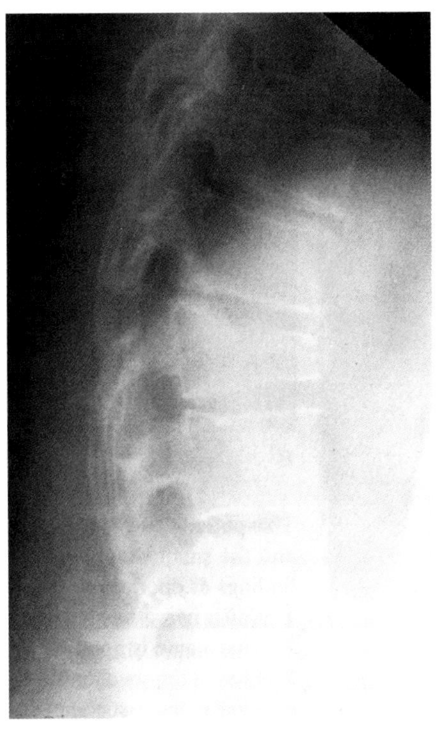

Figure 37.1

A construction worker aged 40 years fell off some scaffolding about 6 m from the ground. He landed on his feet (he was wearing heavy boots), onto the grass verge and lay collapsed. He complained to his mates of severe pain in his back and pointed to his upper lumbar region as the site of this. An ambulance soon arrived; the paramedics immediately established that he was fully conscious and that he could move both legs normally. He was carefully transferred to a stretcher and transported to hospital.

What is the obvious thing to have in mind when you, as the casualty officer, go to assess this patient?

Obviously he has sustained a severe lower back injury. Check if there is evidence of neurological damage. Is there a vertebral fracture and are there any other injuries?

The casualty surgeon removed the patient's boots and socks and confirmed that he had full motor power in the lower limbs and no sensory loss. With the help of the nursing staff, the patient was undressed to allow for full assessment. There was localized bruising, marked tenderness and a slight wedge deformity to detect at the dorsolumbar junction.

What other injuries must be excluded when a patient has fallen on his feet from a height?

From below upwards, the patient may have fractured the calcaneus, fractured through the neck of the talus (sometimes with backward dislocation of the body of the talus), or sustained fractures at the ankle or the tibial or femoral condyles. In this patient, there was no clinical evidence of injury to the legs – possibly because of the protection of his heavy boots.

The patient was transferred to the radiology department where anteroposterior and lateral X-rays were taken of the dorsolumbar spine (Fig. 37.1).

What does the lateral dorsolumbar X-ray show?

A wedge fracture of the 12th thoracic vertebra. The adjacent disc spaces are normal and there is no forward displacement of T12 on the L1 vertebral body. This is therefore classified as a stable injury of the vertebral column.

What type of fracture is likely to produce a spinal cord or spinal nerve root injury, and why is this risk greater in cervical spine fractures than in dorsolumbar injuries?

- An unstable fracture with forward or lateral displacement of the spine is likely to produce a spinal cord or spinal nerve root injury.
- There is a much closer fit of the cervical spinal cord within the cervical part of the vertebral canal compared with the greater space for the conus of the spinal cord (which terminates usually at the level of the first lumbar vertebra) and the cauda equina in the dorsolumbar region.

How should this patient be treated?

The patient is nursed in bed to allow the associated soft tissue injury to heal. During this time, general physiotherapy is used to keep up joint mobility and muscle exercise. This is followed by exercise and active mobilization.

If the fracture is unstable but without spinal cord or nerve root involvement, how is the dorsolumbar vertebral fracture treated?

Operative reduction and plate fixation.

Case 38 A lacerated wrist

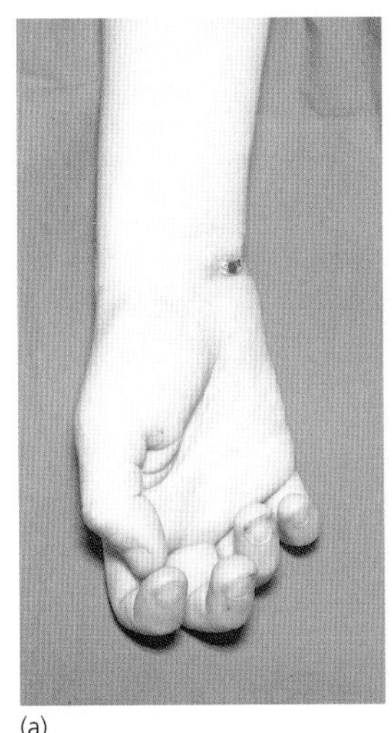

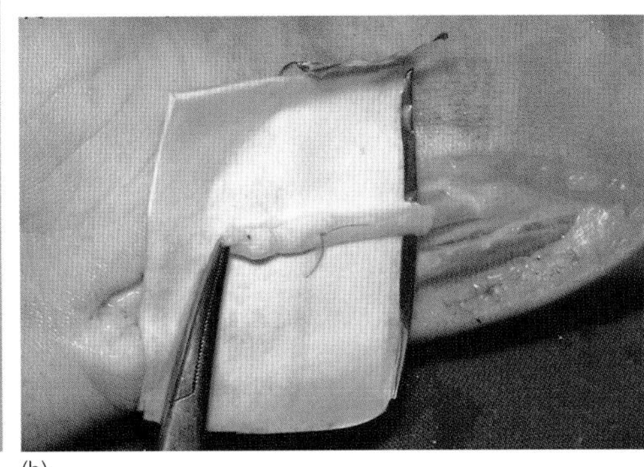

Figure 38.1 (a) (b)

One of our laboratory technicians, a graduate aged 25 years, cut his right wrist on a fragment of broken glass that he had not noticed on the laboratory bench. He pulled out the shard of glass and realized at once that the ulnar part of his hand and his little finger were numb.

Which peripheral nerve must have been injured?

Obviously the ulnar nerve as it lies at the ulnar side of the wrist.

This is the commonest peripheral nerve to be damaged by an open wound; what is the anatomical basis of this fact?

The ulnar nerve lies quite superficially at the wrist, as it emerges to lie immediately on the radial side of the flexor carpi ulnaris tendon, which can be identified as the most ulnar of the tendons palpable and visible at the wrist. The nerve then crosses superficially to the flexor retinaculum (which protects the median nerve as this passes deep to the retinaculum in the carpal tunnel) (Fig. 38.2). The ulnar nerve is accompanied on its radial side by the ulnar artery and its venae comitantes, which can also be lacerated in this type of injury, although fortunately not in this case.

What were the sensory and motor findings when the surgeon examined this young man's hand?

The sensory loss, both to pin-prick and light touch, comprised the ulnar border of the palmar aspect of the right hand and the palmar aspect of the little finger and ulnar border of the ring finger. The patient could not abduct or adduct his extended fingers. This was best demonstrated because he could not grip a piece of paper between any of his fingers with the hand placed flat on the table.

Describe the anatomical basis of these findings

The sensory supply to the hand comprises the following nerves (Fig. 38.3):

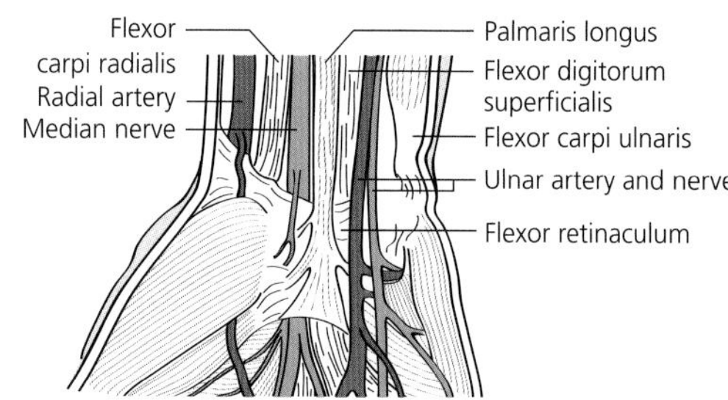

Figure 38.2 Structures on the anterior aspect of the wrist.

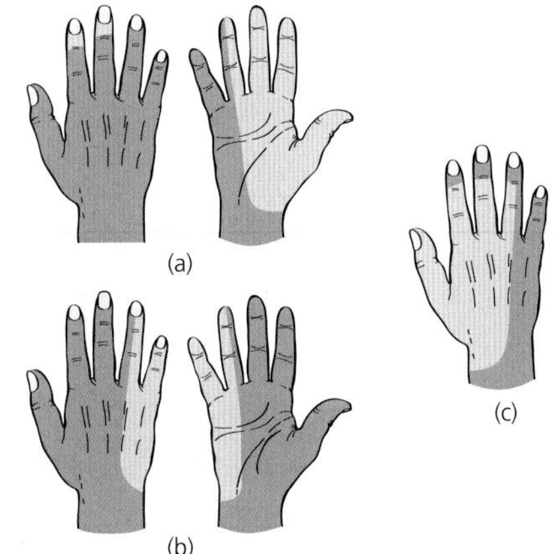

Figure 38.3 The usual cutaneous distribution (shown in pale blue) of (a) median, (b) ulnar and (c) radial nerves in the hand (considerable variations and overlap occur).

• The median nerve, which innervates the skin of the anterior aspects of the three and a half digits on the radial side.
• The radial nerve, which supplies the same distribution on the dorsal aspect.
• The ulnar nerve, which supplies the remaining one and a half digits on both their palmar and dorsal aspects.

However, the branch of the ulnar nerve, which supplies the dorsal aspect of the hand and fingers (the dorsal cutaneous branch), arises from the main trunk of the nerve about a hand's breadth above the wrist, dives beneath the flexor carpi ulnaris and reaches the dorsum of the hand. This branch will escape injury, as in the present case, when the nerve is damaged on the anterior aspect of the wrist.

On the motor side, the median nerve supplies the muscles of the thenar eminence (abductor pollicis brevis, flexor pollicis brevis and opponens pollicis) and the two radial lumbrical muscles. The ulnar nerve supplies all the remaining intrinsic muscles of the hand – the dorsal and palmar interossei, the three muscles of the hypothenar eminence, the adductor pollicis and the radial two lumbricals. (Note that the radial nerve supplies none of the intrinsic muscles of the hand.)

Figure 38.1 shows the hand in the typical deformity produced by this nerve lesion. What is this deformity called and how would you explain its anatomical basis?

Clawed hand (main en griffe). The intrinsic muscles of the fingers not only abduct and adduct the fingers, as in the clinical test described above, but also extend the interphalangeal joints. The fingers therefore lie at rest in the flexed position. However, the two radial lumbricals, supplied by the median nerve, are still functioning, so the deformity is less marked on the radial side.

The patient was operated on later the same day by an orthopaedic surgeon with a special interest in peripheral nerve injuries. The ulnar nerve was exposed through a longitudinal incision and found to be completely divided, as shown in Fig. 38.1b. Its ends were freshened and it was repaired using fine (9/0) nylon interrupted sutures to tack the epineural sheath together.

How are peripheral nerve injuries classified with regard to severity of the damage, and what is the rate of nerve regeneration?

The classification is into three degrees of injury:
• *Neurapraxia*: The nerve is contused but the fibres are intact; full recovery is anticipated.
• *Axonotmesis*: The axon and myelin sheath are injured without division of the perineural sheath.
• *Neurotmesis*: Complete division of the nerve; as in the present case.

Nerve regeneration takes place, under favourable conditions, at a rate of 1 mm a day. In this patient, fortunately, full recovery took place.

Case 39 A hand deformity

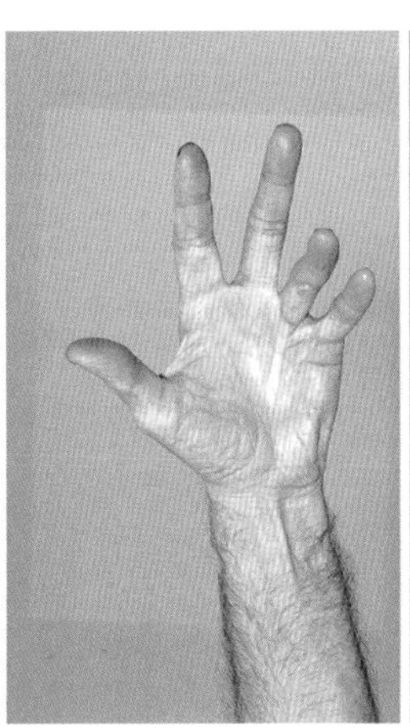
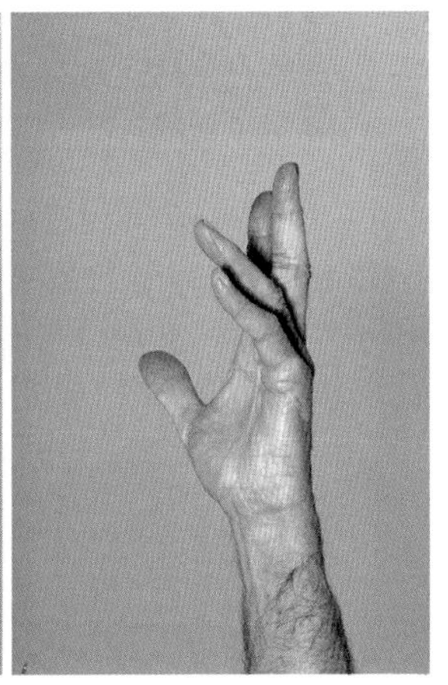

Figure 39.1

Figure 39.1 shows the left hand of a 72-year-old retired bus driver. His right hand was quite normal and general examination showed an otherwise fit old gentleman.

This is a common deformity, mostly occurring in men, but sometimes found in women. What is it called and what produces it?

Dupuytren's contracture.* Dupuytren demonstrated the pathology of this condition by dissecting the hand of a patient with this deformity at postmortem. He demonstrated that the palmar aponeurosis was grossly thickened and contracted, but that the underlying flexor tendons were perfectly normal. Previously it had been held that it was tendon contractures that were the cause of this deformity.

*Baron Guillaume Dupuytren (1777–1835), surgeon at the Hotel Dieu, Paris.

Is anything known of the aetiology of this condition?

It is said to be associated with a wide range of things – smoking, alcohol, epilepsy, diabetes, liver disease, tuberculosis and AIDS (acquired immune deficiency syndrome) – but as it is so common in the general elderly population, perhaps 15% of men over the age of 65, there is little hard evidence to support any of these factors.

Which fingers are usually affected, and which part of the finger always escapes and why?

This condition usually commences in the ring finger, spreads to the little and sometimes the middle finger, but only rarely are the index finger or thumb involved. Since the palmar aponeurosis only extends to the base of the middle phalanx, the distal interphalangeal joint always escapes. Indeed, in an advanced case, the distal joint may actually be hyperextended against the palm of the hand.

Is this condition associated with any other contracture?

About 10% of patients have an associated contracture of the plantar fascia of the foot on one or both sides (Fig. 39.2). Usually the patient is unaware of this, but you will find it if you look! The patient in Fig. 39.2, whose hands were mildly affected, complained that his plantar contracture caused discomfort on walking, 'as if there was a stone in my shoe'.

How is this condition treated?

The majority of patients are not bothered by the condition; others can be reassured that it is only very slowly progressive. If, however, it is interfering with function, the affected fascia is excised (Fig. 39.3).

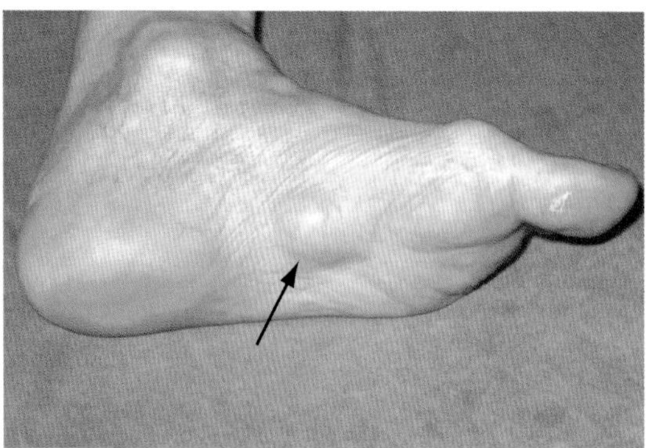

Figure 39.2 Dupuytren's contracture of the plantar fascia (arrowed).

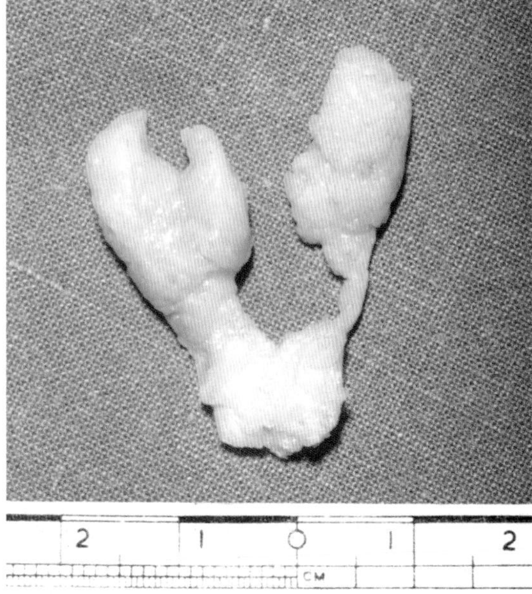

Figure 39.3 A resected specimen of thickened fascia.

Case 40 A deformed finger

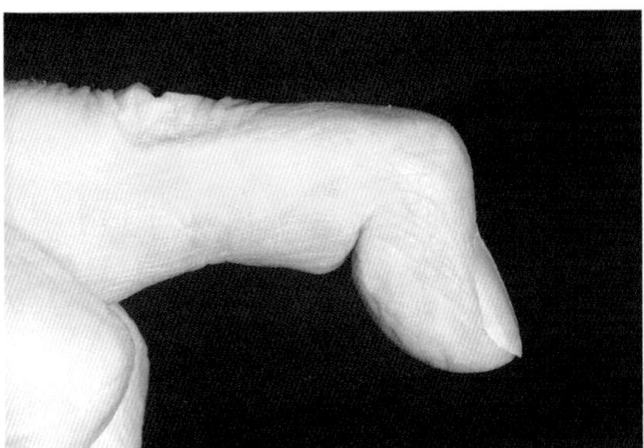

Figure 40.1

This young man has a characteristic deformity of the right index finger.

What is this deformity called?

A mallet finger.

How is it caused?

Either by avulsion of the extensor tendon of the finger at its insertion into the base of the terminal phalanx, or through a flake fracture at the posterior aspect of the base of this phalanx (Fig. 40.2, arrowed).

Which sport is linked to this injury?

Cricket. The hard ball, at speed, forcibly flexes the terminal interphalangeal joint.

How may this condition be treated?

The finger is immobilized with the distal interphalangeal joint extended, using a mallet finger splint (Fig. 40.3). If there is a fracture of the base of the distal phalanx, this can be fixed by means of a pin.

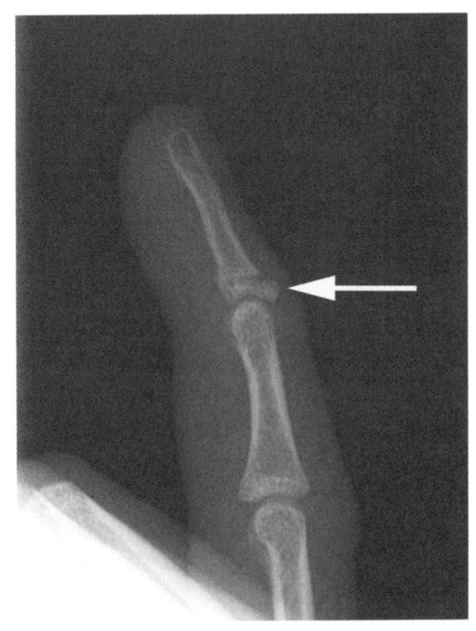

Figure 40.2 X-ray of a mallet fracture.

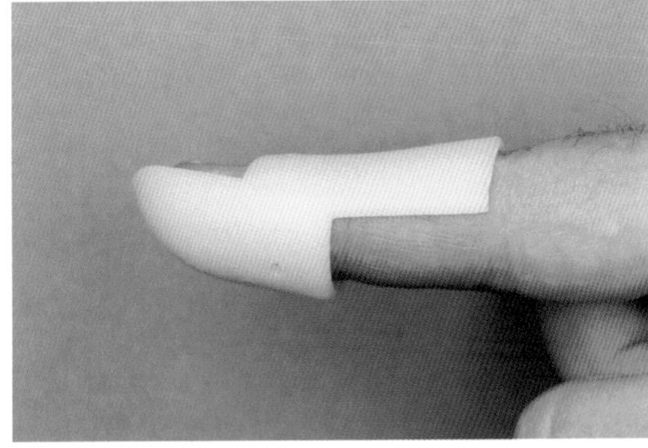

Figure 40.3 A mallet splint.

Case 41 A boy with a droopy eyelid

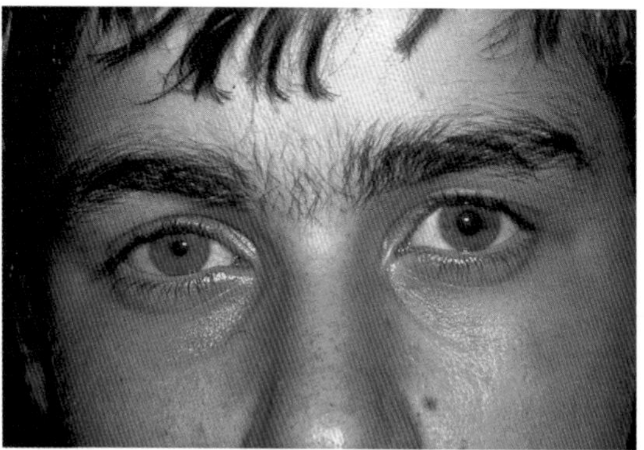

Figure 41.1

Figure 41.1 shows the eyes of a young school boy aged 17 years. Ever since boyhood, from about the age of 6 or so, he had suffered from severe sweating of the hands and, to some extent, of the axillae and feet – the condition of hyperhydrosis. The hand sweating, in particular, had now become an unpleasant nuisance and a social problem. In writing, he found the paper soaked through and the ink ran. His fingers slipped on the word processor, so he found it best to do his school work using a pencil and copious amounts of blotting paper. He avoided shaking hands because people did not like to touch him. Small objects, like coins, would slip out of his wet fingers. The axillae were fairly well controlled with antiperspirants and his sweaty feet were not really a problem to him.

On examination, he was found to be a very pleasant, bright young man, otherwise perfectly well. However, the hands, at normal room temperature, were rather cold and very wet. The axillae and feet were damp. He readily agreed to have a bilateral upper thoracic sympathectomy and was delighted with the result – dry warm hands and cutaneous sweating under control. However, he noticed immediately after his operation (as did his surgeon) the appearance of his right eye.

What do you notice about the right eye and eyelid and what is this condition called?

There is ptosis (drooping) of the right eye and constriction (meiosis) of the right pupil – the condition is termed Horner's syndrome.*

What is the anatomical structure which, when damaged, produces this syndrome?

Either the cervical sympathetic chain itself or, as in this case, the first thoracic sympathetic ganglion, which provides the T1 outflow to the chain.

Explain why sympathetic damage to the head produces these anomalies

The pupil is constricted because of paralysis of the dilator pupillae which is supplied by sympathetic fibres. This leaves intact the constrictor pupillae supplied by the oculomotor (third) cranial nerve. The ptosis is produced by paralysis of the sympathetic fibres, which are transmitted in the oculomotor nerve to supply the levator palpebrae superioris – the elevator of the upper lid.

In the initial phase of this injury, there is also vasodilatation and loss of sweating of the face on the same side, but this is usually transient.

In performing an upper thoracic sympathectomy, the surgeon makes every effort to preserve the T1 ganglion, whose fibres supply the head and neck. The aim is to interrupt the outflow from T2 and T3, which supply the upper limb. In this case T1 was inadvertently injured. Today, this operation is usually performed endoscopically using a thoracoscope. This provides brilliant visualization of the anatomy and reduces still further the risk of T1 injury.

*Johann Horner (1831–1886), Professor of ophthalmology, Zurich.

Can you name some other quite common causes of Horner's syndrome?

It may be seen in tumour invasion of the cervical sympathetic chain, for example from a Pancoast tumour at the lung apex, secondary deposits in the cervical lymph nodes or from invasion by a poorly differentiated thyroid carcinoma. A severe injury of the roots of the brachial plexus may tear the cervical chain at its rami communicantes.

What effect will cervical sympathectomy have on the patient's feet?

There will be a compensatory increase in sweating in the feet. The patient should be warned of this prior to surgery.

Case 42 A lump on the lip

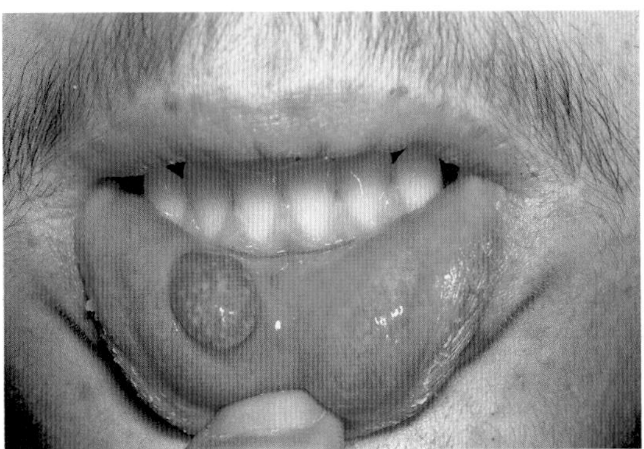

Figure 42.1

Figure 42.1 demonstrates the lips of a 20-year-old engineering student who presented with this painless, blue cystic lesion on the lower lip. He was concerned about its appearance and the fact that he kept biting it.

What is this lesion called?

This is the typical appearance of a mucous retention cyst of the lower lip. It really could not be anything else.

What is its aetiology?

Leakage of mucus beneath the mucosa due to minor trauma to the mucous glands of the lip.

These cysts contain clear, colourless mucus. Why then do they appear blue?

Reflected light – in the same way that the sea appears green or blue.

How do these cysts bother the patient?

Exactly as in this case. Patients do not like their appearance and they get caught between the teeth.

What treatment would you advise?

Surgical excision with suture of the defect using absorbable sutures. This was duly performed on this patient under local anaesthesia in the day surgery unit.

Case 43 A white plaque on the tongue

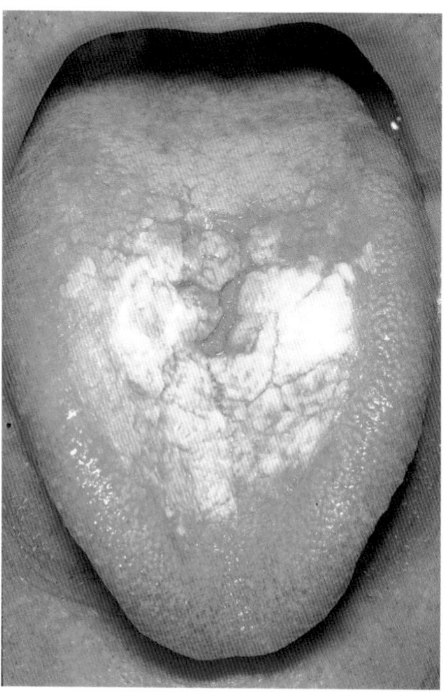

Figure 43.1

Figure 43.1 shows the tongue of a 62-year-old greengrocer who had noticed a small area of white discoloration at the centre of his tongue 3 or 4 years ago. This had gradually enlarged to its present size, but was quite painless. He was a heavy cigarette smoker – 30 a day – a habit that commenced in his teens. He had lost all his teeth by the time he was 40 and, since then, had well-fitting complete upper and lower dentures. He was a 'social drinker', beer only.

On clinical examination, he was a rather overweight but healthy man. The white plaque was slightly thickened, not ulcerated and quite painless to touch. The mouth was otherwise normal and the cervical lymph nodes were impalpable. He was mildly hypertensive (165/95) but apart from this, the full clinical examination was normal.

What name is given to this condition, and what does the word mean?

Leukoplakia, which means white plaque.

Where else may this condition be found?

Anywhere within the oral cavity, but it may affect other mucosal squamous epithelia – the larynx, vulva and lower anal canal.

What does this condition look like under the microscope?

There is hyperkeratosis – increased thickness of the prickle cell layer of the epithelium and retention of the nuclei in the keratinized layer.

What mnemonic covers its aetiological factors?

Although this condition may occur without obvious cause, remember the S's!

- Smoking (as probably in this case): Pipes even more than cigarettes.
- Syphilis: Always carry out serological tests for syphilis in these patients (negative in this case).
- Septic teeth.
- Spirits.
- Spices: It is especially common in the Indian subcontinent and it is estimated that some 20% of betel nut users over the age of 60 have this condition.

What is the importance of this condition?

It is often premalignant. Suspect it if there is local thickening, pain, ulceration, bleeding or local erythema.

Which patients are at particular risk of malignant change?

The danger increases with the age of the lesion and is in the region of 4–5% at 20 years. The risk is greater in patients over the age of 70 (about 7%) than for patients under 50 (about 1%).

How is this condition managed?

• Remove any underlying cause. For example, as in this patient, by stopping smoking, having warned him of his risk of developing a very unpleasant cancer.

• Biopsy any suspicious area for malignancy.

• Surgical excision, with skin graft if necessary. In this patient laser excision was performed.

Case 44 A baby with two gross congenital deformities

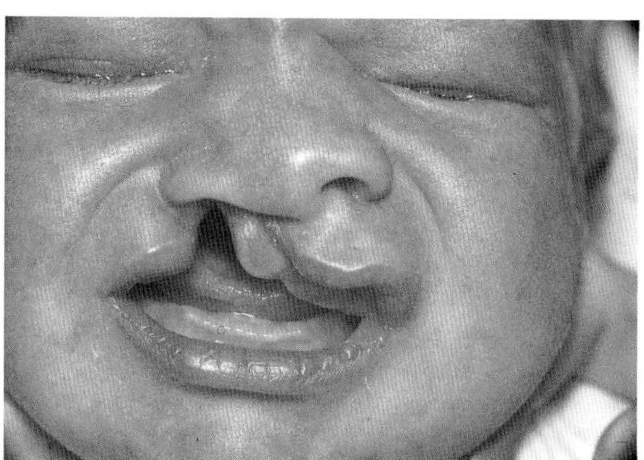

Figure 44.1

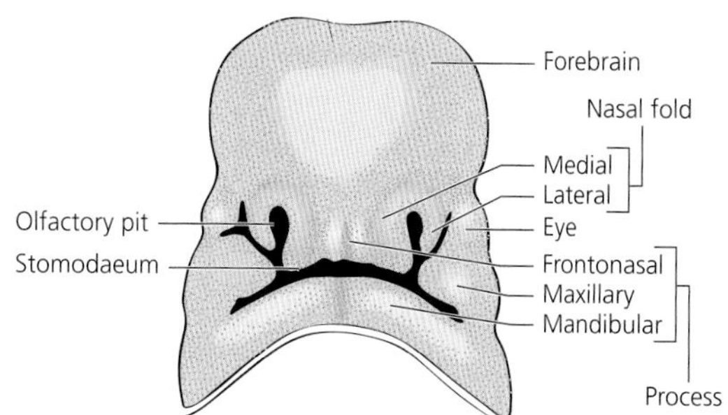

Figure 44.2 The ventral aspect of a fetal head showing the three processes, frontonasal, maxillary and mandibular, from which the face, nose and jaws are derived.

Figure 44.1 shows two obvious abnormalities in this otherwise healthy 2-day-old baby girl.

What are these lesions called?

Cleft lip and cleft palate. This is the commonest congenital facial abnormality in the UK and there are about 1000 babies born each year with one, either or both of these lesions.

How often, as in this case, do they coexist?

In round figures, 50% of babies have both conditions, 25% cleft lip only and 25% cleft palate only.

Why is it important to carry out a detailed clinical examination of this child?

Of course, you carry out a detailed examination of all your patients! However, specifically here it is important to remember that whenever one congenital anomaly is found, whether in a baby or older patient, a search must be made for other congenital lesions. Some diseases are well known to be associated with each other, for example, hydrocephalus and spina bifida (see Case 32, p. 68), duodenal atresia with Down's syndrome,* etc. Babies with a cleft lip and/or cleft palate have some other congenital anomaly in about 10% of cases. Special associations are with spina bifida and with syndactyly (fusion of fingers or toes).

What is the embryological explanation of these two conditions?

- Cleft lip results from different degrees of failure of fusion of the frontonasal and maxillary processes (Fig. 44.2).
- Cleft palate results from various degrees of failure of fusion of the palatine processes of the maxilla and the premaxilla – that part which bears the four incisor teeth (Fig. 44.3).

What is the immediate problem presented by this palatal defect?

Interference with the normal sucking mechanism. Breastfeeding is unlikely to be successful. A soft plastic bottle is

*John Langdon Down (1828–1896), medical superintendent, Earlswood Asylum, Redhill, and physician, London Hospital.

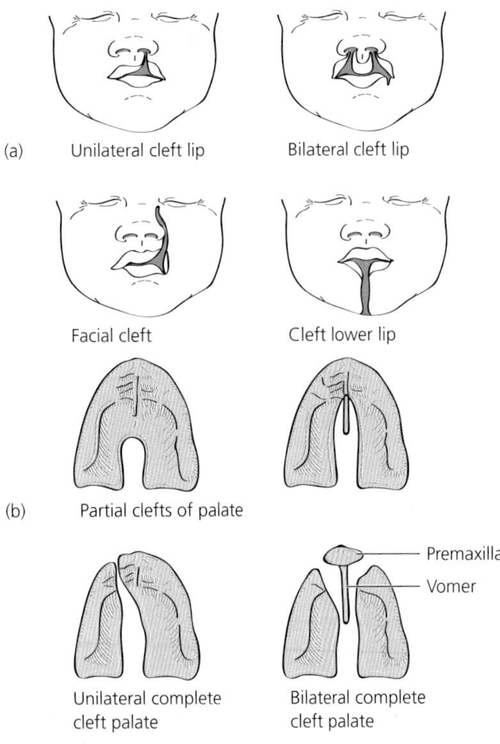

Figure 44.3 Types of (a) cleft lip and (b) cleft palate.

used to squirt the feed – preferably the mother's expressed breast milk – rhythmically into the baby's mouth. The infant can swallow the milk normally and, if positioned in the semi-upright position, nasal regurgitation through the cleft palate is minimal.

What should be the further management of this baby?

Well over half these babies are diagnosed at antenatal scan so that the surgical team can meet the parents and give them information about these conditions and the repair protocol. This goes some way to diminish the shock on seeing the newborn child. Surgical repair is performed in a specialized paediatric unit at about 3 months of age. Speech therapy and secondary plastic procedures are carried out as the child grows.

Case 45 A painful submandibular swelling

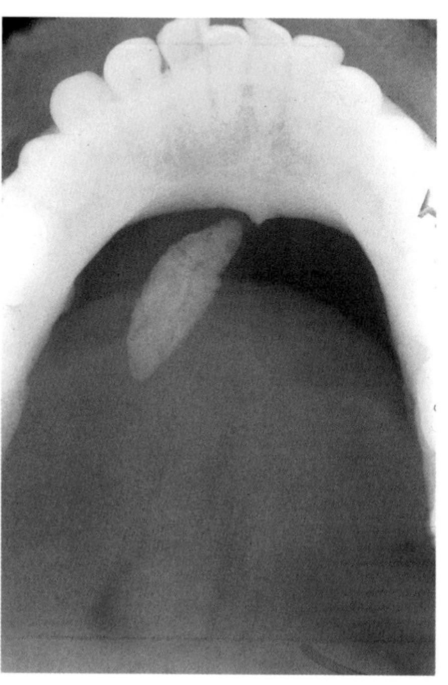

Figure 45.1

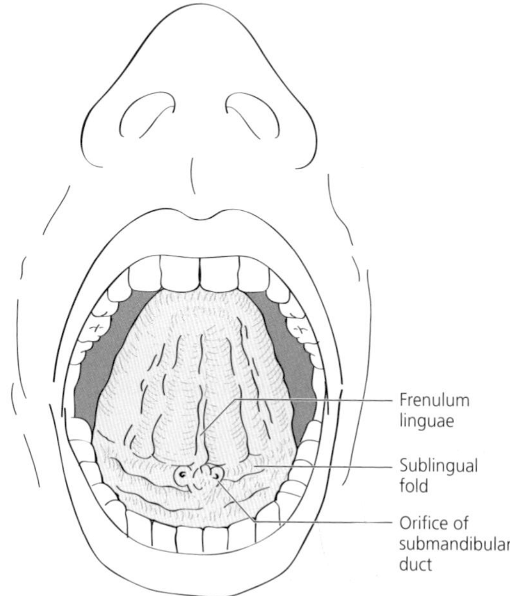

Figure 45.2 View of the open mouth with the tongue elevated.

One of our nurses, aged 23 years, complained of a swelling beneath the angle of her jaw on the right side which became more prominent and distinctly painful whenever she had something to eat – especially if this was spicy or tasty. She was also aware of something in the floor of her mouth on that side. Figure 45.1 is the X-ray we had taken of the floor of her mouth.

What does the film demonstrate?

A radio-opaque calculus in the duct of the right submandibular gland.

How are the submandibular salivary gland and its ducts examined clinically?

First inspect the orifice of the submandibular ducts on either side. These lie on either side of the base of the frenulum linguae (Fig. 45.2). In the case of the normal gland, pressure beneath the angle of the jaw produces a jet of saliva from the duct. Sometimes the calculus can be seen protruding from the duct orifice.

Next palpate the gland on either side bimanually, with one index finger in the floor of the mouth and the other beneath the angle of the jaw. On the normal side, the submandibular gland is felt as a rubbery swelling; on the affected side, the gland is enlarged and tender, and the stone is readily felt in the floor of the mouth (Fig. 45.3).

Do calculi develop in the other salivary glands?

Occasionally in the parotid gland, but never in the sublingual gland, which drains by a series of short ducts into

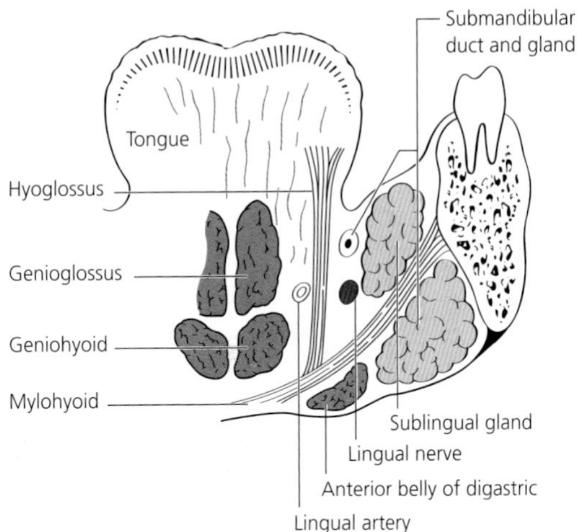

Figure 45.3 Coronal section of the floor of the mouth. N, nerve; A, artery.

the floor of the mouth and into the submandibular duct.

What is the chemical composition of these calculi?

Calcium phosphate and carbonate. The high calcium content is the reason why the great majority of these stones are radio-opaque.

Is anything known about the aetiology of these stones?

The answer is that they are something of a mystery. Unlike what one would imagine, they are always found in patients with clean and healthy mouths and with excellent, healthy teeth. A possible explanation is that the calculi form around minute fragments of tooth paste or even a tooth brush bristle.

How are submandibular calculi treated?

If the stone is seen at the duct orifice, it can sometimes be picked out with a fine pair of forceps. If in the duct itself, as in this nurse, the duct is opened in the floor of the mouth, the calculus removed and the duct left open. Sometimes a clump of stones form in the gland itself, and then the gland requires excision through an incision behind and below the angle of the jaw, carefully avoiding the submandibular branch of the facial nerve (VII).

Care 46 A lump over the angle of the jaw

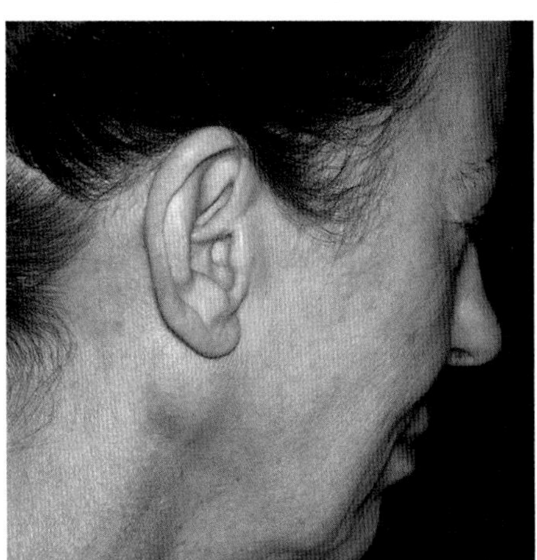

Figure 46.1

Figure 46.1 shows the left side of the face of a housewife and part-time secretary aged 46 years. She had noticed a lump, about the size of a pea, a few years before. As it was quite painless, she did nothing about it. The lump gradually enlarged to its present size and it was her husband who eventually persuaded her to seek medical advice. Apart from the lump she was perfectly well.

With this story, and just looking at the lump, what diagnosis would you have in mind?

The lump is certainly in the region of the parotid gland, so you would think of a parotid tumour. Its slow growth suggests that it is likely to be a benign pleomorphic adenoma (Fig. 46.2).

What must you do now, on examination of the lump, to confirm or refute your very provisional diagnosis?

As with any lump anywhere in the body, your first task is to examine the exact anatomical localization of the lesion. Could this lump be, not in the parotid gland, but in the overlying skin or subcutaneous tissues? Figure 46.3 shows a patient sent to our surgical outpatient clinic by his doctor as having a parotid tumour – however the lump was mobile, obviously tethered to the skin and was a subcutaneous sebaceous cyst!

Rarely, a mass arises in the masseter and will become tethered when this muscle is contracted by clenching the teeth. Tumours, both benign and malignant, can originate in the mandible.

In this patient's case, the lump lay precisely in the parotid itself.

Having examined the lump itself, what other procedures must you perform in the full clinical examination of the parotid gland?

- Inspect the parotid duct, which can be seen to open at the level of the second upper molar tooth.
- Test the facial nerve (VII) (Fig. 46.4): A facial palsy very strongly suggests invasion by a malignant parotid tumour.
- Inspect and palpate the fauces: A parotid tumour may plunge into the pharynx in the region of the tonsil.
- Palpate the cervical lymph nodes.

Does this tumour affect the other salivary glands?

Ninety per cent of tumours of the salivary glands – both benign and malignant – affect the parotid gland. However, they may be found in the submandibular, sublingual or accessory salivary glands scattered over the inside of the mouth and the palate.

What does a pleomorphic adenoma look like under the microscope?

There is a mixture of epithelial and myoepithelial elements in a variable background stroma that may in some cases resemble cartilage (Fig. 46.4).

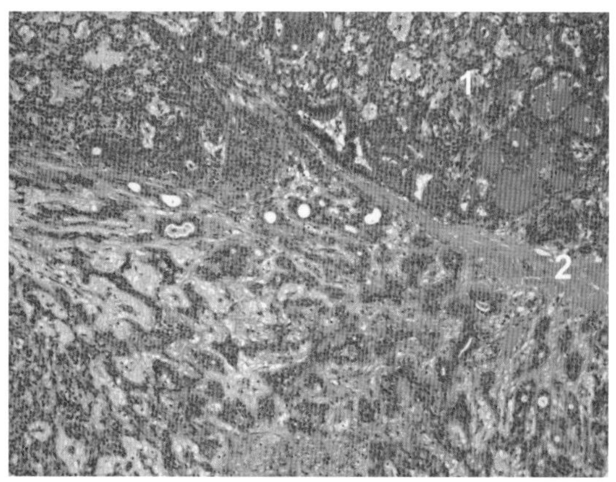

Figure 46.2 Histology photo of a pleomorphic adenoma of the parotid showing glandular acini with a blue-staining stroma showing epithelial (1) and myoepithelial (2) elements (magnification × 10, haematoxylin and eosin stain).

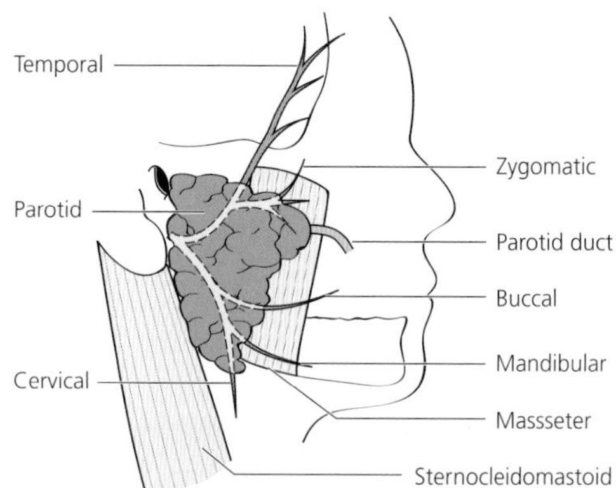

Figure 46.4 The named branches of the facial nerve that traverse the parotid gland.

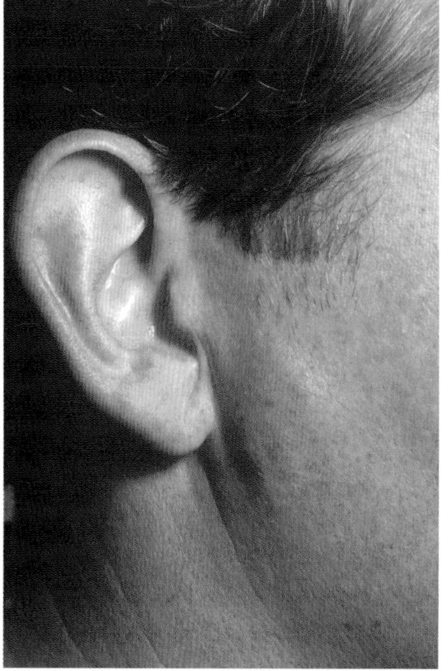

Figure 46.3 A misdiagnosed sebaceous cyst.

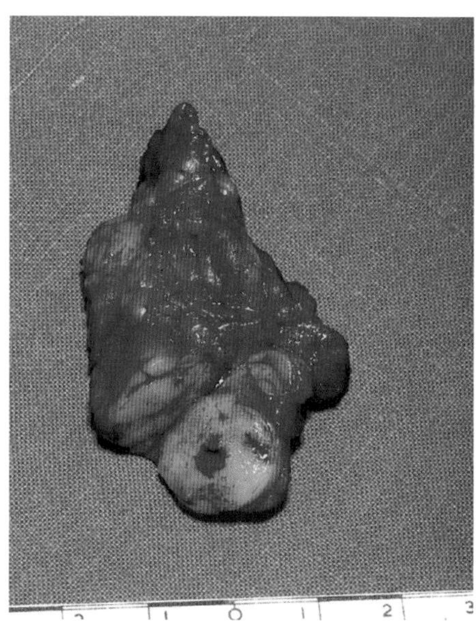

Figure 46.5 Surgically excised tumour.

Figure 46.5 is of the surgically excised specimen in this case. Although the tumour is apparently encapsulated, why has it been removed with a cuff of surrounding gland?

The capsule in these tumours is often breached by 'amoeboid' processes of the tumour. These may be left behind if the tumour is merely shelled out and recurrences will then be inevitable. In this case the facial nerve was identified as it entered the gland and was carefully preserved before excising the tumour.

Case 47 A patient with difficulty swallowing

A 60-year-old civil servant complained of increasing difficulty in swallowing, which had gradually become worse over the past 2 years. At first it was quite mild but was now becoming a real nuisance to him. He found that food, and now even fluids, would tend to stick in his throat. In recent months he found that he might regurgitate food he had just swallowed. The whole affair was quite painless. His weight had not changed, he felt well and there were no other relevant features in his past or present history.

Clinical examination revealed a slim, healthy man, with no abnormal findings. He was given a glass of water to drink, which made him splutter a bit, but nothing could be felt on most careful palpation of the neck.

Difficulty in swallowing, dysphagia, is always a symptom to be considered with the greatest of care. What is your classification of its possible causes?

1 *General causes.* First, do not forget general causes – neurological conditions – that may affect swallowing; these include:

- Myasthenia gravis.
- Bulbar palsy, usually of vascular origin, affecting IX and X cranial nerves.
- Bulbar poliomyelitis and diphtheria may still occur in developing countries. Hysteria, so called 'bulbus hystericus', is extremely rare.

2 *Local causes.* These are classified, in every obstructed tube in the body, into causes in the lumen, causes in the wall, and causes outside the wall. In dysphagia, this list is as follows:

- *Causes in the lumen*: Impacted foreign body, e.g. a bolus of food.
- *Causes in the wall*:
  - Congenital atresia.
  - Caustic stricture.
  - Inflammatory stricture secondary to reflux oesophagitis.
  - Achalasia of the cardia.
  - Plummer–Vinson syndrome with pharyngeal web.
  - Tumours of the oesophagus or cardia of stomach.
  - Pharyngeal pouch.
- *Causes outside the wall*:
  - Pressure of enlarged lymph nodes (secondaries or lymphoma).
  - Bronchial carcinoma.
  - Aortic thoracic aneurysm.
  - Retrosternal thyroid.

Your clinical examination being entirely normal, as is a full routine blood count, what would be the first special investigation you would order?

An oesophago-gastro-duodenoscopy (upper gastro-intestinal endoscopy). This has the added benefit of being able to perform a biopsy and make a tissue diagnosis. However, in this case a barium swallow was performed since it is a safe investigation; it is commonly used as a first-line investigation where endoscopy is not readily available. Three of the images in the series are demonstrated in Fig. 47.1.

The appearance was constant on the series of films that were obtained. What condition does it show?

A pharyngeal pouch.

Where is the pouch situated anatomically and what is its presumed aetiology?

It is a protrusion of mucosa between the two parts of the inferior pharyngeal sphincter, the thyropharyngeus and cricopharyngeus (Killian's dehiscence*), as shown in Fig. 47.2. It is believed to result from spasm of the

*Gustav Killian (1860–1921), Professor of otorhinolaryngology, Freiburg and Berlin.

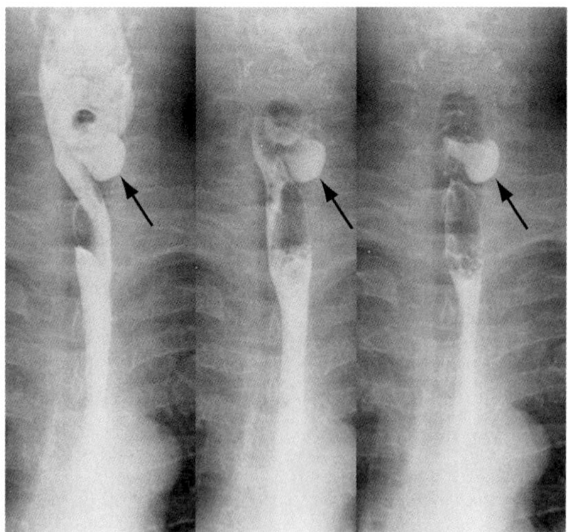

Figure 47.1 Barium swallow illustrating a pharyngeal pouch (arrowed).

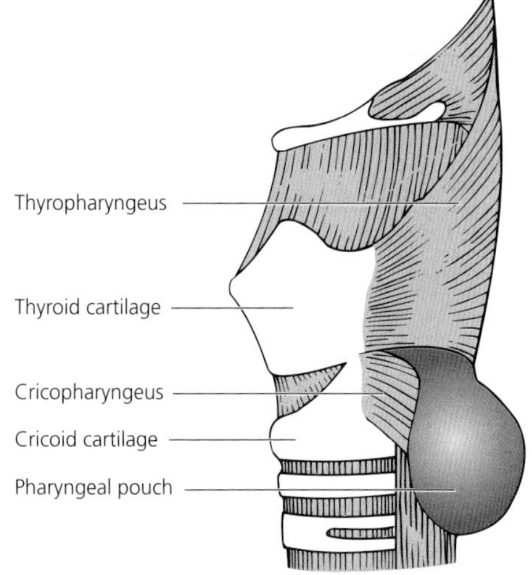

Figure 47.2 A pharyngeal pouch emerging between the two components of the inferior constrictor muscle.

cricopharyngeus, although why this should occur is not understood.

As the pouch gradually enlarges, what does it do to the oesophagus, and why is this important?

As the pouch enlarges, it displaces the oesophagus laterally. This means that an oesophageal catheter or bougie

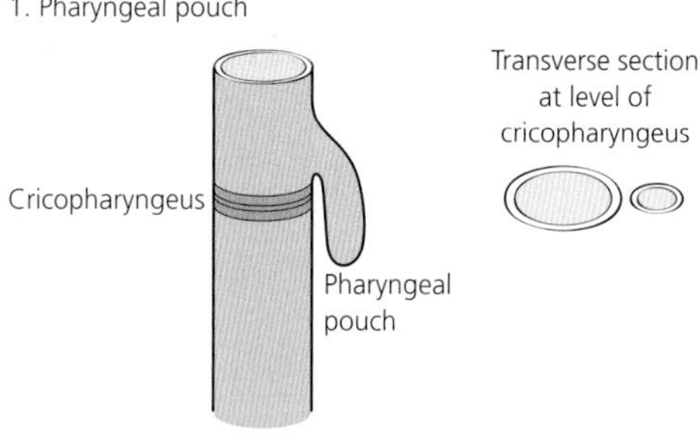

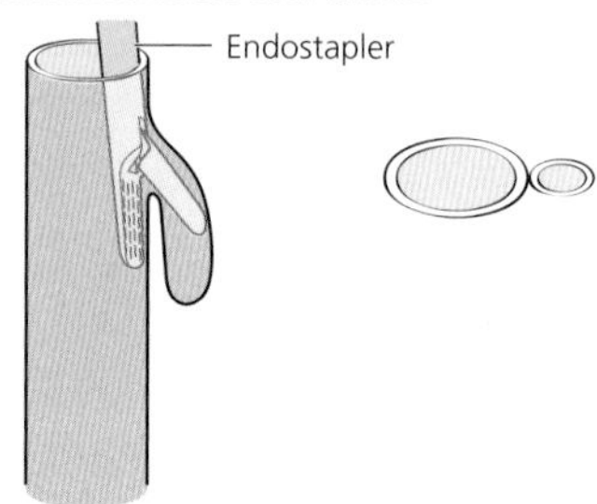

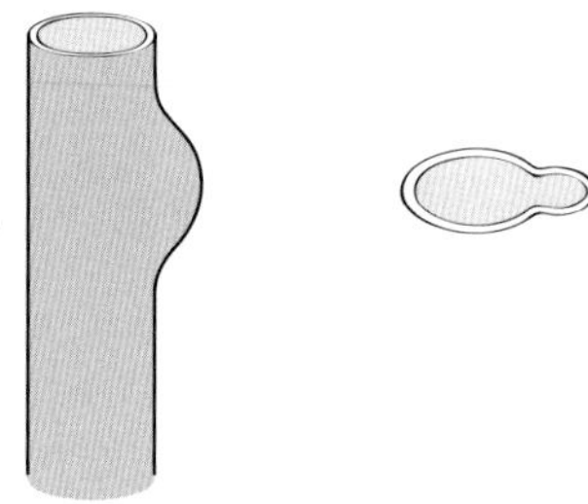

Figure 47.3 Endoluminal surgery.

or oesophagoscope will tend to enter the pouch itself rather than sliding down the lumen of the oesophagus. The pouch may thus be accidentally perforated, with the resultant risk of mediastinitis. Suspicion of a pharyngeal pouch is a good indication to proceed to barium swallow rather than endoscopy as the first-line investigation.

What is the standard treatment of this condition?

Surgical excision of the pouch with longitudinal division of the cricopharyngeus part of the inferior constrictor (myotomy). This was performed on this patient with a highly satisfactory result. Nowadays this procedure may be performed endoscopically by stapling across the two lumina (pouch and oesophagus), thus dividing the cricopharyngeus (Fig. 47.3).

Case 48 Another patient with difficulty in swallowing

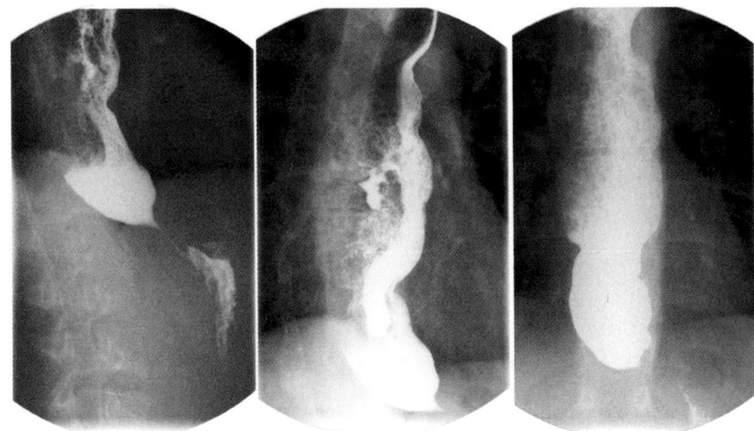

Figure 48.1

A married canteen waitress aged 55 years consulted her family practitioner with a history of difficulty in swallowing. This she had noticed 3 or 4 years previously. Food seemed to stick behind the sternum, but as there was no pain and it was not very severe, she put this down to 'indigestion'. However, it was now a real nuisance and she was worried that something serious was going on. She said that the difficulty was especially marked if she swallowed food she had not chewed well and that, although at first fluids gave no problem, she was now having some difficulty swallowing her drinks. She had not lost her appetite and, as far as she could tell, her weight was steady and she was otherwise healthy and active. She had had two normal pregnancies and no serious previous illnesses. She pointed to the middle of her sternum as the location of her problem.

When her doctor examined her, she was a healthy woman of average build, with no evidence of weight loss or clinical anaemia. There were no masses to feel in the abdomen or the neck. She was given an urgent appointment to the surgical outpatient clinic. The surgeon confirmed the GP's history and clinical findings and ordered a full blood count, which was within normal limits, and a barium swallow X-ray. Typical films of the series are shown in Fig. 48.1.

Describe what the X-ray shows, and what is your diagnosis?

There is gross dilatation and tortuosity of the oesophagus, which leads to a narrowed segment at its lower end. As well as barium, the oesophagus contains a good

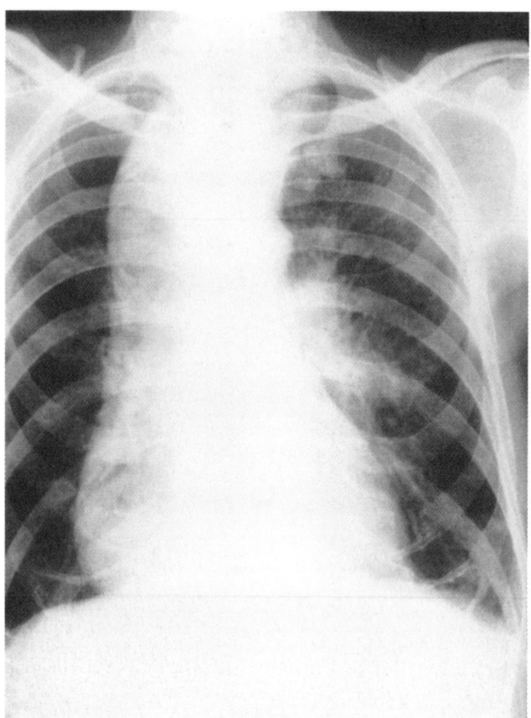

Figure 48.2 Chest X-ray illustrating a grossly dilated oesophagus.

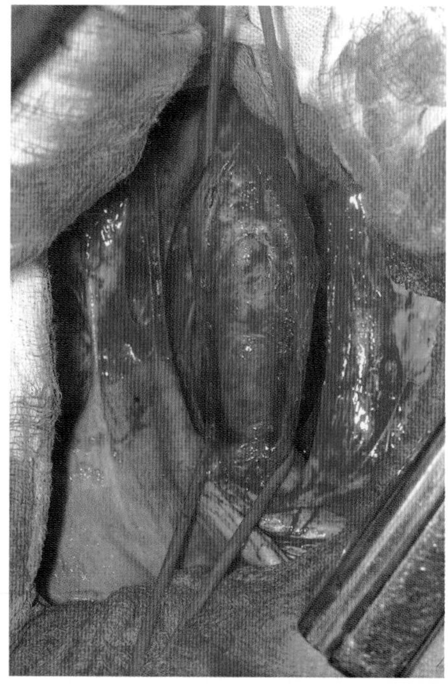

Figure 48.3 Heller's operation.

deal of solid food debris, shown by the filling defects in the pool of barium. These appearances are typical of achalasia of the oesophagus.

What is the aetiology of this condition?

There is neuromuscular failure of relaxation of the lower end of the oesophagus with incoordination of peristalsis of the oesophageal muscles. This leads to progressive dilatation, hypertrophy and tortuosity of the oesophagus above the cardia. Oesophageal motility studies show simultaneous, low amplitude contractions of the oesophagus with impaired relaxation of the lower oesophageal sphincter. Histology shows loss of myenteric plexus nerve cells. The aetiology of this condition remains unknown. It may commence at any age, but particularly in the thirties and forties, and is commoner in women. It is indistinguishable from Chagas' disease,* which occurs in South America and is caused by *Trypanosoma cruzi*; this parasite destroys the intermuscular ganglion cells of the oesophagus.

*Carlos Chagas (1879–1934), Professor of tropical medicine, Rio de Janeiro, Brazil.

What may a plain X-ray of the chest show in an advanced case, allowing the diagnosis to be made on this simple investigation alone?

The grossly dilated oesophagus, full of food debris, may produce the appearance of a mediastinal mass and there may be evidence of pneumonitis from repeated aspiration of oesophageal contents. This plain postero-anterior X-ray of the chest shows just such a case (Fig. 48.2): the patient was an old gentleman of 80, whose main complaint was of repeated attacks of 'bronchitis' – cough, fever and purulent sputum. Only on direct questioning did he admit to many years of difficulty in swallowing.

This patient referred the site of her dysphagia to the middle of her chest, yet the obstruction was at the oesophago-gastric junction – was this unusual?

Patients with an obstruction in the lower pharynx or cervical part of the oesophagus localize the level of the lesion quite precisely in the neck (vagal innervation). However, the thoracic and abdominal segments of the oesophagus and the cardia have sensory innervation from autonomic (sympathetic) afferents. Pain from these sites is poorly localized. The majority of patients, as in this woman, localize the obstruction, pain or discomfort rather vaguely to the mid body of the sternum. If you have ever had an attack of 'heartburn' you will have noticed how difficult it is to define the site of the pain.

How is this condition treated?

Heller's operation† is performed – cardiomyotomy, with the muscle of the lower end of the oesophagus right down to the cardia split down to the mucosa. This was carried out successfully in the present case and Fig. 48.3 shows the lower oesophagus and cardia held between rubber slings immediately after the muscle wall was divided.

In many centres the operation is now performed thoracoscopically. The same effect may be achieved by forcible dilatation of the oesophago-gastric junction by means of a hydrostatic bag at endoscopy. Although this avoids open operation, there is a risk of rupture of the oesophagus.

†Ernst Heller (1877–1964), surgeon, Leipzig, Germany.

Case 49 A third patient with dysphagia

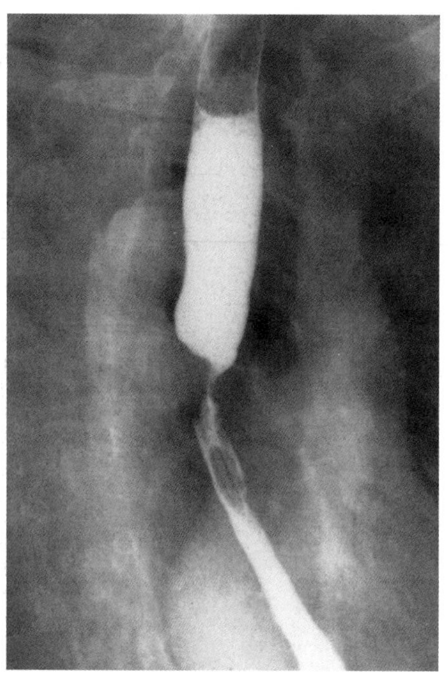

Figure 49.1

The X-ray in Fig. 49.1 shows one plate of a barium swallow series of a 68-year-old retired civil servant, who complained of difficulty in swallowing. He noted that solid foods, but not liquids, were seeming to stick at the lower end of his chest (he pointed to just above his xiphisternum), and this had been getting worse over the past couple of months. There was discomfort when he swallowed, but no actual pain. He had started to avoid eating and believed he had lost several pounds in weight over this time. He smoked 15 cigarettes a day, had a 'smoker's cough' with some mucoid sputum, was a social drinker and had had no serious past illnesses.

Clinical examination in the outpatient department revealed a rather thin anxious man with signs of weight loss. There were crepitations at both lung bases, but nothing abnormal to find on examination of the abdomen or supraclavicular region. A chest X-ray and full blood count were normal.

Describe the X-ray appearance and give the, almost certain, diagnosis

There is a severe obstruction of the mid oesophagus, which is slightly distended above the occlusion. A streak of contrast trickles through the block, to produce a 'rat's tail' deformity. This is the classical appearance of a carcinoma of the middle third of the oesophagus.

How is this diagnosis confirmed?

Fibre-optic oesophagoscopy is performed and a biopsy taken of the lesion.

What is the likely histology of this tumour?

Carcinoma of the oesophagus, until recently, was typically a stratified squamous carcinoma arising in the stratified squamous oesophageal musoca. For no apparent reason the incidence of adenocarcinoma of the lower end of the oesophagus has rapidly increased in the past 25 years and now accounts for about 65% of oesophageal cancers in this country and the developed world. This type of tumour occurs where the specialized squamous epithelium at the lower end of the oesophagus has undergone metaplasia to columnar epithelium as a result of chronic reflux of acid and bile (Fig. 49.2), producing the so-called Barrett's oesophagus (see Case 50, p. 102). The risk of adenocarcinoma is also linked to cigarette smoking, alcohol and obesity.

What is the curative treatment for carcinoma of the oesophagus?

Only surgery offers the chance of cure. However, this is a major operation, with something like a 5% hospital mortality rate. Assessment of fitness for surgery will include pulmonary function tests, electrocardiogram (ECG), etc., while contrast-enhanced CT and endoscopic ultrasound are required to determine the stage and spread of the tumour and to avoid unnecessary surgical exploration.

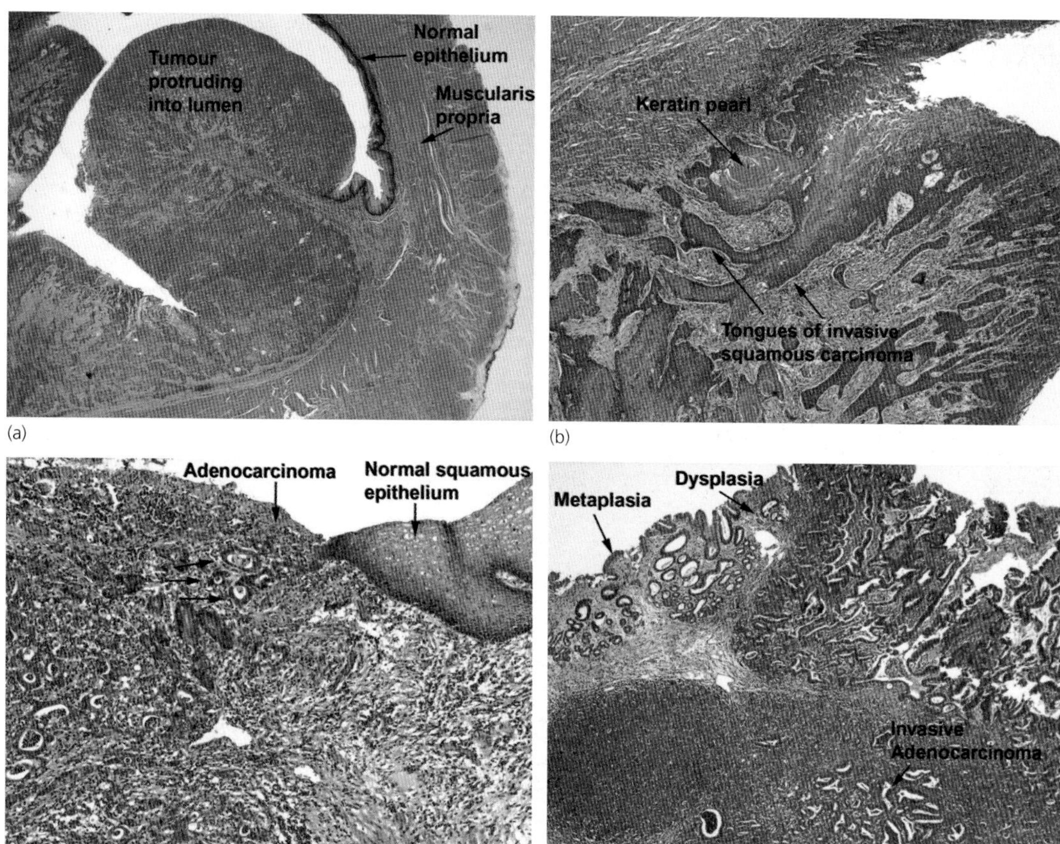

Figure 49.2 Histology of squamous and adenocarcinoma of oesophagus. Squamous carcinoma at a magnification of × 2 (a) and × 4 (b). Note the tumour protruding into the lumen, and the keratin deposits typical of squamous cancers. (c) Adenocarcinoma of the oesophagus where tumour can be seen to arise from adjacent normal squamous epithelium and to posses the typical glandular structures (arrowed) of an adenocarcinoma (magnification × 10). (d) A different tumour showing evidence of mucosal metaplasia with adjacent dysplastic areas and invasive tumour (magnification × 10). This is typical of Barrett's oesophagus.

What about palliative treatment?

This is required in patients with local disease not considered fit for major surgery, those with advanced local disease or with evidence of metastatic spread, and those who have undergone radical surgery but return with recurrent disease.

It is extremely important to relieve the misery of dysphagia in these patients, and this can often be achieved by the insertion of an expandable metal stent. Palliative cytotoxic therapy and radiotherapy may also be employed.

Case 50 Heartburn

A 50-year-old housewife consulted her family practitioner with the request for something to relieve her severe heartburn. When the doctor took a detailed history, this revealed that the patient had been experiencing a burning pain for several years, which she localized to about the middle of the body of the sternum. There was no radiation of the pain. She had been self-medicating, with some success until recently, using a whole variety of proprietary indigestion and antacid tablets and medicines. The pain would come on shortly after her meals, especially her evening dinner, the main meal of the day. She also had her sleep disturbed by the pain and had noticed that this was less likely to happen if she slept propped up with pillows. She also found that the pain might come on if she stooped down, for instance to pick something up from the floor. Occasionally at night or on stooping she had noticed regurgitation of bitter-tasting fluid into her mouth, and this she had found to be particularly unpleasant, but she had never actually vomited.

On direct questioning, she had never noticed the food sticking in the chest on swallowing, i.e. there was no evidence of actual dysphagia. Apart from these symptoms she was well, her appetite good and her bowels acted normally. She had had three children and had gained a lot of weight after the third pregnancy and was now quite obese. Functional enquiry was otherwise normal.

Apart from her obesity and moderate hypertension (blood pressure 160/110), clinical examination was normal.

What is the likely clinical diagnosis based on these findings?

The symptoms are quite typical of a sliding hiatus hernia with gastro-oesophageal reflux. Acid regurgitation into the lower oesophagus produces the pain, which typically occurs after meals (with consequent acid secretion by the stomach) and on lying down, when the cardia of the stomach herniates through the dilated oesophageal hiatus in the diaphragm.

What is the first-line special investigation to carry out in order to confirm or refute this clinical diagnosis?

Upper gastrointestinal endoscopy is now the investigation of choice when it is available locally. On this occasion the family practitioner referred the patient for a barium swallow and meal examination (Fig. 50.1).

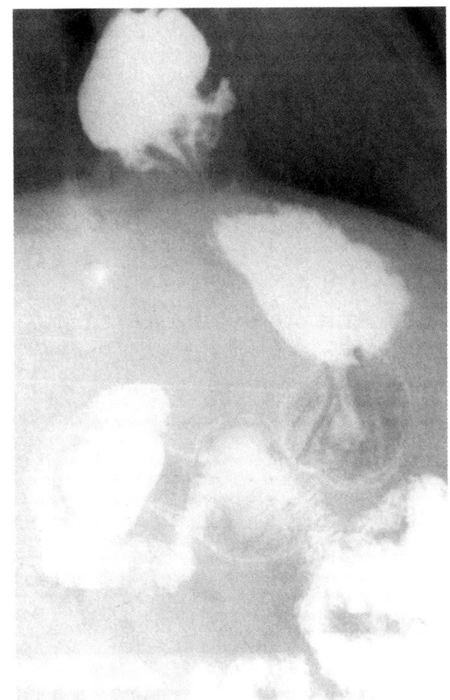

Figure 50.1 Barium swallow and meal examination of the patient.

The deformity shown was constant on a series of films. What does it demonstrate?

There is a large sliding hiatus hernia. The fundus and upper body of the stomach are seen to lie above the crescentic border of the left hemidiaphragm.

What position has the patient been placed in this film?

In order to demonstrate the hernia, the patient has been tipped head-downwards, and is lying on her left side. Note that, in this position, the fundus of the stomach is filled with barium, whereas in the usual erect position of a barium meal examination the fluid level of the gastric air bubble is seen.

In what sort of person is this condition particularly common?

This is the classical case – a middle-aged, obese female.

What symptoms may be associated with a hiatus hernia?

The condition may be entirely symptomless and is discovered when a barium meal or endoscopy is performed for some other cause or when it is found at laparotomy or laparoscopy for some other pathology. Associated oesophageal reflux results in symptoms similar to the present case – burning epigastric or retrosternal pain, which is aggravated by lying down or stooping. Sometimes the chest pain may mimic angina. Longstanding acid reflux may result in stricture formation and bleeding. Barrett's oesophagus* (mucosal gastric metaplasia) may occur in longstanding cases, with the risk of development of adenocarcinoma. A very large hernia may produce mechanical effects – particularly cough and breathlessness.

*Norman Barrett (1903–1979), thoracic surgeon, St Thomas's Hospital, London.

Case 51 Vomiting in a baby

A baby boy aged 3 weeks was brought to the children's accident and emergency department of a teaching hospital and the parents gave the following history: he was their second child and his sister, aged 4, was perfectly well. He had had a normal delivery, at full term, and mother and child left hospital the following day. He was being breastfed and had no problem until 4 days previously, when he began to be sick after his feeds. He would suck avidly then appear to be in discomfort and would then vomit the unchanged feed, which would 'shoot out'. The milk was never green or discoloured in any way.

What is your first clinical impression on hearing this story?

It sounds very suspicious that this baby has infantile hypertrophic pyloric stenosis. This typically presents between 2 and 8 weeks from birth; presentation later than 12 weeks is very unusual.

On examination, the baby had the classical clinical findings of this condition. What would you expect to find?

Boys are affected much more often than girls (80%) and they are often the first born. The condition may occur in siblings; the mother of one of our patients diagnosed the condition correctly in her second baby on his first vomit – she remembered his elder brother's symptoms so vividly!

The patient shows signs of dehydration and the anterior fontanelle may be depressed, although this sign is only evident at a fairly advanced stage. If a test feed of warm water is given, the baby drinks avidly but shortly after he vomits. This is often 'projectile' and shoots out of the baby's mouth. The vomit is the fluid just taken and is free from bile staining.

On inspection of the abdomen, visible peristalsis may be seen immediately after the feed, passing from left to right across the upper abdomen. Much more commonly – in about 95% of cases – the hypertrophied pylorus is felt as a distinct mass, 'the pyloric tumour'. Feeling this, in a fretful infant, requires a good deal of clinical skill. The baby is either put to the mother's breast or given a bottle and examined in the mother's arms. The warmed hand is gently insinuated over the baby's abdomen and the index and middle fingers placed over the right upper quadrant. Whatever you do, do not dig! The pyloric tumour is an olive-shaped mass about 1 cm in diameter. This finding is diagnostic.

In a doubtful case, the tumour can be picked up on ultrasonography.

What is known about the aetiology of this condition?

Amazingly little! Apart from the family history risk and its preponderance in males, as already noted, and the fact that it is commoner in north European and American Caucasians than in other races, with an incidence in the UK of about three per 1000 live births, its origin is obscure. A similar condition has been produced in puppies by administering pentagastrin to pregnant dogs.

The baby was given intravenous fluid replacement and operated upon the next morning. Some photographs were taken at surgery (Fig. 51.1).

What do they demonstrate?

Figure 51.1a shows the index finger and thumb of the left hand of the surgeon holding the stomach out of the wound. The hypertrophied pylorus is seen just beyond these. Figure 51.1b shows the incision made across the pylorus. This will be carried down to the gastric mucosa, with care being taken not to puncture the mucosal layer (Ramstedt's operation*) (Fig. 51.2).

---

*Conrad Ramstedt (1867–1963), surgeon, Munster, Germany.

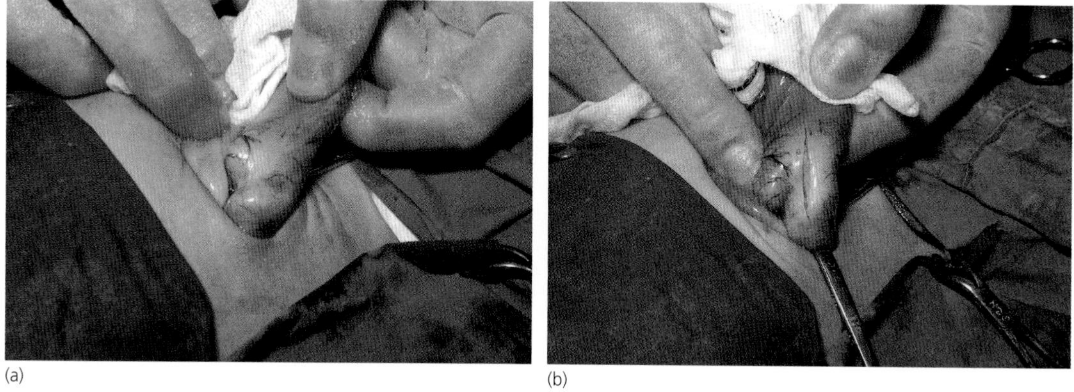

Figure 51.1 Ramstedt's pyloromyotomy. The stomach and proximal duodenum are delivered through the wound (a), and an incision made through the serosa across the pylorus (b).

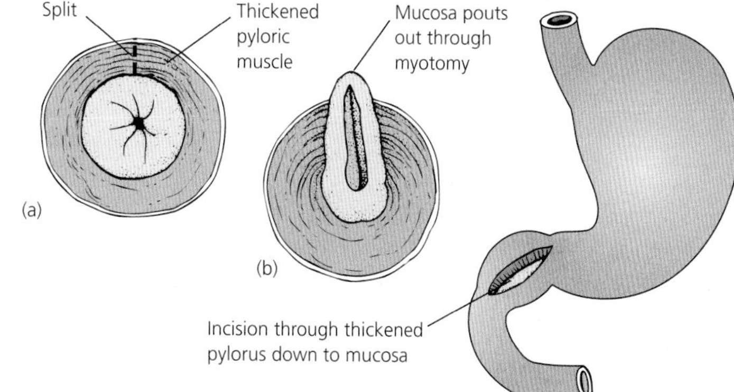

Figure 51.2 Ramstedt's pyloromyotomy, showing the pathology (a) and operative procedure in transverse section (b). The thickened muscle at the pylorus is split down to the mucosa.

What is the prognosis in such a case?

The mortality approaches zero and the long-term results are excellent.

Case 52 A gastric ulcer

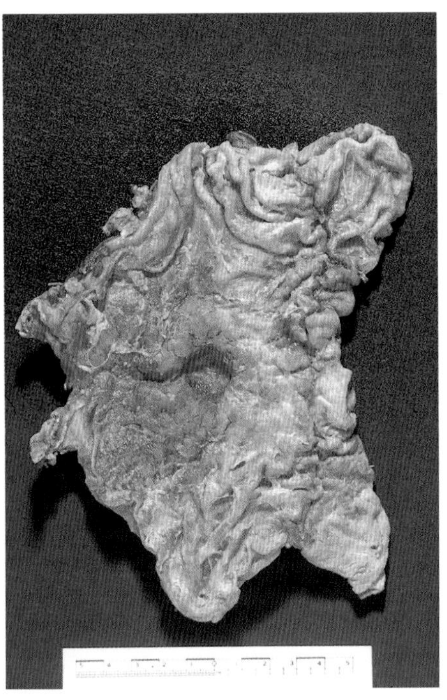

Figure 52.1

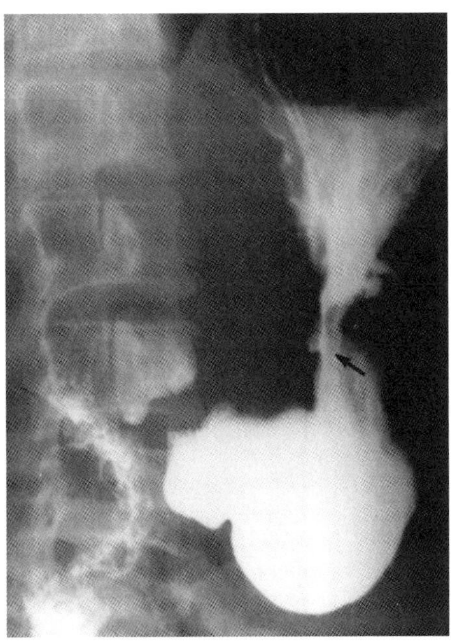

Figure 52.2 Barium meal illustrating the niche of the gastric ulcer on the lesser curve (arrowed).

Figure 52.1 shows an old specimen resected from the stomach of a 57-year-old publican. He had a long history of epigastric pain, but was reluctant to attend his family doctor for fear of being lectured about his smoking and drinking habits. Nevertheless he had slowly been losing weight, with the pain being exacerbated on eating. He had tried antacids but they gave only short-term relief, and his sleep was regularly disturbed by the pain.

What is the most likely diagnosis?

This is a gastric ulcer. There is no thickening or heaping up of the edges so it is likely to be a benign ulcer.

This ulcer was diagnosed on a barium meal (see Fig. 52.2) and is indicated on the lesser curve of the stomach by an arrow. How would a patient with these symptoms be investigated today and why?

Endoscopy is the investigation of choice, and would have diagnosed the presence of this ulcer and enabled biopsies to be taken to look for evidence of malignancy.

Gastrectomy for peptic ulcers used to be commonplace, but they are infrequently performed nowadays. It was once believed that peptic ulcers were related to excess acid production in the stomach. What is now known to be the aetiology?

It is now recognized that the commonest cause of peptic ulceration is infection with *Helicobacter pylori*, an organism that was not recognized until the pioneering work by Marshall and Warren* in Australia in 1979. Treatment is with antibiotics, and not surgery.

How is infection with *Helicobacter pylori* diagnosed?

The organism possesses a urease enzyme that converts urea into ammonia and carbon dioxide. This is the basis of two diagnostic tests. In the first a biopsy of the stomach is placed in a solution of urea together with a pH indicator; a change to alkali pH gives a rapid confirmation of the diagnosis. Alternatively the patient is given 14C-labelled urea to drink. The *Helicobacter* breaks down the urea liberating $14CO_2$ which is exhaled and can be detected on the breath. Lastly, serum *Helicobacter* antibodies indicate past infection.

*Barry Marshall (b. 1951), gastroenterologist, Royal Perth Hospital, Australia; J. Robin Warren (b. 1937), pathologist, Royal Perth Hospital. They won a Nobel Prize for their work in 2005.

Case 53 A bloody vomit

A 67-year-old retired schoolteacher with rheumatoid arthritis presented in shock following a brisk haematemesis during which she vomited coffee grounds and fresh blood with clots. She had no previous history of indigestion, but on direct questioning had been passing melaena for the previous 2 days.

Her rheumatoid arthritis had been difficult to control and affected her hands and wrists the most. She had required gold injections in addition to regular ibuprofen for pain. On examination she was pale with a pulse of 120 and blood pressure of 90/50 mmHg. Her abdomen was soft with some epigastric tenderness and there was melaena on the examining glove on rectal examination.

What should the initial management comprise?

The patient needs aggressive resuscitation. Oxygen should be commenced by face mask, and venous access gained with large bore cannulae. Intravenous fluids, such as Hartmann's solution or Gelefusin should be given to restore a normal blood pressure, and blood sent for cross-matching. A bladder catheter is essential to monitor urine output, particularly in patients who are volume depleted following haemorrhage and on a non-steroidal anti-inflammatory drug (NSAID), which increases the risk of acute renal failure. In elderly patients the rate and amount of fluid administration needs to be carefully monitored lest pulmonary oedema is precipitated. Once resuscitation is underway an assessment is made to establish whether bleeding is ongoing – continued vomiting, melaena or failure to respond to fluid replacement.

What is the likely diagnosis and how should it be proven?

The patient is likely to have a bleeding peptic ulcer. Diagnosis is by endoscopy which, in the presence of bleeding, should be performed without delay.

How should a bleeding duodenal ulcer be managed? What are the indications for surgery, and what non-surgical options are available in patients unfit for surgery?

- Therapeutic endoscopy is now the first line of treatment. The ulcer base, and any visible vessel, is injected with 1:10 000 epinephrine (adrenaline) to stop the bleeding. Endoscopic clips or thermal, laser or argon plasma coagulation may be used where available. A high dose infusion of a proton pump inhibitor, such as intravenous omeprazole, is commenced, given as an 80 mg bolus followed by 8 mg/h infusion for 72 h. Endoscopy can be repeated after 24 h to further treat the ulcer.
- The indications for surgery have changed since the advent of therapeutic endoscopy and improved results with intravenous proton pump inhibitors. Factors suggesting that surgery may be indicated include continued bleeding in spite of endoscopic treatment, a visible vessel at the ulcer base, transfusion requirements in excess of 4 units in 24 h in a patient over 60, or 8 units in a younger patient. The nature of the surgical intervention has also changed; under-running of the bleeding vessel in the base of the ulcer being preferred to gastrectomy, combined with full medical management including treatment for *Helicobacter*.
- In patients unfit for surgery, or where surgery is not desirable, mesenteric angiography with embolization of the gastroduodenal artery may be appropriate.

Case 54 An acute abdominal emergency

A retired merchant seaman, while enjoying a glass of beer with his friends one evening, suddenly collapsed with extremely severe general abdominal pain. An ambulance was called and he arrived at the local A&E department about half an hour after the onset of the pain.

The surgeon on duty took a rapid brief history. The patient had suffered from episodes of 'indigestion' for many years but never went to the doctor about this, merely dosing himself with proprietary indigestion tablets. These pains were epigastric in location, would come on after meals and might wake him at night. However, this present attack was quite different – very much worse, diffuse over the abdomen and, on direct questioning, he admitted to feeling pain over the right shoulder. He had not vomited but was feeling sick. He was a heavy cigarette smoker and a moderate beer drinker.

On examination, the patient lay absolutely still on the trolley, with his legs drawn up; the slightest movement aggravated the pain. He was pale, clammy and breathing with rapid short breaths. His pulse was 90/min, temperature 37°C and blood pressure 130/70 mmHg.

The abdomen was held rigidly tense, and was uniformly tender; it was silent on auscultation. The normal liver dullness over the lower right chest was replaced by undoubted resonance to percussion.

If you encountered this situation, what would be your clinical diagnosis?

The previous history is very suggestive of a chronic peptic ulcer. The patient now has the classical features of a general peritonitis of sudden onset. Putting the two together makes perforation of a chronic peptic ulcer into the peritoneal cavity the obvious first choice.

An X-ray of the chest and upper abdomen was obtained in the A&E department and is shown in Fig. 54.1.

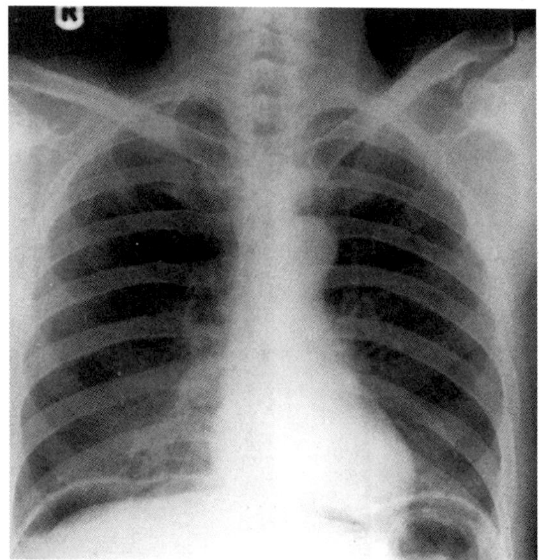

Figure 54.1 X-ray of the chest and upper abdomen.

What does the film demonstrate?

The lung fields are clear. There is obvious free gas under both hemi-diaphragms.

This is a typical finding after perforation of a peptic ulcer, as gastric gas escapes into the peritoneal cavity, but is it a constant finding in this condition?

Radiological evidence of free air on a plain chest X-ray is only present in about 70% of cases, but it is a serious error to discount the clinical diagnosis because of a negative X-ray. CT will confirm free intraperitoneal gas where doubt exists.

The patient complained of pain over the tip of the right shoulder – why so?

This is referred pain via the phrenic nerve (C3, C4 and C5), which supplies the diaphragm, to the corresponding dermatomes. In the majority of cases it is necessary to ask the patient directly about this distribution of the pain. The patient knows there is something seriously wrong inside his belly and often thinks his aching shoulder is irrelevant!

What is the management of this patient?

Reassurance; intravenous opiate, analgesia and antibiotic therapy is commenced together with intravenous fluid replacement. Surgical repair of the perforation is followed by medical therapy.

Case 55 A fateful vomit

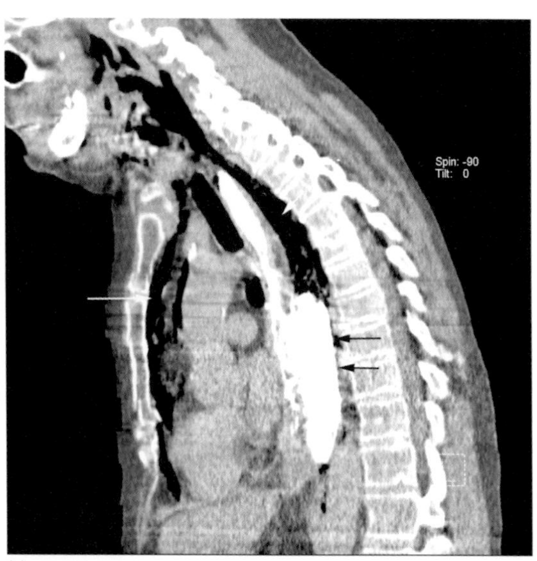

(a)

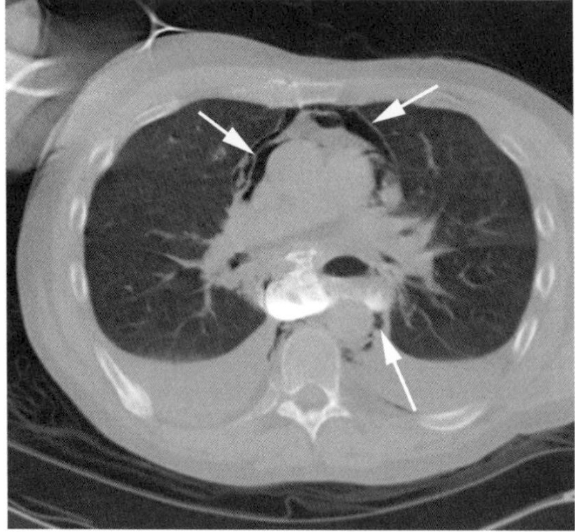
(b)

Figure 55.1

A town counsellor collapsed at home shortly after returning home from the annual Mayoral banquet where he had overindulged. He had developed a crushing central chest pain shortly after vomiting back a good deal of the banquet. There was no blood in the vomitus. Over the next couple of hours the pain increased in severity, and he also developed left shoulder tip pain. His general practitioner referred him into the admitting physicians as a probable myocardial infarction, and indeed there were ischaemic changes on the electrocardiograph that was performed when he arrived in hospital.

On arrival he was pale, cold and clammy, with a blood pressure of 90/60 mmHg and a tachycardia of 110/min. The examining resident elicited subcutaneous crepitus (surgical emphysema) over the upper chest, a finding for which he could find no explanation. The admission chest X-ray confirmed air in the tissues and fluid in the left subphrenic space. A thoracic CT scan was then undertaken as the patient swallowed soluble contrast. Figure 55.1 shows a transverse and sagittal section through the chest.

What is the most likely diagnosis?

The patient has sustained a rupture of the oesophagus. This usually occurs at the hiatus and extends proximally for a varying distance, and the history is typical. Subcutaenous crepitus may extend up to the face, and is a response to the pneumomediastinum. ECG changes are common, and reflect the ensuing chemical and bacterial mediastinitis. The CT images show contrast leaking out of the oesophagus (Fig. 55.1a, black arrows) and air in the mediastinum on both the sagittal and transverse sections (white arrows on Fig. 55.1a, b).

After whom is it named, and in whom was it described?

This is Boerhaave's syndrome,* named after the physi-

*Hermann Boerhaave (1668–1738), physician, Leiden, the Netherlands.

cian who described it at the autopsy of the Grand Admiral of the Dutch Fleet.

What is the appropriate investigation to confirm the diagnosis?

A contrast swallow, using a water-soluble contrast medium. While barium gives better pictures it is very difficult to remove from the mediastinum and pleura since it is barely water soluble, so Gastrografin or a similar water-soluble contrast agent is used.

What treatment is required?

Surgery is required to repair the tear and wash out the mediastinum and chest. Broad spectrum antibiotics are appropriate, and a jejunostomy is fashioned for enteral feeding while the repair heals. Repairing the tear may involve wrapping the fundus of the stomach around the repair, but large tears may require a resection and primary anastomosis with mobilized stomach. Large bore chest drains are placed, and will give an early indication of a leak from the anastomosis.

What is the likely outcome, and on what does this depend?

The prognosis depends on the delay between rupture and surgery, since the longer the delay the poorer the tissues are to repair. Good postoperative nutritional support is vital.

Case 56 A serious gastric lesion

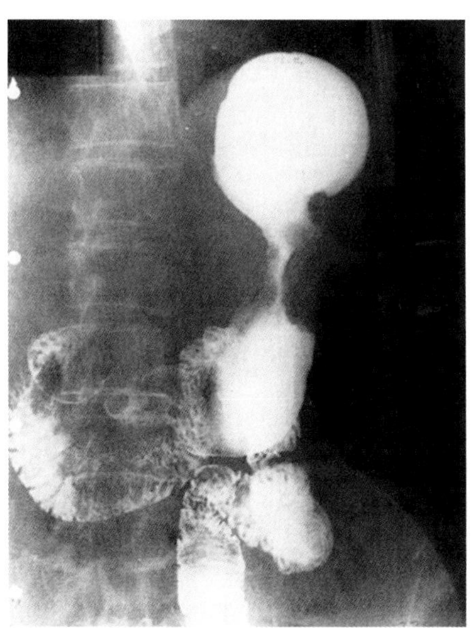

Figure 56.1

A 59-year-old supermarket manager presented with a short history – 4 or 5 months – of epigastric discomfort after meals, loss of appetite and loss of weight, which had dropped from its normal 75 kg to 68 kg. He had no discomfort at night. He had tried various proprietary indigestion remedies, but none had helped him. When examined by his medical practitioner, he looked pale and had obviously lost weight. Examination of the abdomen revealed some epigastric tenderness, but no masses could be felt. There was no hepatomegaly or clinical ascites. The supraclavicular nodes were impalpable and rectal examination was clear. The physician arranged for his patient to have an urgent barium meal examination. The appearances of the deformity in Fig. 56.1 were constant throughout the X-ray series.

Describe what this patient's X-ray demonstrates

There is a constant elongated narrowing, or stricture, occupying the body of the stomach. The fundus appears normal and there is free flow of barium into the duodenal loop.

Putting the clinical features and the X-ray appearances together, what is your working diagnosis?

Carcinoma of the body of the stomach.

What is the obvious next step to be carried out in the investigation of this patient to confirm or refute this diagnosis?

Urgent gastroscopy and biopsy of any suspicious area seen. This was done, and a malignant ulcer seen, almost encircling the body of the stomach. Examination of the multiple biopsy specimens taken showed a rather poorly differentiated adenocarcinoma.

Note that nowadays fibreoptic oesophago-gastric endoscopy is the screening investigation of choice in patients such as this, where a peptic ulcer or malignancy is suspected clinically. It is an interventional and uncomfortable investigation with a small risk of complications, such as perforation, compared with merely swallowing some flavoured clear fluid, but it has a high degree of sensitivity and specificity and allows an immediate biopsy to be taken of any suspicious lesion.

What clinical evidence would you seek of lymphatic spread of this tumour?

Palpation of the supraclavicular fossa for enlarged supraclavicular nodes spread along the thoracic duct (Troisier's sign,* signifying involvement of Virchow's

*Charles Emil Troisier (1844–1919), Professor of pathology, Paris.

node†). Note that his clinician was careful to perform this step in his examination of the patient.

What abdominal signs would you look for that would indicate portal vein and transcoelomic spread?

- *Portal vein spread*: Enlargement of the liver with or without jaundice together with ascites due to raised portal pressure.
- *Transcoelomic spread*: Ascites due to exudation from peritoneal seedings of tumour.

Note, in addition, that in the female patient a pelvic examination may reveal bilateral ovarian masses due to transcoelomic deposits of tumour (Krukenberg's tumour‡).

†Rudolf Virchow (1821–1901), Professor of pathology, Wurzburg and then Berlin.

‡Friedrich Krukenberg (1871–1946), pathologist, Halle, Germany.

Case 57 A surgical specimen of stomach

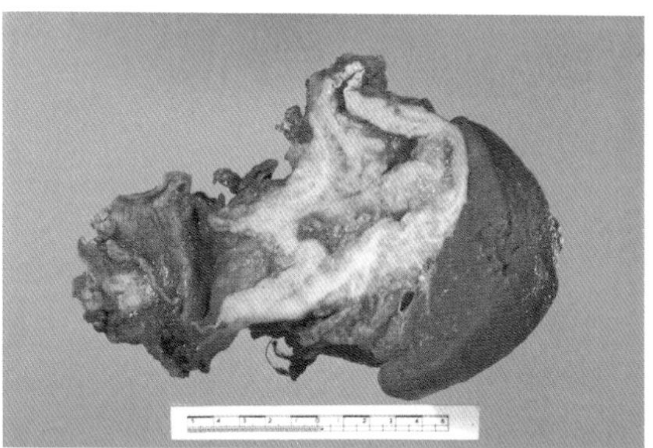

Figure 57.1

The specimen in Fig. 57.1, received by the pathologist from the operating theatre, is of a total gastrectomy and splenectomy performed on a woman of 61 years, who had presented with a short history of anorexia, weight loss and upper abdominal discomfort. She had had considerable difficulty in swallowing.

Examination had revealed a rather wasted patient who was not clinically anaemic, and whose full blood count proved to be normal. No masses, ascites or hepatomegaly were found on abdominal examination and there was no supraclavicular lymphadenopathy. She had been referred for urgent gastroscopy, where the stomach was found to be non-distensible, rendering the examination quite difficult; however, an area of ulceration was seen along the lesser curvature. Several biopsy specimens were taken, all of which revealed adenocarcinoma. She underwent a total gastrectomy and omentectomy, the spleen being removed with the specimen.

What are the names (one English and one Latin) given to this condition where the stomach is converted into a rigid tube by the infiltrating carcinoma?

Leather bottle stomach or linitis plastica.

What produces this appearance?

This is caused by submucous infiltration of the tumour with a marked fibrous reaction. This produces a small, thickened, contracted stomach with or without only superficial ulceration.

How common is carcinoma of the stomach in the UK, and what is happening to its incidence in this country?

Carcinoma of the stomach is the seventh commonest cause of death from cancer in the UK and indeed in most of the developed world (Table 57.1). Over the last half century it has dropped progressively from second place, after carcinoma of the lung, in this invidious 'league table'; the reason for this is the subject of much debate. However, adenocarcinoma of the lower end of the oesophagus has recently shown a remarkable rise in incidence and oesophageal cancer is now the fifth commonest cause of death (see Case 49, p. 100).

Is anything known about the aetiology of gastric cancer?

There is a link with subjects having blood group A. The incidence is raised in patients with pernicious anaemia and malignant change occasionally is found at the edge of a benign gastric ulcer. There is no definite association with smoking, obesity or alcohol consumption. The disease is far commoner in Japan and in some parts of South America than in Western Europe and the USA.

Smoked food and preservation with salt may be a factor in these high incidence areas, and possibly the fall in consumption of such foods might be a factor in the decline in incidence of gastric cancer elsewhere.

Interestingly, whatever the carcinogenic agent(s) might be, they seem to be important early in life; Japanese migrants retain their life-time risk of developing this tumour after leaving their own country.

Table 57.1 The commonest causes of death from cancer in the UK, 2005.

Rank	Cancer	Number per 100 000 population
1	Lung	55.8
2	Colorectal	26.8
3	Breast	20.8
4	Prostate	16.7
5	Oesophagus	12.4
6	Pancreas	12.1
7	Stomach	9.4
8	Bladder	7.9
9	Ovary	7.4
10	Non-Hodgkin's lymphoma	7.4

Areas of high incidence of *Helicobacter pylori* infection also have a high incidence of gastric cancer.

What is the prognosis in gastric cancer and on what factors does it depend?

Prognosis in gastric cancer, as with any malignant tumour, depends on the extent of spread of the tumour and its degree of differentiation. Overall the prognosis of gastric cancer is poor in this country because of the advanced stage at which many of these tumours present. Patients with early stage tumours, without lymph node metastases, may have an 80% 5-year postoperative survival. In Japan, where the high incidence of the disease has merited endoscopic screening, high rates of survival are seen. It is to be hoped that the recent establishment of more and more endoscopic units in the UK may also result in improvement in early diagnosis and hence of prognosis.

Case 58 An acutely painful, distended abdomen

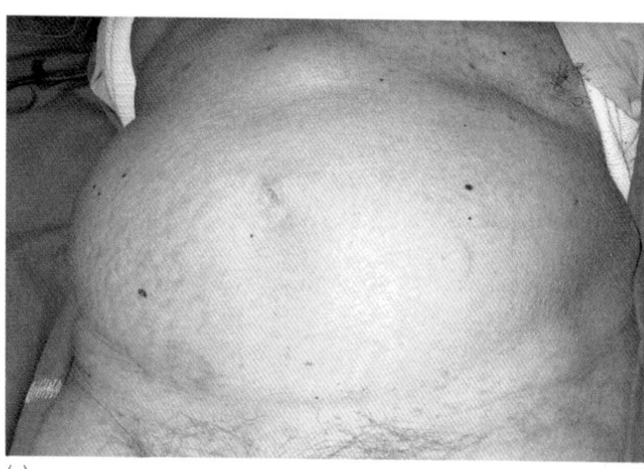
(a)

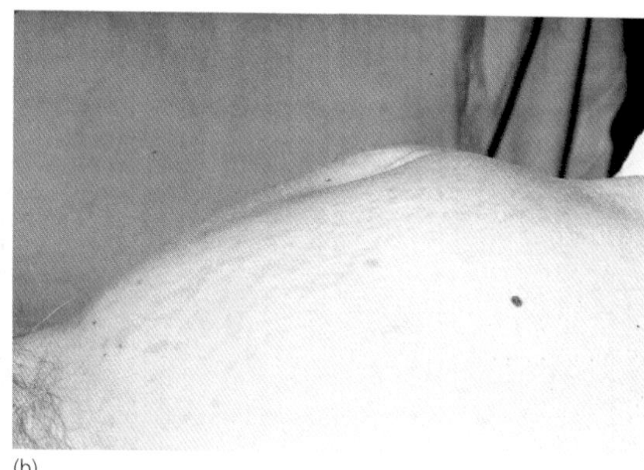
(b)

Figure 58.1

A housewife aged 56 years was admitted to hospital as an acute surgical emergency. Twelve hours before admission, shortly after she had gone to bed, she suddenly experienced acute central abdominal pain and vomited up her supper. The pains recurred every few minutes, were getting worse and made her double up. She vomited several more times, now greenish fluid. Her bowels had not acted and she had not passed flatus since the pain began. Ten years previously she had her appendix removed as an emergency through a right paramedian incision and the surgeon told her afterwards that it was gangrenous and had nearly burst.

Apart from this, she had previously been quite well. She was on hormone replacement therapy and had had three children, all normal deliveries. Until this episode, her bowels had moved normally.

On examination, she was in obvious pain, which was coming on in spasms every few minutes – she said 'like labour pains, but worse'. Her termperature was 37°C, pulse 100 and blood pressure 130/78 mmHg. She was dehydrated with a dry, coated tongue. Inspection of the abdomen revealed the appearance shown in these photographs of the patient (Fig. 58.1).

What are your inspection findings?

The abdomen is grossly distended. There is a well healed, low right paramedian operative scar. There are no obvious herniae at the umbilical, inguinal or femoral orifices. Careful inspection, over a few minutes, detected obvious visible peristalsis, waves of contraction being seen to pass from left to right across the abdomen. Palpation revealed no abdominal masses, but the abdomen was diffusely tender and there was marked guarding. There was no clinical evidence of free fluid on percussion, but noisy bowel sounds were obvious on auscultation. Rectal examination revealed an empty rectum and no masses were felt.

Putting all this information together, what is now your clinical diagnosis?

She has all four of the classical features of acute intestinal obstruction:

- Acute colicky abdominal pain.
- Abdominal distension.
- Vomiting.
- Absolute constipation – i.e. for flatus as well as faeces.

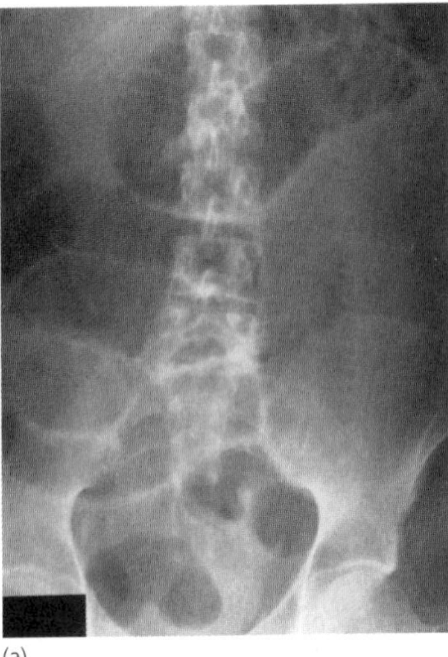
(a)

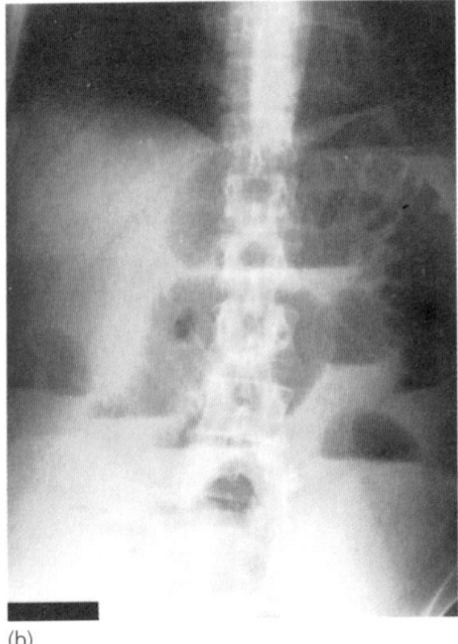
(b)

Figure 58.2 X-ray of the abdomen: (a) supine and (b) erect.

The fact that she has had a previous abdominal operation – no matter how long ago – together with the absence of any evidence of a strangulated hernia at the umbilical, inguinal or femoral orifices – makes obstruction due to adhesions or an adhesive band by far the most likely cause of this emergency.

What radiological investigation is used to help confirm the diagnosis?

A plain X-ray of the abdomen.

This was carried out, and the two films that were taken are shown in Fig. 58.2.

What is the position of the patient in the X-rays and what do these films show?

The patient is supine in Fig. 58.2a and erect in Fig. 58.2b. The first shows dilated loops of bowel in a ladder pattern. The valvulae coniventes can be seen to pass transversely right across the bowel wall, which is typical of small intestine. Figure 58.2b shows multiple fluid levels. The X-rays strongly support the clinical diagnosis of small bowel obstruction.

It is important to note that a small percentage of patients with this condition show no obvious anomaly on plain abdominal X-rays. This is explained by the loops of distended bowel being completely filled by fluid.

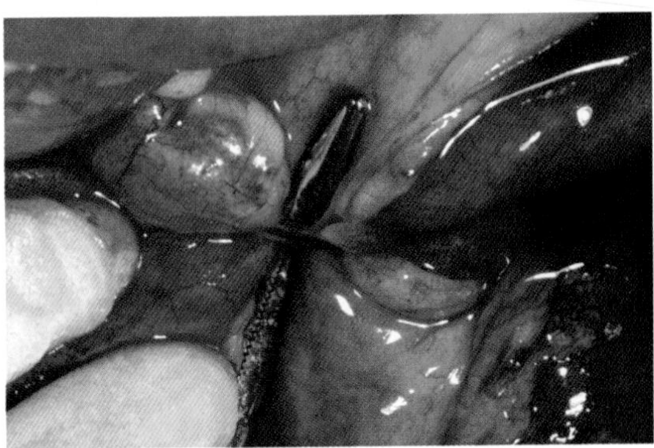

Figure 58.3 A band adhesion is seen in front of the surgical instrument and obstructing the adjacent bowel loops.

Other investigations can be:
- Radiology of the abdomen after injection of water-soluble contrast through a nasogastric tube.
- Abdominal CT scan.
- Abdominal ultrasound.

What is the initial management of this patient?

- Reassurance that she is going to get better – the first thing to do with every emergency patient!
- Relieve the pain with morphine, best given intravenously.

- Nasogastric suction to empty the distended stomach.
- Commence intravenous replacement of fluid and electrolytes.
- Prophylactic antibiotic therapy, such as a combination of metronidazole and a cephalosporin, is indicated if surgery is to be undertaken and is given at the induction of anaesthesia. Otherwise, if the patient is septic, it should be started following culture of blood, urine and sputum (if present).

The patient failed to settle on conservative management and was operated upon 48 h later. The abdomen was explored through a lower midline incision. Distended loops of small intestine were immediately encountered. An adhesive band was found to pass across a loop of small intestine and obstruct it (Fig. 58.3). The band was divided and the patient made a smooth recovery.

Case 59 Neonatal intestinal obstruction

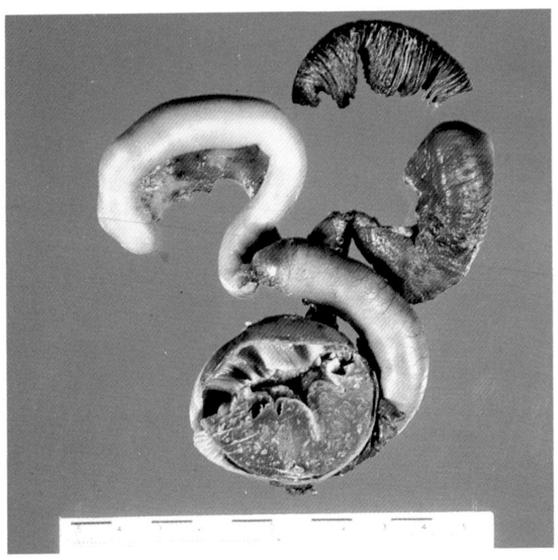

Figure 59.1

This specimen is a segment of terminal ileum removed at emergency surgery on a severely ill premature baby with intestinal obstruction (Fig. 59.1). The lower end of the specimen has been cut across so that you can see the lumen of the bowel and its contents.

Can you make a diagnosis of the cause of the obstruction?

This shows the typical appearance of a fairly rare condition. The cut end of the ileum shows that it is blocked by a mass of inspissated meconium. The bowel immediately proximal to this can be seen to be distended with this material, like a sausage, while the piece of ileum above this, although distended, does not contain meconium. This condition is termed meconium ileus.

What is the underlying pathology that accounts for this condition?

This is the neonatal presentation of 10–15% of infants with cystic fibrosis. Because of the loss of secretion of intestinal mucus and blockage of the pancreatic ducts, with consequent loss of tryptic digestion, the lower ileum of the fetus becomes blocked with inspissated sticky meconium.

What is the typical X-ray appearance of the abdomen in this condition?

There are distended loops of small intestine containing meconium with a characteristic mottled 'ground glass' appearance.

What may happen to the obstructed segment of intestine?

Perforation of the bowel may occur in intrauterine life, producing a (sterile) meconium peritonitis. The impacted distended segment of intestine may develop areas of gangrene from pressure necrosis. Both these complications, of course, greatly increase the morbidity and mortality of this disease.

How is this condition treated?

It may be possible to clear the inspissated plugs of meconium by instillation of Gastrografin (a water-soluble, radio-opaque contrast agent) per rectum under X-ray control. If this fails, or if the bowel has perforated, surgery is required. It may then be possible to open the intestine and remove the inspissated meconium by lavage, but if the impacted bowel cannot be cleared or shows areas of gangrene, as in this case, or has actually perforated, then resection is required.

Case 60 A very constipated small boy

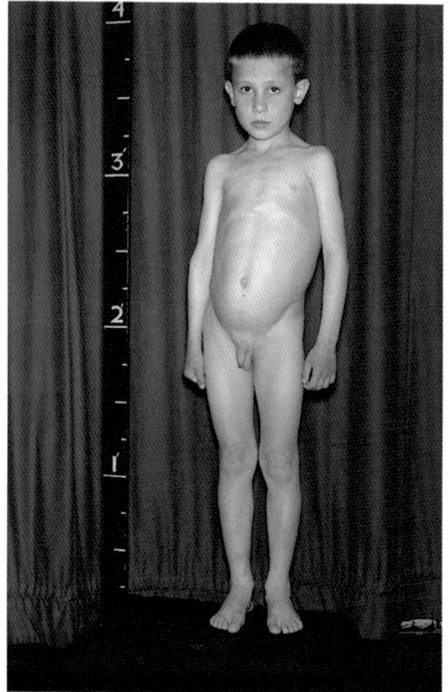

Figure 60.1

This is a boy of 15 years, who looks much younger, and is much smaller than his chronological age would suggest. He was brought to this country from overseas for treatment. His parents gave a history that his abdomen had appeared distended ever since he was a baby. He has been constipated all his life; he might go days or even a week without a bowel movement. His parents had tried a whole range of aperients without success and now his aunt, who was a trained nurse, was giving him an enema once a week. This usually produced a constipated stool. There was no blood seen in the motions at any time.

On examination he was a very bright, intelligent boy, who attended school with children of his own age and easily kept level with them in his school subjects. The abdomen, as can be seen in Fig. 60.1, is grossly distended but not tender. On rectal examination, the anal canal was normal and empty, but a mass of hard faeces could be felt at the tip of the examining finger. The testes were in the normal scrotal position, but he was pre-pubertal, with no genital, facial or axillary hair.

What is your clinical diagnosis? Give both the scientific name and the eponym by which it is commonly called.

Congenital megacolon or Hirschsprung's disease.*

What is the pathological basis of this condition and how is this pathology demonstrated in the laboratory?

There is faulty development of the parasympathetic innervation of the distal bowel in that there is an absence of the ganglion cells of the plexuses of Auerbach† and Meissner‡ in the rectal wall. This defect sometimes extends into the distal colon and may rarely affect the whole of the large bowel. The involved segment of intestine is spastic, with gross proximal distension of the large intestine above the narrowed segment. The diagnostic test is to take a biopsy of the rectal wall, which must include muscle; complete absence of the ganglion cells is confirmed.

---

*Harald Hirschprung (1830–1916), Professor of paediatrics, Queen Louisa Hospial, Copenhagen.

†Leopold Auerbach (1821–1897), Professor of pathology, Breslau.

‡George Meissner (1829–1905), Professor of anatomy, successively in Basle, Freiberg and Gottingen.

What is the sex distribution of this disease?

For some unexplained reason, 80% of these patients are male.

What important differential diagnosis must be made in these cases?

Acquired megacolon. This is a condition of severe constipation which usually commences when the child is 1 or 2 years old; many are mentally subnormal. Rectal examination in these patients is typical – impacted faeces are present right up to the anal verge. If necessary, a biopsy is performed to clinch the diagnosis; normal ganglion cells are present. This condition responds to treatment with regular enemas and aperients.

What are the radiological findings in patients with congenital megacolon?

A plain X-ray of the abdomen shows dilated loops of large bowel in which faecal masses may be seen. A barium enema demonstrates the characteristic narrow rectal segment, above which the colon is dilated and full of faeces.

Outline the treatment of this condition

If a baby is obstructed in the neonatal period, a colostomy may be necessary. Elective surgery should usually be carried out when the infant is 6–9 months old or until 3 months or more have elapsed from establishment of a colostomy. The aganglionic segment is resected and an abdomino-perineal pull-through anastomosis established between normally innervated colon and the anal canal. It is very important at the time of surgery to ensure, by frozen section histological examination, that ganglion cells are present in the remaining colon.

This procedure was indeed carried out successfully in this young patient, but earlier surgery would have saved him years of misery and would probably have allowed normal development to have taken place.

Case 61 A painful distended abdomen in an old man

An 84-year-old retired labourer, a widower, living in a retirement home, was sent into hospital as an emergency by the home's visiting medical officer. The patient gave a history of 3 days of severe generalized abdominal pain, during which time his belly had become grossly swollen. He had not had his bowels open since the start of this episode, nor had he been able to pass flatus. He had not vomited but now felt nauseated and was anorexic.

Previously he had had normal daily bowel actions, with no blood or slime. His weight was steady. He had arthritis of both hips and walked with a stick, had mild prostatic symptoms and a smoker's cough.

On examination his temperature was 37.2°C, pulse 98 and blood pressure 170/90. He was in obvious pain, rather dehydrated, with a dry tongue, but was pretty fit for his age. His fingers were tobacco stained and there were adventitial sounds at both his lung bases. The abdomen was grossly distended and uniformly tender, but there were no scars of previous surgery and the hernial orifices were clear. No masses could be felt in the abdomen and there was no clinical evidence of free fluid. Rectal examination revealed an empty rectum with smooth enlargement of the prostate.

This scenario is typical of an acute intestinal obstruction. Which would be more likely in this case, obstruction of the small or large bowel?

There is no evidence of a previous abdominal operation (as in Case 58, p. 117), nor evidence of a strangulated external hernia – by far the two commonest causes of an acute small bowel obstruction in the UK. Obstruction of the small intestine is usually accompanied by early and profuse vomiting, whereas this tends to be late, or indeed absent, in large bowel obstruction. Because of the size of the large bowel, distension of the abdomen is usually marked.

Clinically, therefore, the picture here suggests a large bowel, or 'low' obstruction.

The patient was reassured, given morphine for his pain, had a nasogastric tube passed, which aspirated 300 ml of greenish fluid, and had an intravenous line inserted. He then had an X-ray of the abdomen performed while in the supine position (Fig. 61.1).

What does the X-ray demonstrate and what is now the likely diagnosis?

There is an enormously distended oval gas shadow, looped on itself to give the typical 'bent inner-tube sign'. The haustrae do not extend across the width of the gas shadow, suggesting that this is large intestine (compare Case 58, p. 117). These appearances are quite typical of volvulus of the sigmoid colon.

This emergency is relatively uncommon in the UK. In which parts of the world is it much more often encountered? Are there any precipitating factors?

Volvulus of the sigmoid colon is commoner in Russia, Scandinavia and Central Africa. Patients tend to be elderly, and men are affected four times more often than women.

Precipitating factors include:

- An abnormally mobile loop of bowel.
- An abnormally loaded loop of bowel – for example, the sigmoid colon in chronic constipation.
- A loop of bowel with a narrow base.
- A loop of bowel fixed at its apex by adhesions.

Note that, although the sigmoid colon is the commonest site to be affected, volvulus of the caecum, small intestine, stomach and gallbladder may all occur.

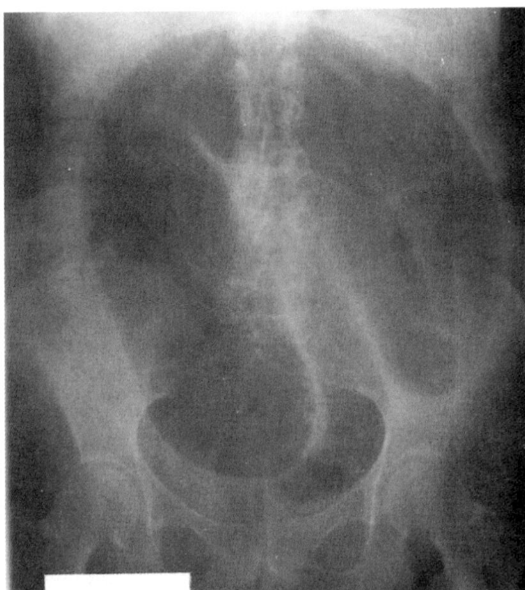

Figure 61.1 Supine X-ray of the abdomen.

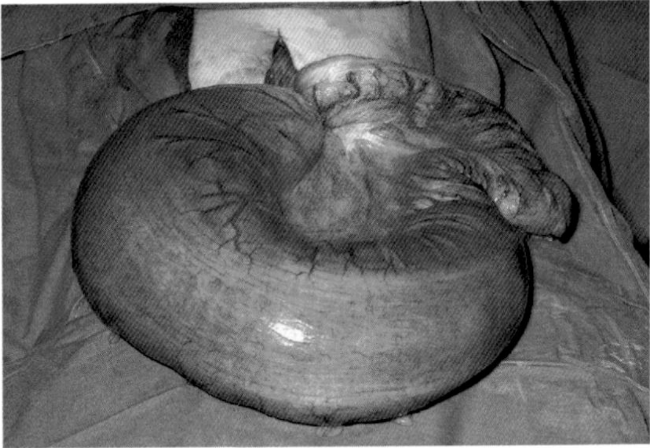

Figure 61.2 Operative photograph showing the hugely distended loop of the sigmoid colon.

What is the conservative measure that is effective in treating the majority of patients with volvulus of the sigmoid colon?

A sigmoidoscope is passed with the patient lying in the left lateral position. A large well lubricated, soft rubber rectal tube is passed along the sigmoidoscope. This usually untwists the volvulus, especially in early cases, with the escape of vast quantities of flatus and liquid faeces. It is then advisable to carry out an elective resection of the redundant sigmoid loop in order to prevent recurrence of the volvulus.

This was tried in the present case, but did not succeed. Left untreated, of course, the loop of sigmoid, with its blood supply cut off by the torsion, would undergo necrosis, so what was the next step in managing this patient?

He was taken to theatre, and under a general anaesthetic the abdomen was opened through a lower midline incision. Figure 61.2 shows the enormously distended and volved sigmoid loop.

The volvulus was untwisted. A rectal tube, which had been placed in the rectum after the patient had been anaesthetized, was then manipulated into the sigmoid loop to evacuate its flatus and faecal contents. A decision was then made to go ahead and resect the redundant sigmoid loop with immediate anastomosis, this being based on the general fitness of the patient.

The alternative would have been to defer definitive resection to a second operation. Apart from a relatively mild episode of postoperative pulmonary collapse (see Case 1, p. 4) the patient made a good recovery.

Case 62 An unusual case of severe rectal bleeding in a child

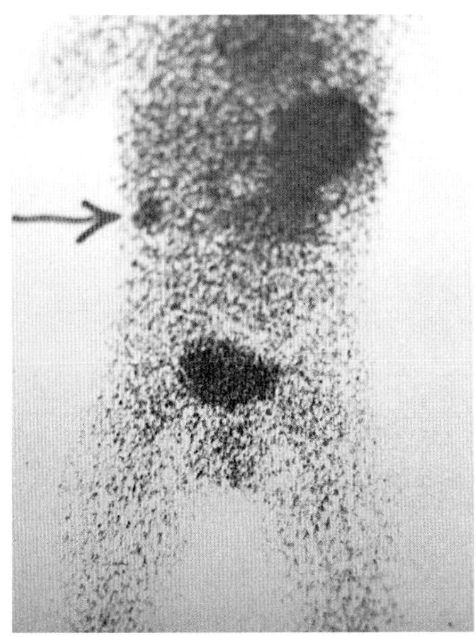

Figure 62.1

A 7-year-old boy was admitted to the paediatric surgical unit as an emergency. The mother gave the history. He was a previously perfectly healthy child, apart from the usual coughs and colds and one episode of otitis media, which had been treated with antibiotics. Early on the morning of admission, he woke up and rushed to the toilet with an urgent desire to defecate. He called his mother, who found him very pale and who saw that they contained a large amount of dark red blood and clots. This had never happened before. The family doctor was called, who arranged his urgent hospital admission.

On examination, the child was frightened and crying but not in any pain. The mucosae were pale. His pulse was 110 and blood pressure 100/70. Abdominal palpation was entirely normal – there was no tenderness or masses. Rectal examination was normal, but the glove was streaked with dark blood.

His condition rapidly returned to normal after a blood transfusion.

In view of these negative findings, an urgent radionuclide scan was performed using technetium-99m. The scan is shown in Fig. 62.1 and, to help you with this, the abnormality that was disclosed is labelled with a pointer.

What normal and abnormal structures are demonstrated on the child's scan?

The large shadow in the upper left side of the abdomen is the stomach, where the radionuclide is taken up by the acid-secreting parietal cells in the gastric musoca. The shadow in the pelvis is the bladder, where the radioactive material has been excreted in the urine. The small shadow that has been arrowed is the typical appearance produced by the parietal cells in the ectopic gastric mucosa lining a Meckel's diverticulum.*

What, therefore, was the cause of the child's haemorrhage?

Hydrochloric acid, secreted by the ectopic gastric mucosa in the Meckel's diverticulum, has produced ulceration in the diverticulum or in the adjacent ileum. The haemorrhage has resulted from erosion of a vessel in the ulcer wall.

After restoring the child's condition to normal by the blood transfusion, he underwent laparotomy and the Meckel's diverticulum was excised. This is shown in Fig. 62.2.

What is the embryological origin of a Meckel's diverticulum?

It represents a persistent remnant of the vitello-intestinal duct in the fetus.

---

*Johann Friedrich Meckel (1781–1833), Professor of anatomy, Halle, Germany. His father and grandfather both preceded him as professors of anatomy.

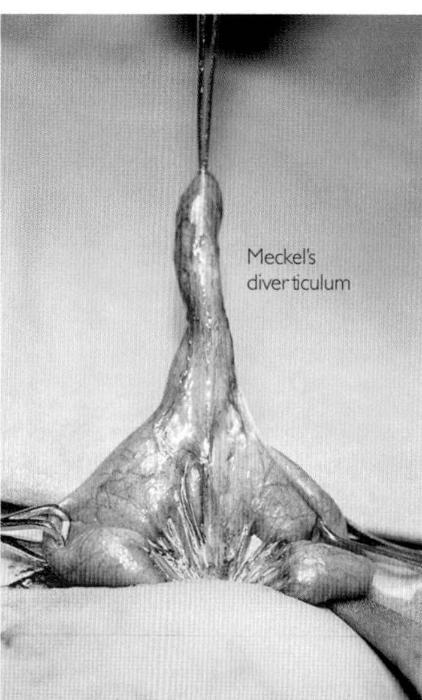

Figure 62.2 Meckel's diverticulum.

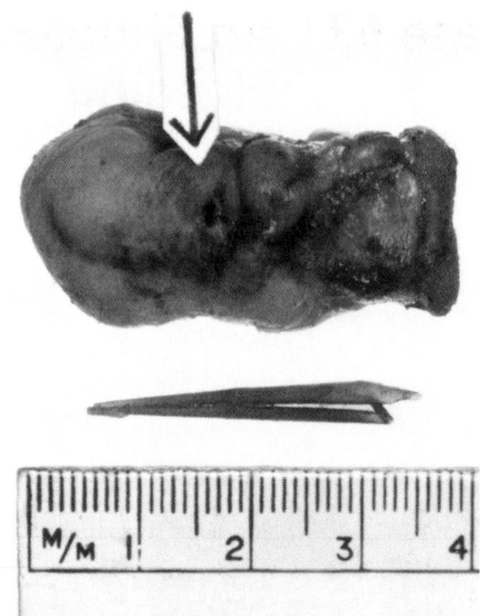

Figure 62.3 A Meckel's diverticulum perforated by a rolled up piece of tomato skin.

Where is it found and how often is it said to occur?

The diverticulum lies on the antimesenteric border of the ileum, about 0.6 m from the ileocaecal junction and occurs in about 2% of the population.

The great majority of these diverticula are symptomless and are only discovered incidentally at laparotomy for some other condition or at autopsy. However, those that do cause trouble may do so in a number of ways, what are these?

- Acute inflammation: Closely mimicking acute appendicitis. If the appendix is found to be normal at operation, the surgeon next looks for a possible Meckel.
- Perforation by a foreign body: A fish bone, chicken bone, toothbrush bristle and many other sharp objects may do this (Fig. 62.3). Again, the preoperative diagnosis is invariably acute appendicitis.
- Diverticulum may invaginate into the ileum and become the head of an intussusception.
- The vitello-intestinal duct may persist right up to the umbilicus, resulting in a small bowel fistula, or the distal end of the duct may present as a 'raspberry tumour' at the umbilicus in the newborn baby.
- A band may pass from the tip of the Meckel to the umbilicus; this band may snare a loop of intestine to produce an acute intestinal obstruction or may act as the apex of a volvulus of the adjacent ileum.
- Peptic ulceration, as in the case of this child, presenting either with haemorrhage or perforation.

Case 63 An abdominal mass in a young man

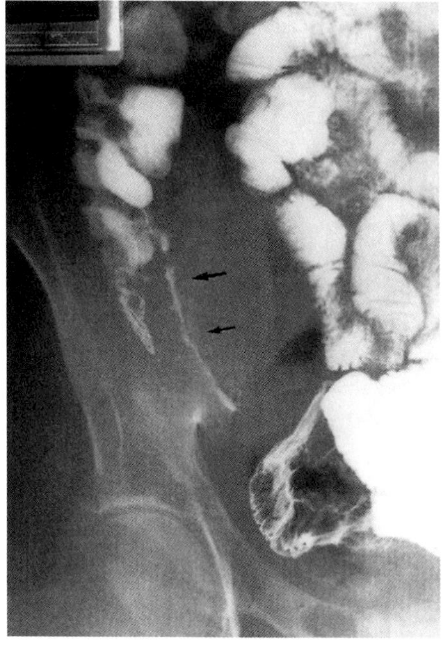

Figure 63.1

A trainee schoolmaster aged 25 years was referred to the gastroenterological medical outpatient clinic by his family practitioner with an urgent appointment. He gave a history of 6 months of attacks of colicky pain in the right iliac fossa, which were accompanied by diarrhoea. The bowels would act up to three or four times a day and would be loose, even watery, but he had never noticed any blood. The attacks were getting more frequent and more intense, and in the last couple of weeks he was in almost constant pain or discomfort and was quite unable to work. His appetite was now very poor and he thought he had lost about 1 kg in weight.

When examined in the clinic he looked ill and anaemic. He was afebrile and his blood pressure was 134/70. Examination of the abdomen revealed a tender mass in the right iliac fossa; there was no abdominal distension or clinical evidence of ascites. Rectal examination was negative, and there was no evidence of perianal disease.

He was admitted urgently to the unit. A battery of investigations was carried out, including a barium meal and follow-through examination. Figure 63.1 shows the long strictured segment of terminal ileum (arrowed).

What is the name given to this appearance, and what disease characteristically produces this change?

The 'string sign' of Kantor.* This, together with the clinical picture, strongly suggests the diagnosis of Crohn's disease.†

What other radiological features may be seen in Crohn's disease?

There may be fine ulceration, which may give the so-called 'rose thorn' appearance of the mucosa, and this can be seen on careful inspection of Fig. 63.1. Several segments of stricturing may be seen, separated by apparently normal bowel ('skip lesions'), and fistulous tracks may be demonstrated into other structures – an adjacent loop of small bowel or large bowel, for example.

Can Crohn's disease affect other parts of the alimentary tract?

Although the terminal ileum is the commonest site for

*John Leonard Kantor (1890–1947), gastroenterologist, Presbyterian Hospital, New York.

†Burrill Bernard Crohn (1884–1983), gastroenterologist, Mount Sinai Hospital, New York. The condition was described by Morgagni (1680–1771).

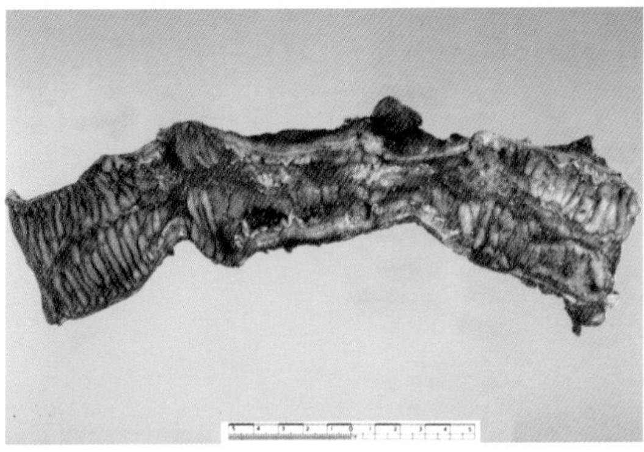

Figure 63.2 Cobblestoning and linear mucosal ulceration in Crohn's disease.

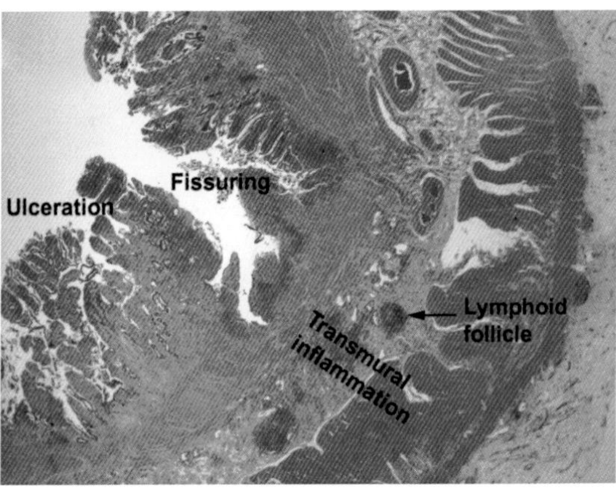

Figure 63.3 Histology of Crohn's disease.

Crohn's disease – hence the common but scientifically inaccurate name of regional ileitis – any part of the alimentary tract from mouth to anal canal may be involved, including the perianal skin. It is associated with severe multiple anal fissures and fistulae (see Cases 75 and 77, pp. 150 and 154).

What are the typical naked eye and histological appearances of the bowel in this disease?

The bowel is bright red and swollen. Mucosal ulceration, which tends to be in a linear direction, and intervening oedema results in a 'cobblestone' appearance of the mucous membrane (Fig. 63.2). The wall of the intestine is greatly thickened, as is the adjacent mesentery, and the regional lymph nodes are enlarged. There may be skip areas of normal intestine between involved segments and there may be fistulae into adjacent structures.

Microscopic examination shows chronic inflammatory infiltrate through the whole thickness of the bowel with non-caseating foci of epithelioid and giant multinucleate cells. Ulceration is present, with typical fissuring ulcers extending deep through the mucosa (Fig. 63.3). These may extend through the bowel wall to form abscesses or may fistulate into adjacent structures.

What is known about the aetiology of this disease?

The simple answer is not all that much! There is a genetic component, in that 20% of patients with Crohn's disease have an affected relative. Recently an association has been described with a genetic mutation in the NOD gene family – these are genes involved in the innate immune response to bacterial antigens within the gut. *Mycobacterium avium* subspecies *paratuberculosis* has also been suggested as a cause, and is known to affect immune signalling. In reality it may be a synthesis of many of these theories, with impaired innate immunity, both genetically and environmentally acquired, affecting the host response to otherwise innocuous gut flora.

What would be your initial non-operative management?

The initial management of an acute Crohn's ileitis involves anti-inflammatory treatment with oral corticosteroids, such as prednisolone (0.5–1 mg/kg/day). As the disease responds, elemental diet is introduced to maintain the remission. This is a liquid diet comprising protein, in the form of amino acids or short chain peptides, as well as carbohydrate, fats, vitamins and minerals. If the ileitis is not severe, elemental diet alone, without oral steroids, may enable disease remission and long-term control of symptoms.

What would be the indication for surgery in this man?

The most likely indication for surgery in this man would be intestinal obstruction secondary to the stricturing. The underlying aim when operating on Crohn's disease is to avoid resecting more bowel than necessary. Many patients may require multiple operations and bowel resections, resulting in short gut syndrome and a dependence on total parenteral nutrition.

There are two main procedures

- For short strictures, the stricture is opened longitudinally and closed transversely, so-called 'strictureplasty'.
- For longer strictures, the affected bowel is resected with an end-to-end anastomosis of the two ends.

Case 64 A striking and diagnostic facial appearance

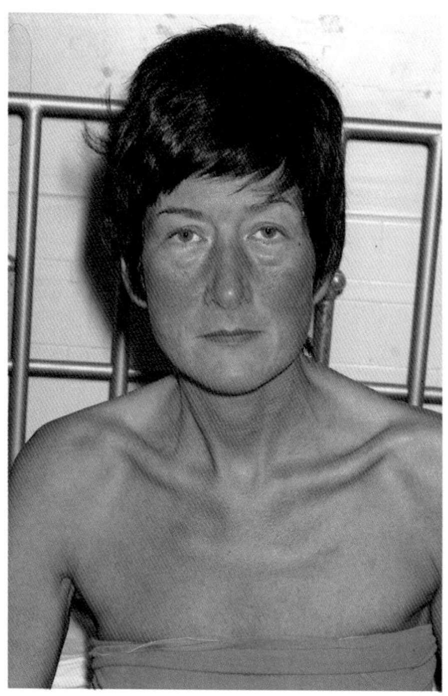

Figure 64.1

Figure 64.1 shows a 42-year-old, married secretary. Five years previously she had presented with a subacute bowel obstruction and a palpable mass in the right iliac fossa. She underwent a laparotomy, when a tumour was found in the terminal ileum, together with enlarged nodes in the adjacent mesentery. The liver was macroscopically entirely normal. The affected segment of bowel and the adjacent mesentery were resected and she made an excellent recovery.

She now has a considerable hepatomegaly, which extends 10 cm below the right costal margin. Together with this, she has a striking appearance of a flushed, reddish blue complexion, which gets even more intense after food or if she has a glass or two of wine.

What is this syndrome, and what is the origin of the tumour that produces it?

The carcinoid syndrome. The primary tumour arises in the Kultschitzky cells* of the intestinal mucosal crypts, which characteristically take up silver stains.

What is the commonest site of the tumour?

The majority are found in the appendix and are found incidentally at laparotomy or present as acute appendicitis. The great majority of these are relatively benign and do not recur after a simple appendicectomy. However, a small percentage, about 4%, develop secondary spread.

More rarely, carcinoid tumours are found in the distal ileum or proximal large bowel, and these typically spread to the regional nodes and to the liver, as in the case of this patient. Rarely they occur in the lung. About 10% are associated with the multiple endocrine neoplasia type 1 (MEN-1) syndrome.

What other clinical features may be found in the carcinoid syndrome?

As well as the enlarged liver and flushing with attacks of cyanosis, there may be diarrhoea with abdominal pain and noisy borborygmi, bronchospasm and pulmonary and tricuspid valve stenosis.

What is the biochemical basis of these features?

The carcinoid tumour secretes 5-hydroxytryptamine (5-HT, also known as serotonin), in addition to a variety of other hormones. The liver is normally able to inactivate these hormones as they reach this organ via the portal vein. However, in the presence of liver metastases, 5-HT

*Nicolae Kultschitzky (1865–1925), Professor of histology, Kharkov, Russia. After the Russian Revolution he became a lecturer in anatomy at University College, London.

is secreted directly into the systemic circulation, with the appearance of the above effects (Fig. 64.1).

What biochemical investigation is used to clinch the diagnosis?

5-HT is excreted in the urine as 5-hydroxyindole acetic acid (5-HIAA). A raised level of this is found in a 24 h urine collection from the patient.

What modalities of treatment are available?

It may be possible to resect the liver metastases if these are not too extensive. If widespread, the deposits can be embolized via a catheter introduced into the femoral artery and guided into the hepatic artery. This was indeed carried out in this patient with a gratifying remission.

In other cases, cytotoxic drugs may be used. Symptoms may be controlled using 5-HT antagonists, e.g. methysergide or octreotide, the latter being a somatostatin analogue that inhibits the release of 5-HT. Even if widespread deposits are present, it is well worthwhile persevering with treatment as the tumour is slow growing and the patient may survive for many years in reasonable health.

Case 65 Acute abdomen in a medical student

A first year medical student was taken to the accident and emergency department of her teaching hospital by a fellow student in her digs. She was seen promptly by the A&E specialist registrar, who obtained the following history. She was quite well until the early hours of that morning, when she was woken up by central, dull, abdominal pain. This got worse as the morning went on and she vomited some of her last night's supper and then some greenish fluid. She then found that the pain had moved to her lower right abdomen, was much worse and hurt her if she moved around in bed – she was best off lying on her side, keeping as still as possible and with her knees bent up.

Her bowels had moved normally the day before, but not since the pain began. Her periods were normal, the last a fortnight before, and there were no urinary symptoms. Apart from chickenpox as a child, she had always been well. She had never had a pain like this before.

On examination, the registrar found that she looked flushed and apprehensive. Her tongue was heavily coated and she had foetor oris. Her temperature was 38.0°C and pulse 96. She was reluctant to move on the trolley, and gingerly shifted herself to lie on her back, but with her knees raised. The abdomen was not distended, but there was marked tenderness in the right iliac fossa with rigidity of the abdominal wall in this area. Bowel sounds were heard, but only after listening for a couple of minutes with a stethoscope.

A rectal examination showed marked tenderness anteriorly and to the right, but no masses were felt. A routine urine examination was normal, including microscopy. A full blood count was sent off, which showed a white cell count total of 13.0 × 10^9/L with a polymorph leucocytosis. A pregnancy test was negative.

This sounds like a 'barn door' case of acute appendicitis and would be the obvious one to make, but what other possibilities enter into your differential diagnosis?

There is a wide spectrum of causes of any abdominal pain – here we will concentrate on the right iliac fossa. Any experienced clinician will tell you that you will encounter many, if not all, of them during your career. Consider the anatomical structures that might be involved and then the possible pathologies affecting them, for example:

- Terminal ileum: Crohn's disease, Meckel's diverticulis.
- Caecum: Carcinoma (in older subjects), solitary diverticulum.
- Mesentery: Mesenteric adenitis.
- Gallbladder: A distended inflamed gallbladder can project downwards into the right iliac fossa.
- Female pelvic organs: Salpingitis, ectopic pregnancy, twisted ovarian cyst.
- Genitourinary tract: Ureteric colic from stone, acute pyelonephritis, referred pain from testis. Consider also referred pain from the chest (basal pleurisy) or CNS (prodromal herpes zoster).

A wise saying is that nothing can be so easy, or so difficult, as the diagnosis of appendicitis!

Does the presence of pus cells in the urine exclude the diagnosis of acute appendicitis? What about the value of a white cell count?

- Although pus cells in the urine suggest a urinary tract infection, an inflamed appendix adherent to the ureter or the bladder may produce microscopic pyuria or haematuria.
- Although the majority of cases of acute appendicitis will have a moderate leucocytosis with predominance of polymorphs, the count may be entirely normal.

Having made a clinical diagnosis, the registrar called the surgeon on take who agreed with the findings, and urgent surgery was deemed necessary. What are the preoperative measures?

- Reassurance.

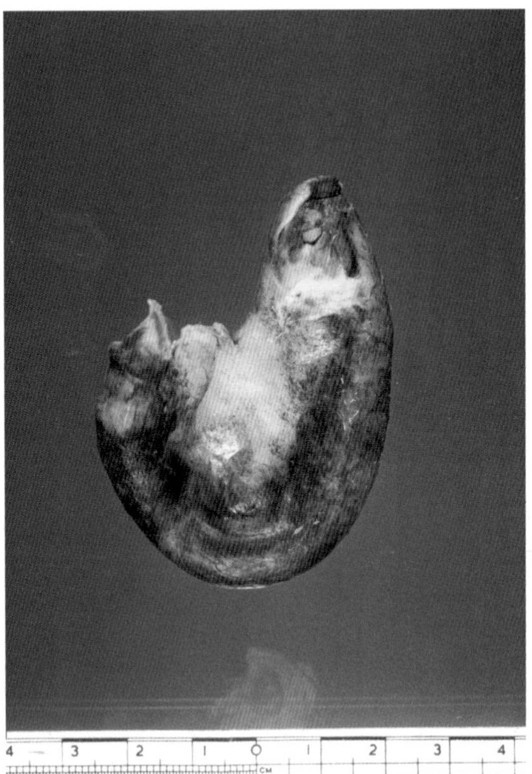

Figure 65.1 Excised inflamed appendix.

• Premedication: 100 mg of pethidine intramuscularly combined with an anti-emetic would be reasonable.

• Commence antibiotic cover, e.g. metronidazole, which can be given as a rectal suppository.

The diagnosis was confirmed at laparoscopy 2 h later, and an acutely inflamed appendix removed (Fig. 65.1).

Left untreated, what might have happened to the patient?

One of three things:

• The acutely inflamed appendix might have become gangrenous and progressed to perforate freely into the peritoneal cavity, producing a general peritonitis.

• The appendix might become walled off to form an appendix mass (see Case 66, p. 133).

• The inflammatory process might resolve, although there is a strong chance of a further attack of appendicitis. It is not uncommon for a patient with acute appendicitis to give a history of having had a similar, although milder, attack weeks or even some months before this episode.

What clinical features would suggest that the acutely inflamed appendix had perforated into the peritoneal cavity?

The temperature and pulse are raised, the patient is flushed and toxic, the abdomen is diffusely tender, with rigidity of the abdominal muscles and with absent bowel sounds – i.e. the clinical picture of a diffuse peritonitis.

Fortunately this medical student made a smooth recovery from her operation and spent her convalescence revising the anatomy of the abdomen.

Case 66 Yet another mass in the right iliac fossa

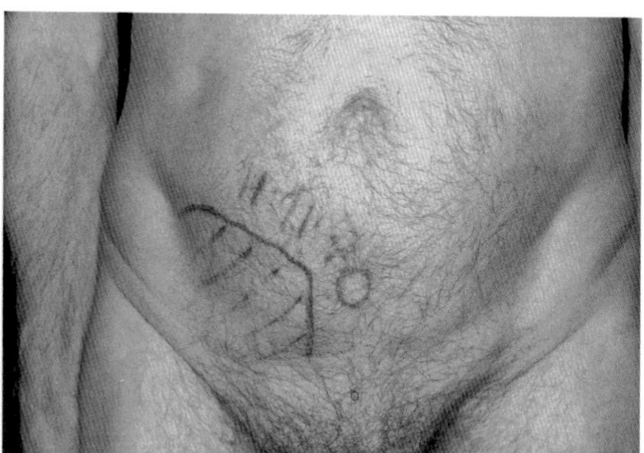

Figure 66.1

A previously healthy young man of 23 years, a supermarket assistant, was brought by taxi to the A&E department with a 5-day history of abdominal pain. When the casualty officer took a detailed history, this revealed that the pain had started in the centre of the abdomen, but had moved to the right lower quadrant after a few hours, and there it had remained. He had felt nauseated and had vomited several times on the first day, but although anorexic, had not vomited or felt sick since then. He had not had a bowel movement although he passed flatus frequently. He had remained in bed at home, looked after by his mother and living on cups of tea. He had put all this down to 'gastric flu' or something he had eaten, but as it did not seem to be getting better, both he and his mother thought they should seek medical advice. Functional enquiry was otherwise negative.

On examination, he was obviously in pain, and did not like moving around on the examination couch, but he looked reasonably well and was not clinically anaemic. His temperature was 38.8°C, pulse 90 and tongue coated and dry. Palpation of the abdomen detected an obvious tender mass in the right iliac fossa, which was marked out with a felt tip pen and is shown in Fig. 66.1. The rest of the abdomen was soft and not tender; normal bowel sounds were present. Rectal examination revealed a loaded rectum, but nothing else.

What is the most likely diagnosis?

The story and physical signs are strongly suggestive of an appendix mass. He had suffered an attack of acute appendicitis, which, fortunately, had been sealed off, probably by omentum and had not perforated into the peritoneal cavity.

How would the story have differed if the mass was due to Crohn's disease of the terminal ileum?

Crohn's disease would need to be considered if there had been a history of previous diarrhoea, often with loss of weight.

What common disease would you have to consider in the differential diagnosis if this patient had been 73 and not 23 years old?

Carcinoma of the caecum, although this rarely occurs in young adults.

What is the management of an appendix mass?

Treatment is initially conservative. Further delineation of the mass can be made using ultrasound or CT (Fig. 66.2). The mass is outlined on the skin, as has been done in this case, and its size is carefully and repeatedly observed, together with the patient's general condition, pulse and temperature. The patient is put on bed rest and allowed fluids only by mouth. Metronidazole is prescribed.

In the majority of cases, about 80%, the mass resolves. In some pyrexia continues and the mass enlarges with abscess formation. Under these circumstances the abscess is drained surgically, either by open operation or

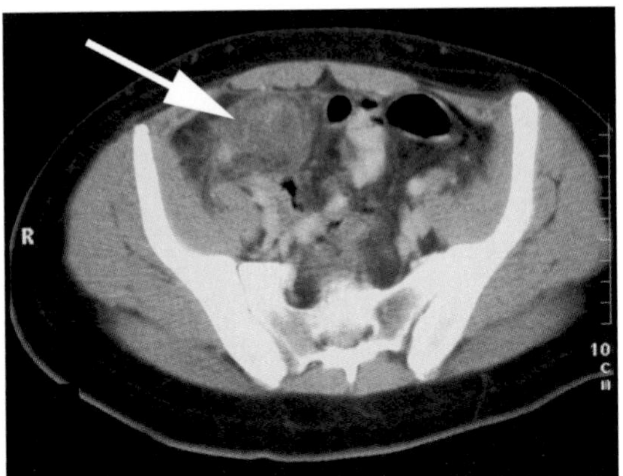

Figure 66.2 CT scan illustrating an appendix mass (arrowed).

percutaneously under imaging control. At this procedure, no attempt is made to remove the appendix, which would be difficult, dangerous and very likely to contaminate the peritoneal cavity.

What subsequent treatment is advised?

Whether resolution occurs or the abscess requires drainage, appendicectomy is carried out 2 or 3 months later – the interval allows the inflammatory condition to settle completely. This is to prevent the risk of a further attack of acute appendicitis.

In this patient, resolution took place quite rapidly over the next few days. Interval appendicectomy removed a small, deformed appendix buried in adjacent omentum.

Case 67 A symptomless finding on a barium enema examination

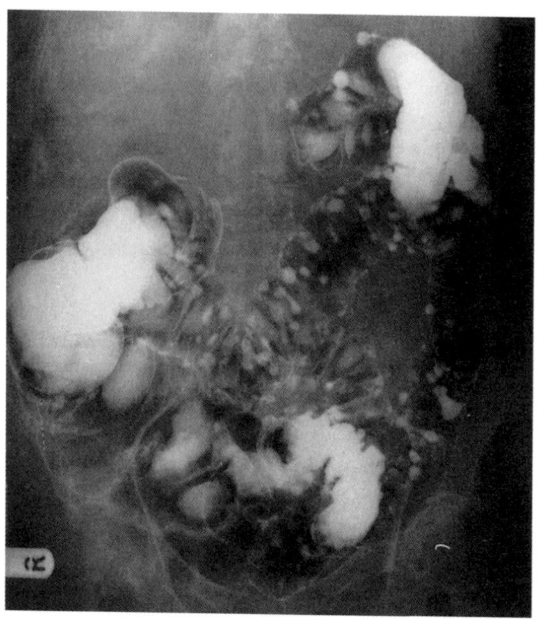

Figure 67.1

A high-powered business man aged 64 years – a health freak who worked out in the gym every day, a non-smoker, non-drinker, who prided himself on being in 'top condition' but who was also a self-confessed hypochondriac – went to a private clinic to have a very complete (and expensive) check up. Not only did this include an exhaustive questionnaire ('bowels regular, once a day, no blood or slime'), a full physical examination (entirely negative), a battery of blood tests (all within the normal range), but also a number of imaging examinations, all of which were normal apart from the barium enema. Figure 67.1 shows a typical image from the study.

What lesion does the X-ray show and how commonly is it found in subjects of this age group?

There are extensive diverticula of the transverse, descending and sigmoid colon. Autopsy studies have shown that colonic diverticula are present in about a third of subjects over the age of 60 in the developed world. They are most commonly found in the sigmoid colon, but may, as in this case, extend into the rest of the left side and the transverse portion of the colon. Occasionally they are found in the right colon. The rectum is never involved.

Is there a known cause of this condition?

Colonic diverticula were rare until the early 20th century and are still uncommon in many parts of Asia and Africa.

The underlying pathology is thickening of the muscular wall of the affected part of the colon due to deposition of, mainly, elastin. The raised intracolonic pressure produces outpouchings of mucosa at the sites of potential weakness of the bowel wall that correspond to the supplying vessels to the colon, as shown in Fig. 67.2. Figure 67.3 shows a close-up of an opened segment of colon with diverticula, which demonstrates faecoliths (arrowed) within the diverticula and marked hypertrophy of the wall (between the double arrows):

Diets that are low in bulk tend not to distend the bowel wall, resulting in the development of high intramural pressure, which can be shown by manometric studies. It is suggested that the modern low roughage Western diet may be responsible for the marked variation in the geographical distribution of this condition.

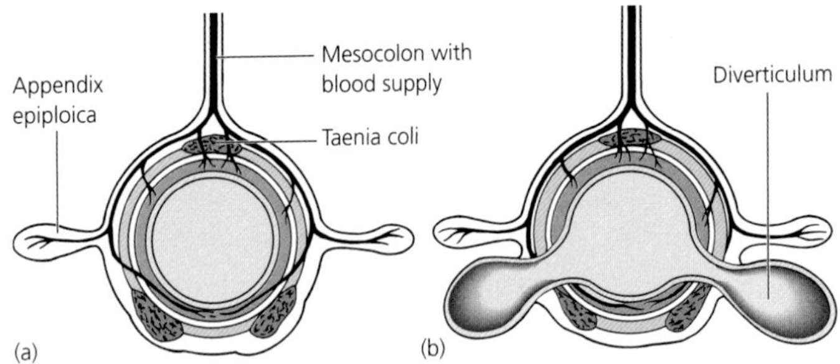

Figure 67.2 The relationship of diverticula of the colon to the taenia coli and to the penetrating blood vessels: (a) normal colon and (b) colon with diverticula; both shown in transverse section.

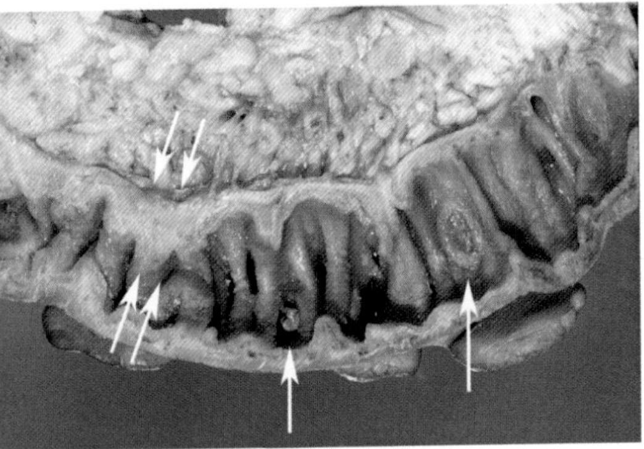

Figure 67.3 A segment of colon with diverticula showing faecoliths (arrowed) and marked hypertrophy of the wall (between double arrows).

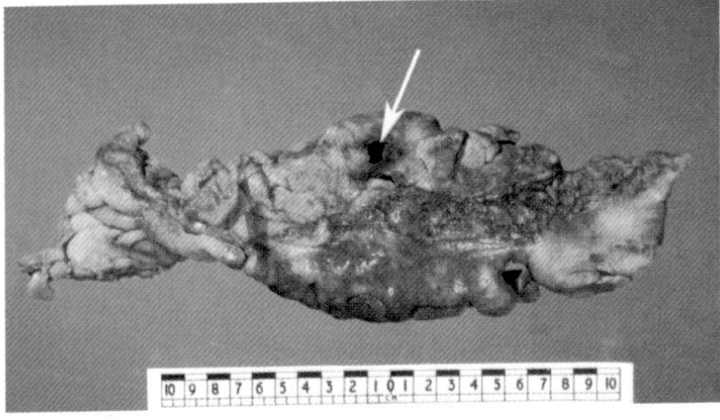

Figure 67.4 A section of sigmoid colon showing a perforated diverticulum (arrowed) at autopsy on a woman of 82 admitted in a moribund state with a faecal peritonitis. She had died in the emergency department.

What are the complications of colonic diverticula?

- The thickened bowel wall may produce subacute obstruction – constipation, bloating and abdominal discomfort. This is referred to as chronic diverticular disease.
- A diverticulum may become acutely inflamed (acute diverticulitis). This may:
  - Perforate into the general peritoneal cavity (Fig. 67.4).
  - Form a localized pericolic abscess.
  - Fistulate into an adjacent organ (the commonest cause of a vesicocolic fistula).
  - Erode a blood vessel in the neck of the diverticulum to produce acute bright red rectal bleeding.

All these complications are seen quite frequently in the surgical wards, yet the great majority of patients with colonic diverticulosis remain symptom-free throughout their lives.

Is there any advice you would give to this patient?

Poor fellow, he is going to be very upset. Explain that he has a very common condition, which probably will never give him trouble and which 30% of his business friends probably have. It would be reasonable to advise a high roughage diet.

Case 68 Ulcerative colitis

A 25-year-old doctor presented to the gastroenterologist of the hospital in which he had just started working with a long history of bloody diarrhoea. He had previously been investigated as a student by flexible sigmoidoscopy and commenced on a course of prednisolone enemas for proctitis. Initially this had reduced his diarrhoea but in the 3 weeks since moving to start a new hospital job he was opening his bowels 12 times a day and passing diarrhoea covered in blood and mucus. He also complained of crampy lower abdominal pain, and a recent weight loss of 8 kg.

On examination, he was pale, pyrexial (temperature 38°C) and tender in the left iliac fossa. No masses were palpable. On rectal examination, there was a granular feel to the mucosa with fresh blood and mucus on the examining finger. A full blood count revealed him to be anaemic (haemoglobin 9.8 g/dl) and hypoalbuminaemic (21 g/L) with a raised C-reactive protein (120 mg/L).

What is the first course of management?

Initial management should aim to make a diagnosis and provide symptomatic relief. Diagnosis requires tissue, which was obtained at rigid sigmoidoscopy and revealed ulceration with blood and mucus in the bowel lumen. Biopsy of the posterior rectal wall was performed. The extent of the disease can be assessed either by colonoscopy or barium enema. Stool culture should also be taken to exclude infective causes, but the previous history of proctitis suggests this was not infective in origin.

What features would suggest this is ulcerative colitis rather than colitis due to Crohn's disease?

Table 68.1 shows the differences between Crohn's colitis and ulcerative colitis. This patient was diagnosed as having typical ulcerative colitis.

What are the complications of this condition?

When considering the complications of any condition it is useful to categorize them into local and general (or systemic).

1 *Local*:

- Toxic dilatation – the colon dilates in fulminant colitis leading to:
- Perforation.
- Stricture.
- Malignant change – usually with longstanding disease affecting the whole bowel.
- Perineal disease, while more common in Crohn's colitis, can occur in ulcerative colitis manifesting with fissure in ano, for example.

2 *General*:

- Weight loss, anaemia and hypoalbuminaemia.
- Seronegative arthropathy, such as ankylosing spondylitis.
- Uveitis – both this and the arthropathy occur in patients who have the B27 human leucocyte antigen (HLA B27).
- Skin complications – pyoderma gangrenosum.
- Primary sclerosing cholangitis, which may precede the onset of colitis and which is also associated with Crohn's disease.

What initial medical therapy would be appropriate?

The doctor was commenced on high dose corticosteroids and his anaemia corrected by blood transfusion. Nevertheless his condition worsened and he underwent a total colectomy (Fig. 68.1).

What are the indications for total colectomy in ulcerative colitis?

- Fulminating disease not responding to medical therapy – with the passage of more than six stools per day with persistent fever, tachycardia and hypoalbuminaemia.
- Chronic disease, not responding to medical treatment.

Table 68.1 Differences between Crohn's colitis and ulcerative colitis.

	Crohn's colitis	Ulcerative colitis
Clinical features	Perianal disease common, e.g. fissure in ano and fistula in ano	Perianal disease rare
	Gross bleeding uncommon	Often profuse haemorrhage
	Small bowel may also be affected	Small bowel not affected
Pathology		
Macroscopic differences	Any part of the colon may be involved (skip lesions)	Disease extends proximally from the rectum
	Transmural involvement	Mucosal involvement only
	Fistulae in adjacent viscera	No fistulae
	No polyps	Pseudopolyps of regenerating mucosa
	Thickened bowel wall	No thickening of bowel wall
	Malignant change rare	Malignant change common in longstanding cases
Microscopic differences	Granulomas present	No granulomas

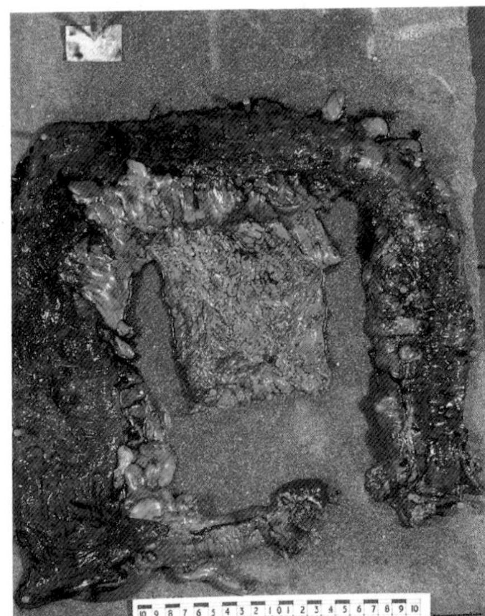

Figure 68.1 Total colectomy.

- Longstanding disease, where colectomy is performed as prophylaxis against malignancy.
- For the local complications mentioned above.

It is often said that patients accept surgery better in fulminant disease, when they perceive anything – including a stoma – as being better than a life spent on the toilet passing bloody stools.

What surgical options are open to this patient?

Total colectomy with excision of the rectal stump is the usual procedure. The remaining small bowel may either be exteriorized as a terminal ileostomy, or continence restored by a ileoanal anastomosis with an interposed ileal pouch (a Park's pouch*). Where the anal disease is controlled an ileorectal anastomosis can be performed, but this will require continued surveillance for malignancy.

*Sir Alan Guyatt Parks (1920–1982), surgeon, St Marks Hospital, London.

Case 69 A complication of longstanding ulcerative colitis

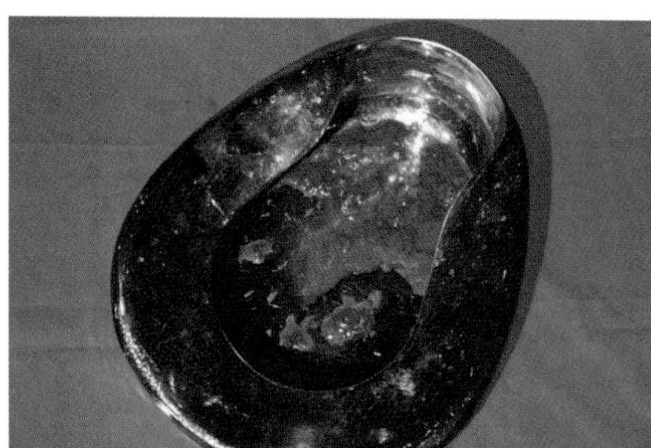

Figure 69.1

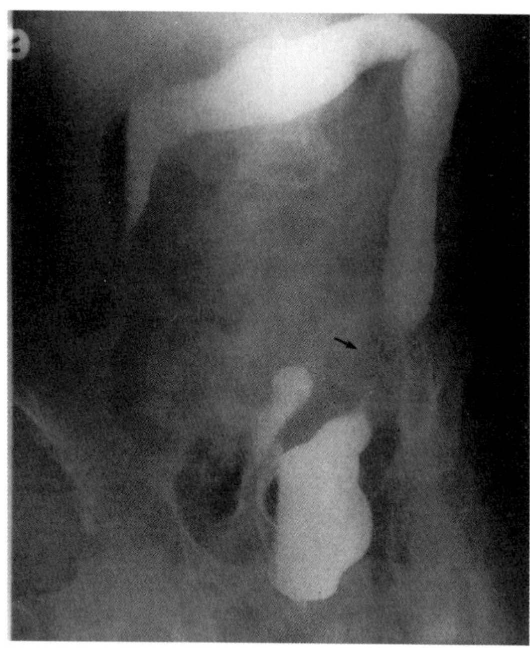

Figure 69.2 Barium enema (see text).

A man of 48 years, a self-employed grocer, has been under the care of his family practitioner and the gastroenterology clinic of the local hospital for his ulcerative colitis since he was 25 years old, with intermittent admissions for exacerbations of his disease. Over the years there have been repeated episodes of bloody diarrhoea, with bright red stools and accompanied by mucus. Figure 69.1 shows a typical example of his stool in a bed pan during such an attack, during which he might pass up to 12 stools in the 24 h.

Severe episodes have been accompanied by profound loss of weight, anorexia and anaemia, which often necessitated blood transfusions. Over the years he has been treated with courses of steroids and with sulphasalazine (sulphonamide/salicylate in combination). Over the past 4 or 5 years he has enjoyed a long remission – his bowels acting only two or sometimes three times a day, semiformed and free of obvious blood. If the bowels became looser, he has simply take some codeine phosphate. His appetite has been good and his weight steady.

However, over the past 3 months his symptoms have flared up again – diarrhoea, bleeding, mucus, weight loss and loss of appetite. Both he and the GP assumed that this was just another tedious recurrence of his colitis. He was sent back to the clinic by his family doctor to have this sorted out.

When seen by his gastroenterologist he did not look at all well – pale and thin. Abdominal palpation revealed a generally tender abdomen, but no muscle guarding. There was a definite tender mass felt in the lower left quadrant of the abdomen, about the size of a cricket ball. Rectal examination showed bright blood and mucus on the glove but no mass was detected. A sigmoidoscopy was performed in the clinic to 15 cm and this showed a red granular, bleeding mucosa. An urgent barium enema examination was ordered and Fig. 69.2 shows one of the films obtained. The appearance of the arrowed segment was constant on all the films and on the screening.

What observations can you make on this X-ray? Together with the clinical features described, what diagnosis (or rather diagnoses) can you make?

The whole length of the colon has lost its normal haustrations and the lumen is narrowed throughout the so-called 'drain-pipe colon'. Fine ulcerations can be seen along the edge of the ascending and part of the transverse colon. There is a long stricture in the lower descending colon.

All this fits with the diagnosis of chronic ulcerative colitis, with carcinomatous change in the strictured segment. Although it is true that non-malignant strictures may occur in longstanding colitis, the presence of a mass on abdominal palpation strongly suggests a tumour.

What further investigation will be necessary to confirm or refute these two pathologies?

Colonoscopy. This was performed under sedation. Serial biopsies were taken of the rectal and colonic mucosa.

> *An ulcerating tumour was seen at 50 cm from the anal verge. A biopsy of this was reported as a poorly differentiated adenocarcinoma. The biopsies taken from other parts of the colon and the rectum showed mucosal ulceration and small abscesses within the mucosal crypts ('crypt abscesses'), together with polymorph and round cell infiltration of the ulcer bases. No giant cell systems were seen. These appearances are typical of chronic ulcerative colitis.*

Which patients with ulcerative colitis are at particular risk of developing carcinomatous change in the mucosa of the large bowel?

The risk is greatest in chronic, total colitis – it does not occur when the inflammatory disease is confined to the rectum (ulcerative proctitis). It may occur irrespective of whether the disease is quiescent or active and may be multifocal. It is especially likely to take place if the disease commences in childhood or adolescence – but then these are the patients who are likely to have longstanding disease. It is estimated that 12% of patients with colitis of 20 years or more duration may develop malignant change.

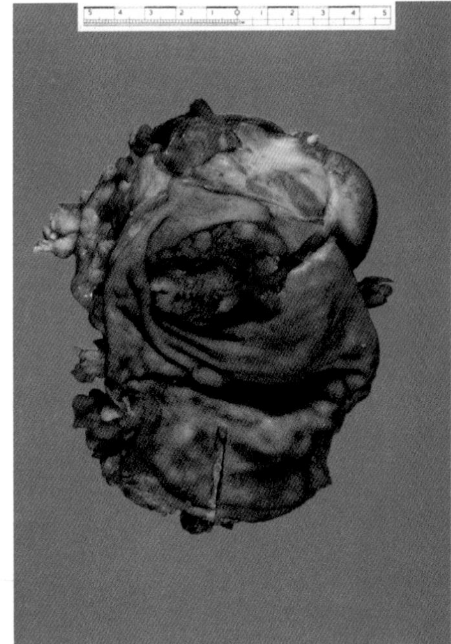

Figure 69.3 Mucosal surface of the tumour-bearing segment of colon.

Outline how you expect this patient was managed

He was admitted urgently under the care of the colorectal surgical team. His blood count revealed profound microcytic anaemia and he received a blood transfusion. Ultrasonography of the abdomen showed no evidence of ascites or hepatomegaly and his liver function tests were normal; a chest X-ray was also normal.

At laparotomy, a tumour was found in the lower descending colon with enlarged local lymph nodes. The rest of the large bowel showed thickening and narrowing. A total colectomy and rectal excision was performed with ileoanal stapled anastomosis, using an ileal pouch. The mucosal surface of the portion of colon containing the tumour is shown in Fig. 69.3.

Histological examination of the tumour showed this to be a poorly differentiated adenocarcinoma (as suggested by the biopsy), completely penetrating the muscle wall of the bowel. Of the 18 lymph nodes dissected out of the adjacent mesocolon, 12 showed tumour deposits (Dukes' stage C).

Case 70 A very old woman with an abdominal mass

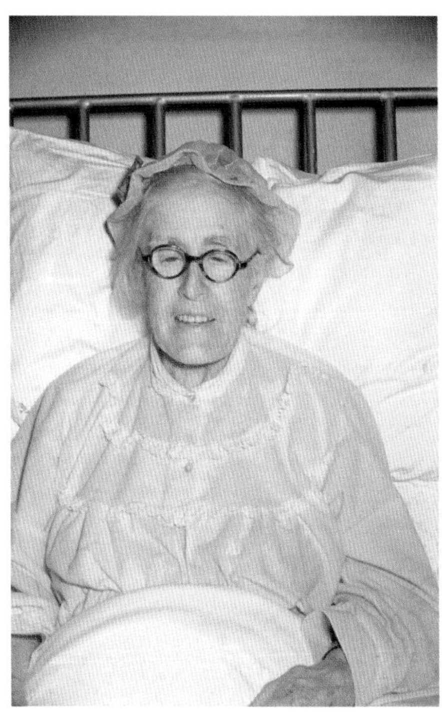

Figure 70.1

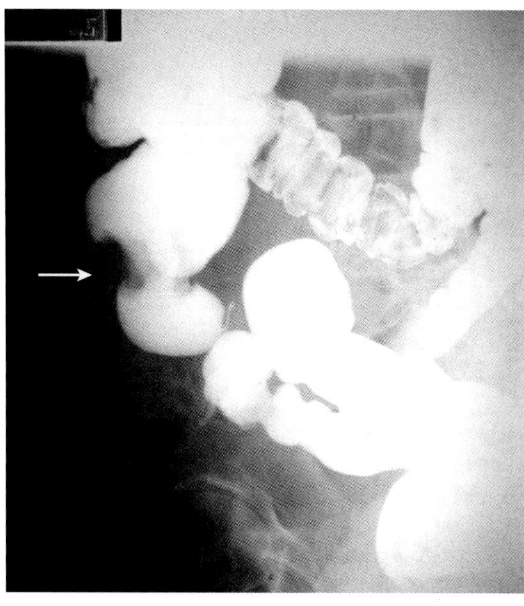

Figure 70.2 Barium enema demonstrating a filling defect in the caecum (arrowed).

Figure 70.1 shows a splendid old woman, a spinster aged 90 years and a former schoolteacher, taken 4 days after her major operation.

She consulted her family doctor, who had looked after her for many years, saying that she had become progressively weaker and more tired over the past few months and that she was no longer her usual active self. Apart from this, she had no other complaints. Her appetite had not changed, her weight remained the same and, in particular, she had noticed no change in her regular bowel habit. Her stools, she said, were quite normal and she had not noticed any blood or slime therein.

When her doctor examined her, he was immediately alarmed by how pale she had become since he had last seen her, about 6 months previously. He gave her a thorough examination and detected a large, slightly tender mass just to the right of, and below, the umbilicus. A rectal examination was clear, but he did an 'occult blood test' on the faecal smear on the glove, which was positive. She was referred urgently to hospital.

In surgical outpatients, the doctor's findings were confirmed; there was undoubtedly a mass in the right iliac fossa. Her haemoglobin was found to be 6 g/dl. She was admitted for a blood transfusion and then had a barium enema performed. One of the plates is shown in Fig. 70.2.

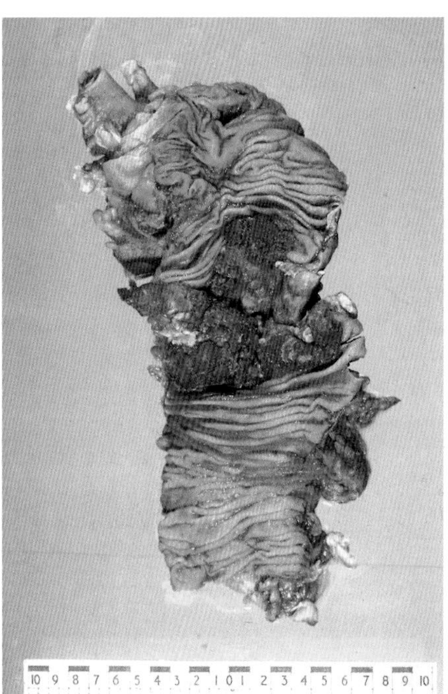

Figure 70.3 A right hemicolectomy specimen from the patient showing the caecal carcinoma.

What lesion can you see in Fig. 70.2, indicated by the arrow?

There is a filling defect in the caecum, which together with the history and clinical findings, is strongly suspicious of a tumour mass.

Surgical exploration was indicated as a matter of some urgency. It was decided against performing a colonoscopy – the mass would need removal whatever its exact pathology. At laparotomy, a tumour mass was found in the caecum. The regional nodes were not enlarged, the liver was clear and, apart from small fibroids in the uterus, no other abnormalities were found. A right hemicolectomy was performed and the specimen shown in Fig. 70.3.

How would you describe this pathology, and what is its likely histological appearance?

There is a papilliferous tumour of the caecum with an ulcerated surface. It is likely to be an adenocarcinoma.

The patient made an entirely smooth recovery from her operation and was soon home. When I asked her, on the students' ward round on her fourth postoperative day, to what she attributed her wonderful good health, she replied: 'I have never smoked, I have never touched alcohol and I have had nothing to do with men'!

How do tumours of the caecum and the right side of the colon commonly present?

On the right side of the large bowel the stools are semi-liquid and the tumours are usually proliferative and therefore obstructive symptoms and signs are relatively uncommon. These patients tend to present 'silently', as in the present case, with features of anaemia due to chronic blood loss and loss of weight.

How do these features differ typically from patients with tumours of the left colon?

Usually tumours of the left side of the colon are constricting growths and the contained stool is solid. There are commonly symptoms of bowel disturbance – constipation, bleeding, passage of altered blood and slime, and/or features of subacute or complete intestinal obstruction.

Describe the possible pathways of spread of a carcinoma of the caecum

- Local: Encircling the bowel wall, invading its wall and then the adjacent viscera.
- Lymphatic: To the regional lymph nodes, with possible late involvement of the supraclavicular nodes via the thoracic duct (Troisier's sign*).
- Blood stream: Via the portal vein to the liver, thence to the lungs.
- Transcoelomic: With deposits of nodules throughout the peritoneal cavity and with ascites. Deposits on the ovaries (Krukenberg tumour†), and rarely a deposit at the umbilicus (Sister Joseph's nodule‡).

---

*Charles Emil Troisier, see Case 56, p. 113.

†Friedrich Krukenberg (1871–1946), pathologist, Halle.

‡Sister Mary Joseph Dempsey (1856–1939), Mayo Clinic, Rochester, Minnesota. She was the ward sister of Dr William Mayo and imparted this gem of clinical wisdom to him.

Case 71 A patient with subacute obstruction

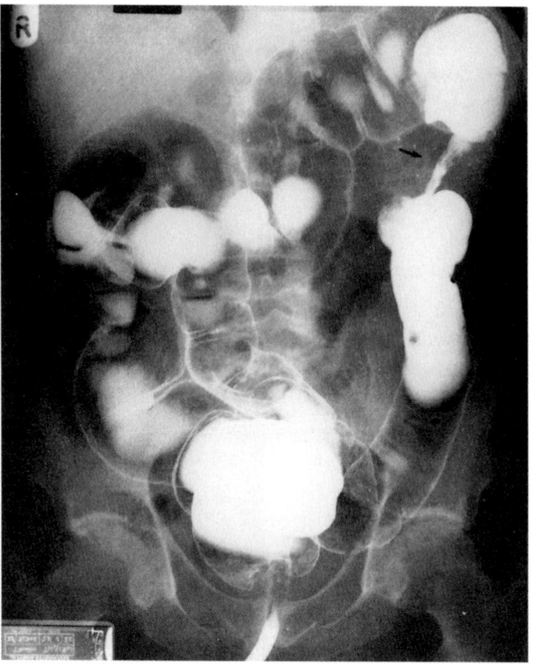

Figure 71.1

A retired electrical engineer aged 69 years was referred urgently to the surgical outpatients. Here he gave a history of a month or more of attacks of colicky central abdominal pain, increasing constipation and a feeling of abdominal distension. The pains at first were mild, but were now quite severe, would come on several times a day, last for up to an hour and would sometimes double him up. His bowels, previously perfectly regular, were now acting only every 2 or 3 days and this with the help of various proprietary laxatives – the stools were hard, but he had not noticed any blood or slime. He had not vomited or felt sick. His appetite had greatly diminished and his wife thought that he had definitely lost some weight. Apart from some mild prostatic symptoms, with nocturia ×1-2, he was otherwise well. There had been no serious illnesses in the past. There was no family history of bowel or other cancers.

Examination revealed a quite healthy, rather overweight patient. His colour was normal. The abdomen was distended with general slight tenderness – he really did not like being palpated – and there was a suggestion of a vague mass to feel in the left upper quadrant. The liver was not enlarged, there was no clinical evidence of ascites and the supraclavicular nodes could not be felt. On rectal examination, the prostate was moderately enlarged but of normal consistency. There were hard faecal pellets in the rectum and the faecal occult blood test was positive.

An urgent barium enema examination was ordered and Fig. 71.1 shows a typical film from the series. The arrow points to a constant abnormality.

What is the likely pathology shown here?

A constricting carcinoma of the descending colon.

What would be the next steps in investigating this patient and in particular establishing the diagnosis?

A full blood count and liver function tests were normal. Chest CT scans showed no evidence of secondary deposits and abdominal CT scan demonstrated a normal liver appearance with no evidence of free fluid.

Colonoscopy was performed under sedation. The tumour was visualized and biopsy specimens were obtained, which histologically showed a moderately differentiated adenocarcinoma. Two small polyps were seen in the sigmoid loop; they were removed and proved to be benign adenomas.

How common is this tumour in the UK; in particular, how does it figure in causes of death from cancer?

Carcinoma of the large bowel (caecum, colon and rectum together) is the second commonest cause of death from cancer, second only to carcinoma of the lung. Incidentally, breast cancer is third, and the commonest cause of death from cancer in women in the UK. Carcinoma of the prostate is fourth (see Table 57.1, p. 116, for the full top 10 'league table').

What predisposing factors may lead to this condition?

Predisposing factors include longstanding ulcerative colitis (see Case 68, p. 137), pre-existing polyps (one or more polyps are found in resected specimens of bowel cancer in about 70% of cases), familial adenomatous polyposis (polyposis coli, which untreated will invariably undergo malignant change) and a hereditary non-polyposis colon cancer (HNPCC) genotype.

What common emergency may result from this disease?

This is the commonest cause in the UK of large bowel obstruction, either acute or chronic; indeed, this patient was heading towards the latter. A less common emergency is perforation, either into the general peritoneal cavity (with dangerous faecal peritonitis) or locally to form a pericolic abscess. Occasionally, fistulation into the bladder, small intestine or, in the female, the vault of the vagina may occur.

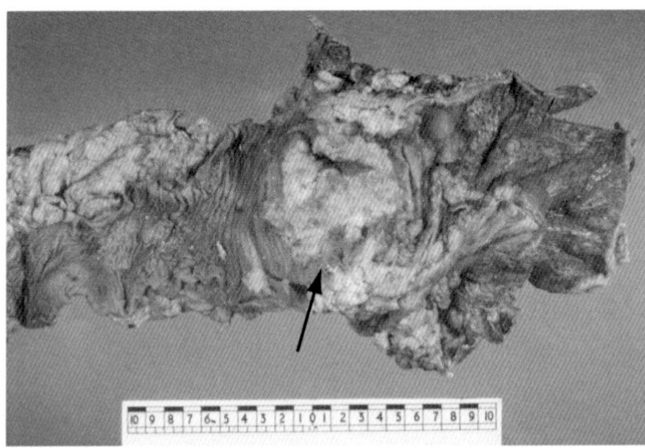

Figure 71.2 Constricting tumour of the descending colon (arrowed).

The patient underwent a left hemicolectomy and, apart from postoperative pulmonary collapse, treated by vigorous physiotherapy, made an excellent recovery. Figure 71.2 shows the appearance of the constricting tumour on its mucosal aspect (arrowed). Histological examination showed it to be a moderately well differentiated adenocarcinoma. Three of the 16 lymph nodes recovered from the specimen showed metastatic deposits (Dukes' stage C). He went on to receive a course of chemotherapy with 5-fluorouracil (indicated in patients with Dukes' C tumours).

Case 72 A pathological anal verge

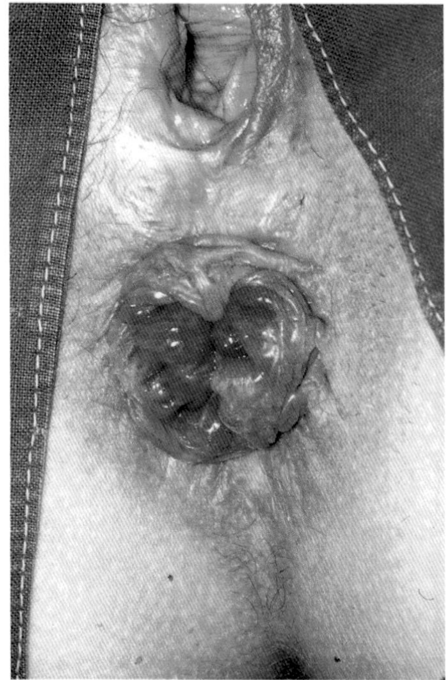

Figure 72.1

Figure 72.1 demonstrates the perineum of a woman aged 50 years, who has been anaesthetized and placed in the lithotomy position on the operating table prior to surgery.

What pathology is demonstrated in Fig. 72.1?

The patient has third degree haemorrhoids or piles. The two words are synonymous, the first derived from the Greek, the second from old English.

What is the anatomical basis of this condition?

Haemorrhoids are dilatations of the venous cushions of the anal canal, which are the commencements of the superior rectal (haemorrhoidal) veins. These drain into the inferior mesenteric vein, then into the splenic vein and finally the portal vein.

There are usually three of these veins arranged roughly at the 3, 7 and 11 o'clock positions, as can be seen in Fig. 72.1. Inferiorly, these veins anastomose with the inferior rectal veins, which drain into the internal iliac veins, and hence form part of the portocaval anastomosis system (see Case 88, p. 179)

How are haemorrhoids classified, and what stage have they reached in this patient?

- *First degree*: The haemorrhoids remain in the anal canal; they may bleed, but do not prolapse.
- *Second degree*: The haemorrhoids prolapse on defaecation, but then return within the anal canal.
- *Third degree*: The haemorrhoids, as in this case, are permanently prolapsed.

What symptoms may trouble the patient with haemorrhoids?

The commonest is rectal bleeding, usually on defaecation. The blood is bright red, due to arteriovenous anastomoses in these veins. Other symptoms are prolapse, mucous discharge, pruritis ani; if the bleeding is heavy or persistent, the patient may present with anaemia – sometimes severe enough to require a blood transfusion.

The only time that haemorrhoids are painful is if they become strangulated. This may follow straining at stool, when the haemorrhoidal mass prolapses and is trapped by spasm of the anal sphincter (see Case 73, p. 147).

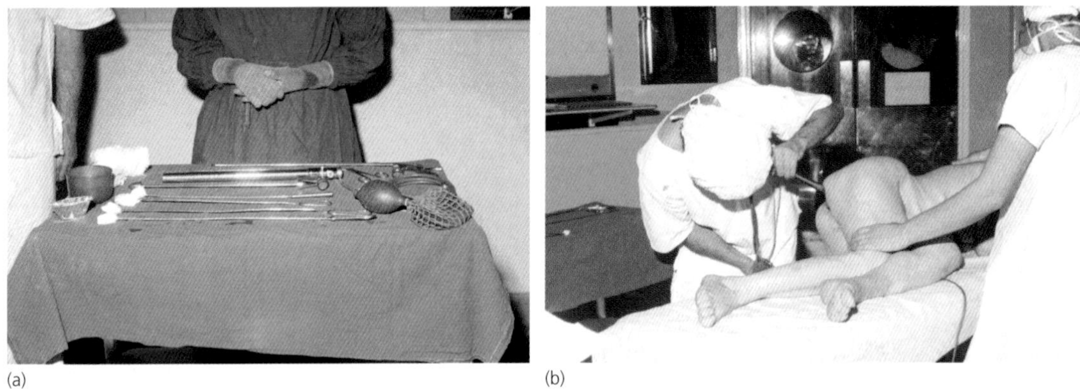

(a) (b)

Figure 72.2 Sigmoidoscopy: (a) instruments and (b) patient position for the procedure.

Rectal bleeding is an early feature of a rectal carcinoma. It is obviously extremely important to exclude this diagnosis in a patient with haemorrhoids. Indeed, not uncommonly the two conditions coexist. How was this done in this patient?

A careful history was taken and a full clinical examination carried out, including, of course, a digital rectal examination. This was followed by sigmoidoscopy using a rigid sigmoidoscope (Fig. 72.2a), which enabled visual examination of the whole of the rectum to be carried out. The patient is placed in the left lateral position with the knees drawn up to the chest (Fig. 72.2b). It is a painless – although uncomfortable – procedure and sedation is only required in very anxious patients.

If there is any suspicion of a lesion higher in the large bowel, a fibreoptic sigmoidoscopy and/or barium enema examination may be indicated.

How are haemorrhoids treated?

First and second degree haemorrhoids can be treated on an outpatient basis by injection of a sclerosant agent, such as 5% phenol in almond oil, or by elastic banding. An advanced case, such as this, is treated by surgical excision – haemorrhoidectomy.

What serious complication may occur in the early days following haemorrhoidectomy?

- Haemorrhage – usually in the first 24 h postoperatively but sometimes delayed for a week to 10 days following surgery.
- Other common complications include urinary retention in men, and constipation due to fear of opening bowels – a mixture of osmotic and lubricant laxatives is usually given, such as lactulose and Milpar.

Case 73 A painful mass at the anal verge

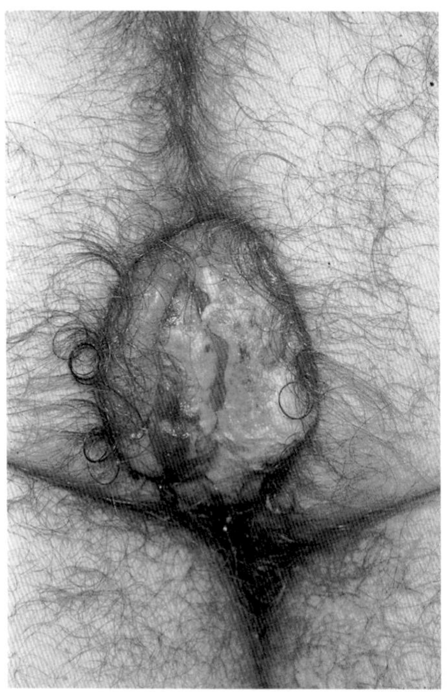

Figure 73.1

Figure 73.1 shows the anal verge of a 60-year-old man who had put up with his prolapsing and bleeding piles for a number of years without bothering to seek medical help. Instead, he used various 'haemorrhoid ointments' without much success and kept a cotton wool pad within his underpants.

Two days before admission to hospital, while straining at stool, a large mass prolapsed out of his anal verge and bled, and, for the first time, his piles became extremely painful.

He tried to push the mass back, but without any success, even when lying in a hot bath. Eventually the severe pain and now a nasty smell made him report to his doctor, who sent him straight to the A&E department.

What is this complication of haemorrhoids called?

Prolapsed strangulated piles.

What is the cause of this complication of haemorrhoids?

The piles have prolapsed and become gripped by the anal sphincter, the venous return has become occluded and thrombosis has occurred. Suppuration and even ulceration of the thrombosed mass will follow.

What is the diagnostic symptom?

The pain – it is only in this complication that haemorrhoids cause anal pain.

What is the standard management of this condition?

Give opiate analgesia for the severe pain. Standard oral medication is insufficient. Put the patient to bed with the foot of the bed elevated and apply cold compresses.

What would be the outcome of this management and is there any alternative, more radical treatment?

The piles fibrose, often with complete or partial cure. However, the process may take 2 or 3 weeks and many surgeons carry out an emergency haemorrhoidectomy for this condition.

Case 74 Another painful mass at the anal verge

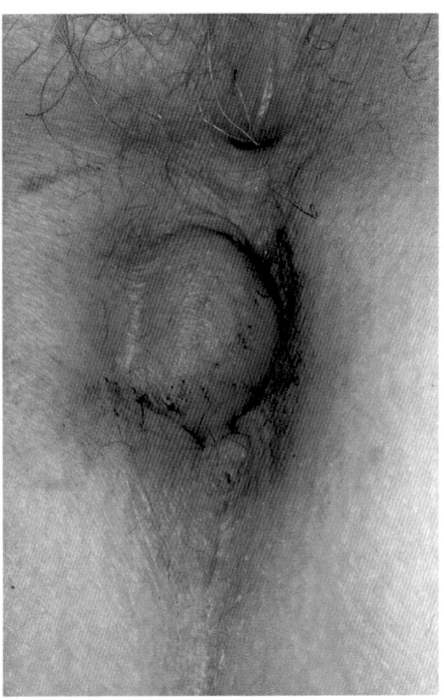

Figure 74.1

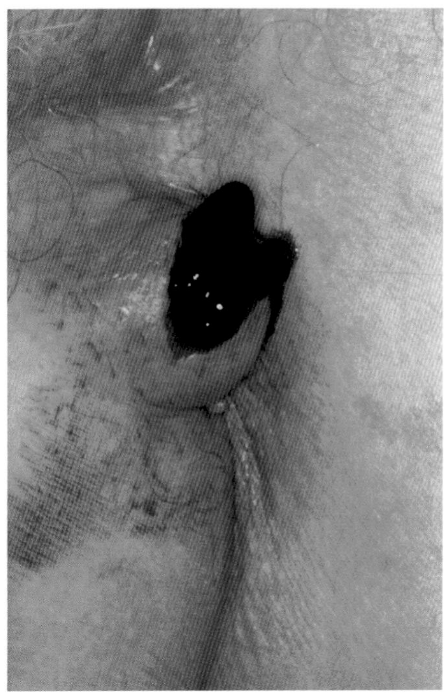

Figure 74.2 Following incision, the perianal lesion reveals its contents (see text).

This patient, a 30-year-old female office worker, hobbled into the accident and emergency department complaining of an acutely painful 'attack of piles'. She said that she had been perfectly well, with no anal problems until the evening before when a very painful lump had suddenly appeared at the anal verge as she was straining to pass a constipated stool. She had been up all night because of the pain.

What condition is shown in Fig. 74.1?

A perianal haematoma.

What produces this pathology?

Rupture of a tributary of one of the inferior rectal veins, usually as a result, as in this case, of straining at stool.

Why is this condition so painful?

The lower anal canal and the anal verge are richly supplied with somatic innervation (the inferior rectal branch of the pudendal nerve S2, S3 and S4) and is sensitive to severe stretching. This is also the basis of the pain experienced in strangulated haemorrhoids (see Case 73, p. 147) and fissure in ano (see Case 75, p. 150)

How did the surgeon immediately relieve the patient's agony?

He injected a little local anaesthetic into the skin over the mass and nicked the lump with the tip of the scalpel. This released the clot, as shown in Fig. 74.2. Any residual clot was then wiped away and a pad dressing applied. This is one of the most dramatic, satisfying and pain-relieving minor operations in the whole repertoire of surgery!

Left untreated, what may happen?

Quite often the haematoma ruptures spontaneously; it may be necessary to just evacuate any residual clot. Small haematomas may slowly absorb, usually leaving a residual skin tag.

Having evacuated the clot, what is the follow-up management of this patient?

A dressing is applied – more to protect the patient's under clothes than anything else – and hot baths prescribed. The small wound rapidly heals over the next few days.

Case 75 An agonizing anal verge

A 40-year-old man attended the rectal clinic complaining of 'painful piles'. When a careful history was taken, this revealed that his symptoms were of 6 weeks of excruciating pain every time he opened his bowels. This was often accompanied by a few drops of bright red blood seen on the lavatory paper. The pain was so bad that he tried to avoid evacuating his bowels, but this just made things worse. Now he had become constipated and passing the resultant hard stools was agonizing.

Apart from a right-sided hernia repair 5 years before, he was otherwise well and had never previously had any bowel symptoms.

When a patient complains of severe anal pain, what common conditions must you consider in your differential diagnosis?

- Fissure in ano.
- Strangulated haemorrhoids (see Case 73, p. 147).
- Perianal haematoma (see Case 74, p. 148).
- Perianal abscess (see Case 76, p. 152).
- Carcinoma of the anal verge (see Case 80, p. 162).

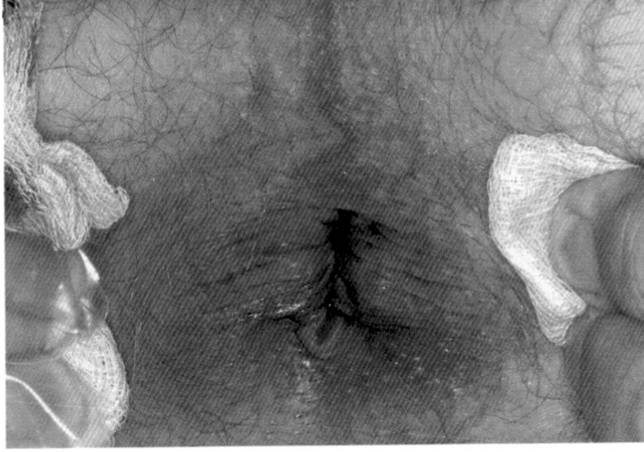

Figure 75.1 A fissure in ano.

- Proctalgia fugax – attacks of severe anal pain without obvious pathology.

The surgeon now proceeded to examine the patient. Apart from a well healed scar from a right inguinal hernia repair, there was nothing to find on general examination. The surgeon then asked the patient to lie in the left lateral position with his knees drawn up. When the buttocks were gently drawn aside, the lesion shown in Fig. 75.1 was revealed. The patient was very apprehensive, but the surgeon reassured him that he was only going to inspect the area and was not going to perform a rectal examination.

What pathology has been exposed?

An anal fissure (fissure in ano) – a tear at the anal verge. Note also the associated skin tag (the sentinel pile) which is the torn tag of anal epithelium the 'points' to the fissure. The great majority of these fissures occur, as in this case, in the 6 o'clock position, directed towards the coccyx. Occasionally, especially in the female, it may occur in the 12 o'clock position.

Why did the (kind hearted) surgeon not perform a rectal examination at this stage?

The area is exquisitely tender. Moreover, the external anal sphincter is in marked spasm in this condition and examination would, in any case, be pretty well impossible.

If multiple fissures were seen at the anal verge, what underlying pathology would you suspect?

This is typically encountered in Crohn's disease of the large bowel.

How is this condition treated?

An early small fissure may heal spontaneously. This is aided by relieving pain with an analgesic ointment, giving a lubricant laxative and prescribing hot baths. Relaxation of the internal anal sphincter may be achieved by applying 2% diltiazem or 0.2% glyceryl trinitrate (GTN) cream. If that is unsuccessful then a 'chemical sphincterotomy' with injection of botulinum toxin to relax the sphincter usually allows healing to take place. If these methods fail, internal sphincterotomy can be considered, but carries the risk of incontinence of flatus and faeces, particularly in parous women whose sphincter may have been damaged years before in childbirth.

Case 76 A very painful buttock

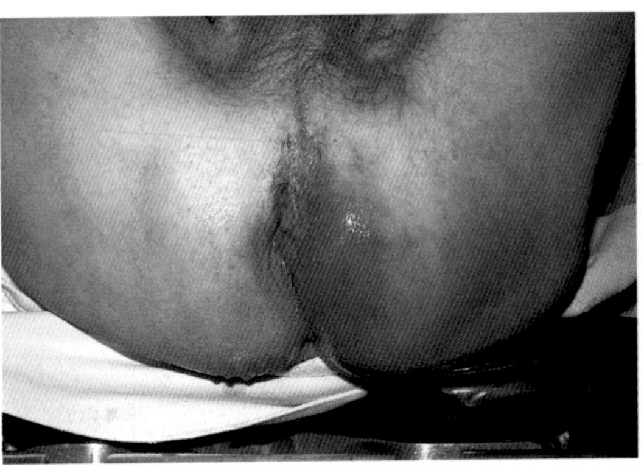

Figure 76.1

A 30-year-old man, a heavy-lorry driver, presented with an intensely painful, swollen, left buttock that had progressively got worse over the last 4 days. He did not feel at all well – hot and sweaty and completely off this food.

On examination in the accident and emergency department he looked ill, his temperature was 38.5°C and pulse 100. Inspection of the perineum revealed the appearance seen in Fig. 76.1 (taken with the patient anaesthetized in the operating theatre).

What is this condition called and what is its precise anatomical location?

A perianal abscess situated in the ischio-anal fossa. This fossa is bounded laterally by the fascia over the obturator internus (i.e. the side wall of the pelvis), medially by the external anal sphincter and the fascia covering the levator ani, anteriorly by the urogenital perineum, and posterially by the sacrotuberous ligament covered behind by the gluteus maximus. The floor of the fossa is perianal skin and subcutaneous fat and the fossa itself is filled with fat (Fig. 76.2).

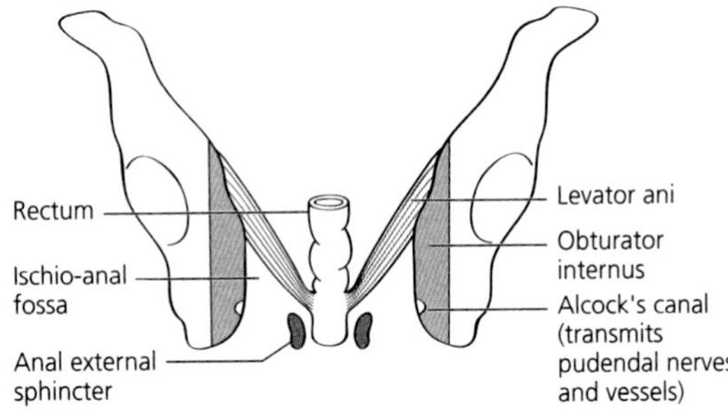

Figure 76.2 The ischio-anal fossa.

Until quite recently this clinically important space was called the 'ischio-rectal fossa' and the abscess called an 'ischio-rectal abscess'. It will be seen from this diagram that both these terms are misnomers.

What is the definition of an abscess?

An abscess is a localized collection of pus. Pus itself is defined as 'living and dead white cells – usually polymorphs – usually, but not always, with living and dead bacteria'. Occasionally pus may be sterile.

What are the classical four features of an abscess?

These were described by Celsus as long ago as the first century AD – pain, heat, swelling and redness (in Latin as *dolor*, *calor*, *tumor* and *rubor*).

How does infection reach the ischio-anal fossa?

There are four possible routes of entry:

• *Perianal*: From an infected hair follicle, sebaceous gland or perianal haematoma (see Case 74, p. 148). This is usually a relatively superficial infection.

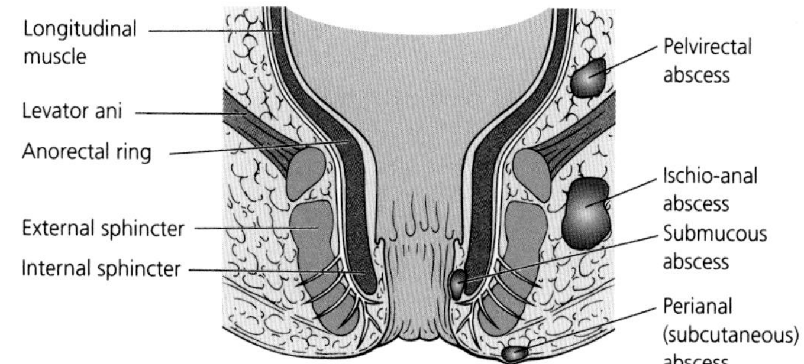

Figure 76.3 The anatomy of perianal abscesses.

- *Submucous*: From an infected fissure in ano (see Case 75, p. 150) or from a laceration of the anal canal.
- *Ischio-anal*: From infection of one of the anal glands that lead from the anal canal into the submucosa (probably the commonest cause) or penetration of the fossa by a foreign body, for example a swallowed fragment of bone. The abscess may track in a horseshoe manner behind the anal canal to the opposite fossa.
- *Pelvic*: Spread inferiorly from a pelvic abscess (rare).

The location of these abscesses is shown in Fig. 76.3.

How is this condition treated?

Early surgical drainage under a general anaesthetic. This gives immediate relief and also prevents possible rupture into the anal canal with a resultant fistula in ano (see Case 77, p. 154).

Case 77 A patient with recurrent perianal sepsis

The patient, a 30-year-old schoolmaster, attended surgical outpatients with the following history – about 3 years previously he developed an abscess on his left buttock. This was drained as a day case at another hospital and healed up. However, since then, there have been repeated episodes of infection; a couple had been drained under anaesthetic at the same hospital and three more had burst spontaneously after sitting repeatedly – and painfully – in a very hot bath. Between these very acute episodes, he usually noticed a discharge of smelly, sticky material near the anal verge and he had to keep a pad of cotton wool within his underpants to prevent his clothes from being soiled. On several occasions he had the impression that flatus was escaping at the site of these infections.

Just on this story you should be able to make a provisional diagnosis of what the condition is

A fistula in ano.

What is the definition of a fistula?

A fistula is a pathological communication between two epithelial surfaces. This may be between two hollow viscera, for example a tracheo-oesophageal fistula or a vesico-colic fistula, or between a hollow viscus and the skin, as in this case or an intestinal fistula onto the abdominal wall.

The patient was admitted semi-urgently for operative treatment. Figure 77.1 shows the patient's perineum as he lies anaesthetized on the operating table in the lithotomy position. What is demonstrated?

In Fig. 77.1a a fine probe has been passed from the external opening of the fistula at the 5 o'clock position and is seen to emerge from the anal canal. In Fig. 77.1b a self-retaining anal retractor has been inserted and the internal opening of the fistula can be seen in the midline (the 6

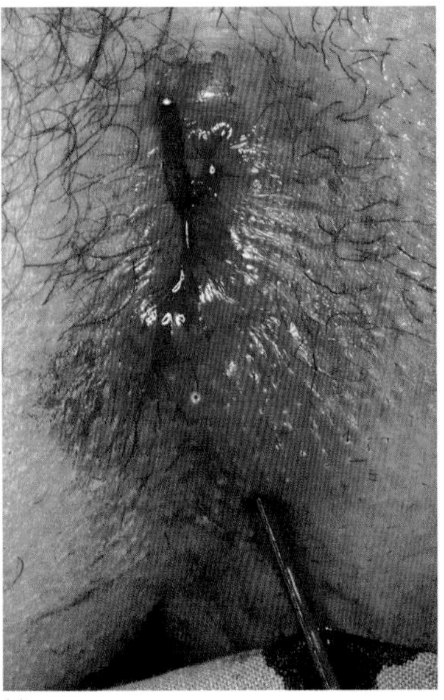

(a)

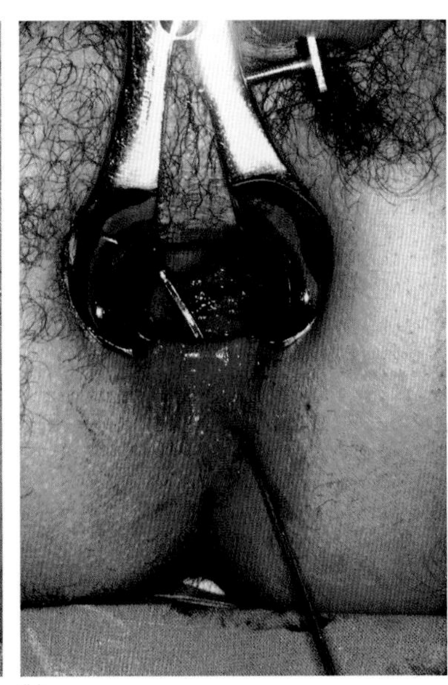

(b)

Figure 77.1 Operative photographs of the patient's perineum.

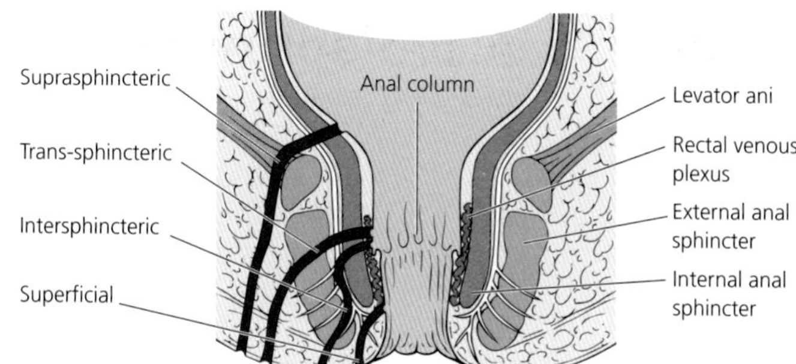

Figure 77.2 The anatomy of perianal fistulae.

o'clock position) fairly low down the wall of the anal canal.

What is the common underlying cause of this condition and what are the rarer causes?

The great majority result from an initial ischio-anal abscess, which ruptures onto the perianal skin and into the anal canal. This was obviously the underlying cause in the present case (see Case 76, p. 152). Rarely, fistulae may be associated with Crohn's disease (where they are often multiple), ulcerative colitis, tuberculosis and advanced carcinoma of the rectum.

How are fistulae in ano classified?

Anal fistulae are classified according to their position and relationship to the internal and external anal sphincters:

- *Superficial*:
  - Submucous.
  - Subcutaneous.
- *Low anal*:
  - Intersphincteric.
  - Trans-sphincteric.
- *High anal*:
  - Suprasphincteric.
- *Anorectal.*

These are demonstrated in Fig. 77.2. The superficial and low anal fistulae are by far the commonest.

What is the treatment of fistulae in ano?

This is invariably surgical. Superficial and low level anal fistulae are laid open along their length and are allowed to heal by granulation. Because no sphincter, or only the subcutaneous parts of the internal and external sphincters, is divided in this procedure, there is no danger of loss of anal continence. Fistulae can only be treated in this manner when they quite definitely lie below the level of the anorectal ring. Careful assessment of the level of the internal opening of the fistula must therefore be made preoperatively and if there is any clinical doubt about the level, endo-anal ultrasound examination must be carried out using an anal probe. This gives a very accurate localization of the track in relation to the sphincters.

In the case of high fistulae (suprasphincteric or high intrasphincteric close to the anorectal ring) only the lower part of the sphincter is laid open. A non-absorbable strong ligature, usually nylon, is passed through the upper part of the tract and is left in place for 2 or 3 weeks so that the deep part of the sphincter becomes fixed by scar tissue – this ligature is called a seton.

When the upper part of the fistulous tract is subsequently divided, the tethered sphincter does not retract and incontinence is prevented.

Case 78 A prolapsing anal mass

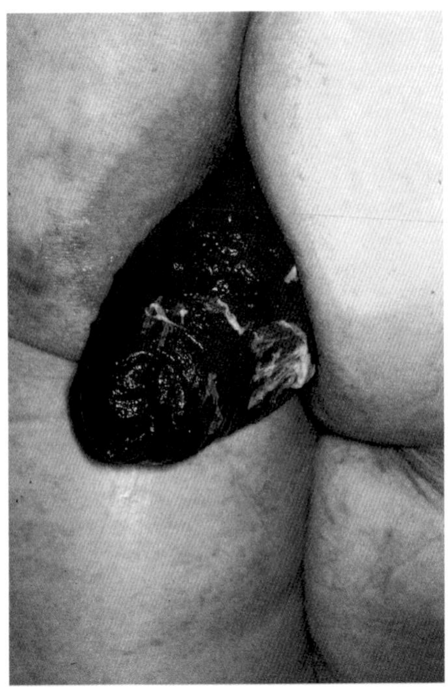

Figure 78.1

The patient, a woman aged 73 years, a retired office worker, attended the colorectal clinic complaining of 'something coming down from the back passage' on every act of defaecation. This she had noticed for the past 2 years but it had become much worse in recent months. The whole affair is quite painless, but it now takes some time for her to push the lump back into her back passage. Two other things are troubling her – in recent weeks she has experienced some incontinence of faeces so that she now keeps a big pad of cotton wool inside her underpants and she is now bothered by some slimy discharge from the rectum, although she has not noticed any blood on her stools or the toilet paper. She is a spinster, has never had a child and is otherwise very well, with no significant past medical history. She does not drink or smoke.

On examination she proved to be an obese lady, with a blood pressure of 160/90, but full clinical examination was otherwise normal apart from her perineum. When she was placed in the left lateral position and asked to strain down behind, the mass shown in Fig. 78.1 emerged from the anal canal. It could be reduced again quite easily by gentle pressure. When a rectal examination was performed, the anal sphincter was patulous, but contracted quite well when the patient was asked to 'tighten up the back passage'.

What is this condition called?

She has a complete prolapse of the rectum associated with some degree of anal incontinence.

What is a partial rectal prolapse?

Partial rectal prolapse comprises few centimetres of prolapsed rectal mucosa.

What types of patient get this condition of partial prolapse?

It is not rare in otherwise perfectly normal babies. It is a frightening sight to the parents, but they can be reassured that it is an entirely self-curing condition. It is also seen in patients with large, extensively prolapsing piles (see Case 72, p. 145).

Give the features of complete rectal prolapse

Complete prolapse, in contrast to the above, involves all layers of the rectal wall. It is usually found in elderly patients, in females far more often than in males and often, as in the present case, in nulliparous women. Apart from the discomfort and the embarrassment of this condition, there may be faecal incontinence due to stretching of the anal sphincter mechanism and there may be discharge of mucus, and sometimes blood, from the exposed mucosal surface.

What is the treatment of this condition?

The patient is fit and her symptoms fully justify surgical treatment. Two operations are commonly performed:

- The first technique is to fix the rectum in the pelvis by means of an abdominal approach such as mobilizing the rectum and wrapping it in polyvinyl sponge. This produces a brisk fibrous reaction, which welds the rectum to the pelvic tissues.
- An alternative is the Delorme operation,* a perianal approach with excision of the rectal mucosa and bunching of its muscle wall to produce a doughnut-like ring. This holds the rectum within the pelvis, rather like the way a ring pessary controls a vaginal prolapse.

In patients who are at high risk of major surgery, the Thiersch procedure† may be used. A nylon suture is passed around the anal orifice to narrow it and keep the prolapse reduced.

*Edmond Delorme (1847–1929), Professor of surgery, Val-de-Grâce, Paris.

†Karl Thiersch (1822–1895), Professor of surgery, Erlangen and then Leipzig. He devised the split-skin graft.

Case 79 An ulcer in the rectum

A civil servant, aged 59 years, consulted his family practitioner complaining that he had 'piles'. When his doctor took a careful history, this revealed that the patient had noted bright red blood in the lavatory pan and on the toilet paper pretty well after every act of defaecation over the past 6 or 7 months. He also noticed slimy material in his motions and quite often had two or three bowel actions a day, something that was unusual for him, since he had prided himself on his regular normal bowel habit. Recently he noticed a feeling of incomplete evacuation and would spend frustrating time in the toilet trying to empty his bowel fully. He was not particularly worried because the whole affair was painless and he was feeling quite well. His weight was steady and his appetite unaffected.

In the past he had had a right-sided hernia repaired 15 years before and an appendicectomy as a young man.

His doctor examined the patient carefully. He looked well and was not clinically anaemic. He examined the abdomen carefully – nothing abnormal was detected apart from the well healed scars of his two previous operations. He meticulously palpated both supraclavicular fossae; no masses were detected. After some protest from the patient, he submitted him to a rectal examination in the left lateral position. A large, firm ulcerated mass was easily felt low in the rectum, and there was blood and mucus on the examining finger. An urgent appointment was made for the patient to be seen in the colorectal clinic.

What would the clinical diagnosis be?

The story and clinical findings strongly suggest a carcinoma of the lower rectum. A large adenoma would be a possibility, but these do not ulcerate. Note that patients nearly always attribute bright red rectal bleeding to piles or haemorrhoids – the two words are synonymous. Indeed, this pathology accounts for a good 90% of such cases. However, this diagnosis must never be made without full clinical assessment.

This very good and conscientious doctor, suspecting the diagnosis of a malignancy in the rectum, carefully examined his patient's abdomen and supraclavicular fossae. What evidence of metastatic spread of the tumour might be picked up by this examination?

- Hepatomegaly, perhaps with jaundice: Evidence of liver deposits.
- Ascites: Evidence of peritoneal seedlings.
- A nodule at the umbilicus (Sister Joseph's nodule*): Also indicative of peritoneal spread.
- Palpable, hard supraclavicular nodes: Advanced lymphatic spread (Troisier's sign†).

At the colorectal clinic, the surgeon confirmed the clinical features described above. What investigation did he then perform in the clinic to establish the diagnosis without question?

A sigmoidoscopy, using a rigid sigmoidoscope (see Case 72, p. 145). This can be carried out with minimal discomfort and without bowel preparation in the great majority of patients. The ulcerating tumour was visualized, its lower level being 4 cm from the anal verge, and a biopsy painlessly obtained using punch forceps.

What type of tumour would be revealed on histological examination of the biopsy material?

The rectum and upper half of the anal canal, like the rest of the alimentary canal up to the level of the oesophagogastric junction, is lined by a columnar epithelium with

---

*Sister Mary Joseph Dempsey, see Case 70, p. 141.

†Charles Emil Troisier, see Case 56, p. 113.

goblet (mucus-secreting) cells (Fig. 79.1). The tumour is therefore an adenocarcinoma. The pathologist can not only confirm the diagnosis but give some help to prognosis on this examination. He grades the tumour into well differentiated, moderately differentiated and poorly differentiated (or anaplastic) depending on the cell pattern and appearance; prognosis becomes worse as these deviate more from normal histology.

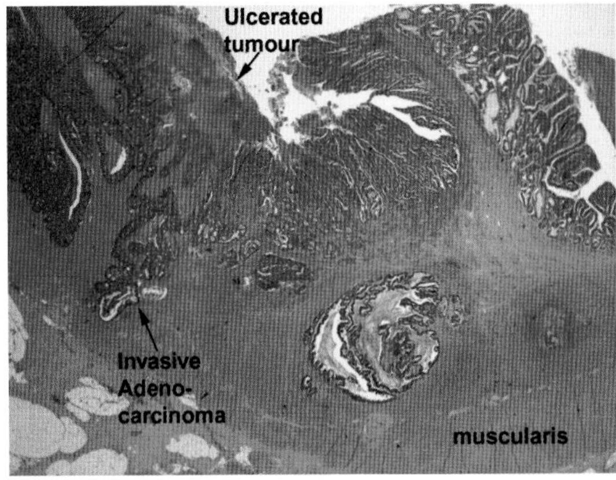

Figure 79.1 Histology slide of a rectal tumour.

What special investigations should now be ordered to assess the patient and stage the tumour?

- *A full blood count*: To check whether the bleeding has resulted in anaemia.
- *Liver function tests*: To check if the patient is affected by possible liver metastases, when typically the alkaline phosphatase rises.
- *CT scans of the chest and abdomen*: To look for metastatic spread, particularly in the chest and liver.
- *Pelvic MR imaging*: To assess the size of the tumour and whether it has spread laterally to the mesorectum.
- *Colonoscopy*: To check for the presence of polyps or a second primary in the more proximal large bowel.

The laboratory and imaging findings in this patient were within normal limits and colonoscopy was clear apart from the rectal tumour. Because of the low level of the tumour, in the lower third of the rectum, resection of the tumour with preservation of the anal sphincter was impossible, so an abdomino-perineal excision of the rectum was performed with the formation of a left iliac fossa colostomy (Figs 79.2 and 79.3). At operation, a full laparotomy was first performed showing no evidence of ascites or hepatic metastases. Figure 79.4 demonstrates the excised specimen.

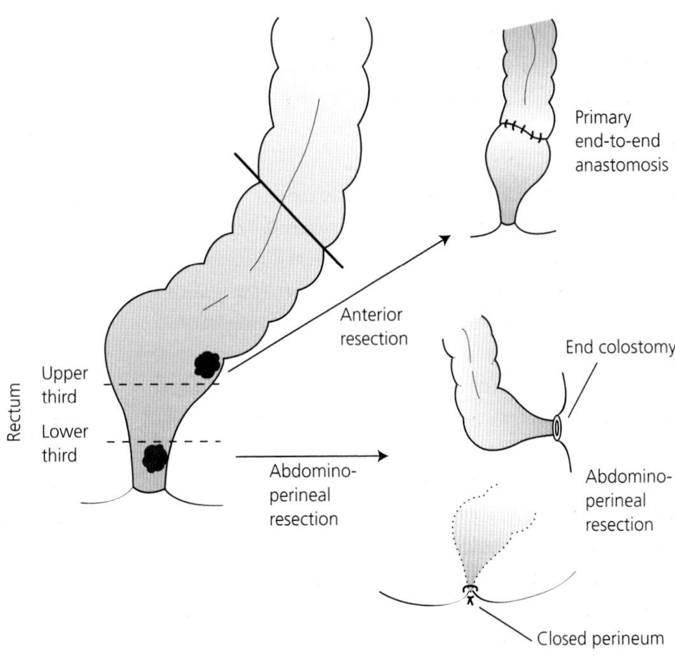

Figure 79.2 Surgical procedures for carcinoma of rectum.

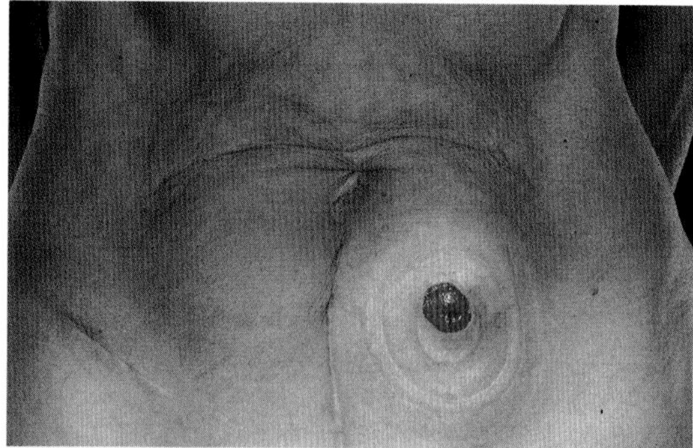

Figure 79.3 An abdomen with healed scar and left iliac fossa colostomy.

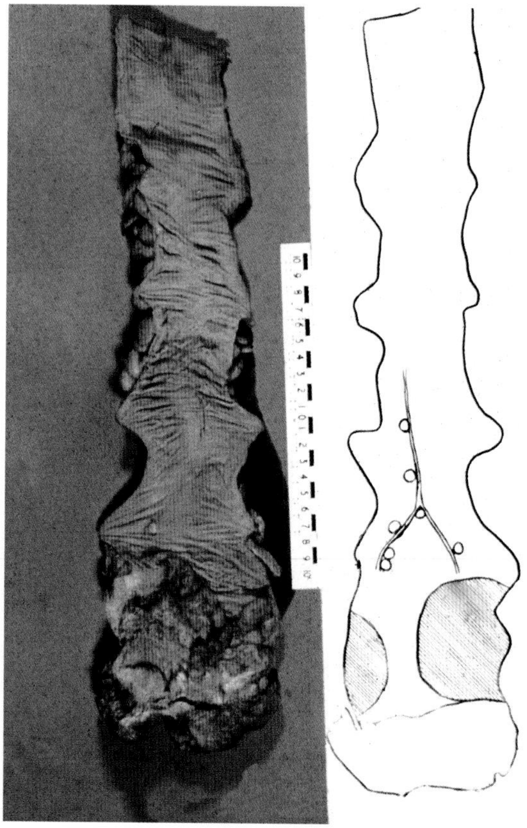

> *Before his operation, the patient was visited by the stomatherapy nurse who was going to train him in colostomy management and also by an ex-patient volunteer, who had undergone the same operation 4 years previously and who now performed a valuable service by encouraging stoma patients in the pre- and postoperative period.*

In addition to the information the pathologist can provide about prognosis from his grading of the tumour, what further information can he now derive from his examination of the excised specimen?

The pathologist studies the depth of penetration of the tumour through the bowel wall and examines the lymph nodes in the specimen. He can now stage the tumour according to Dukes' staging system‡ (Fig. 79.5):

A The tumour is confined to the mucosa and submucosa and has not involved the muscle wall.

B The tumour involves the underlying muscle.

C The tumour has metastasized to the regional nodes.

D There are distant metastases, e.g. to the liver.

The pathologist also searches for evidence of invasion of the draining veins in the specimen.

Figure 79.4 Excised carcinoma of the lower rectum.

Prognosis, i.e. 5-year survival, closely correlates with the degree of differentiation of the tumour (its grade), its Dukes' stage and the presence or absence of venous invasion. The final report in this patient was a moderately differentiated adenocarcinoma, Dukes' stage B, with no evidence of venous involvement.

The subsequent treatment of patients with rectal carcinoma depends on the extent of the tumour. Prior to abdomino-perineal resection, a short course of local radiotherapy is given to reduce the incidence of local recurrence. If the tumour is found to be Dukes' stage C (lymph node involvement) or an advanced Dukes' B (TNM stage 4, invading other organs or structures), the patient receives a long course of radiotherapy and chemotherapy with 5-fluorouracil. If the tumour is Dukes' A or non-advanced Dukes' B, then no adjuvant treatment is indicated.

---

‡Cuthbert Esquire Dukes (1890–1977), pathologist, St Mark's Hospital, London.

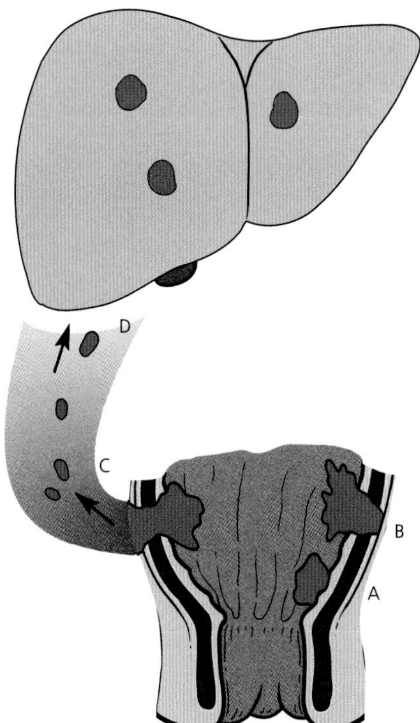

Figure 79.5 Dukes' classification of tumours of the large bowel: A, confined to the bowel wall; B, penetrating the wall; C, involving regional lymph nodes; and D, distant spread.

Case 80 An ulcer at the anal verge

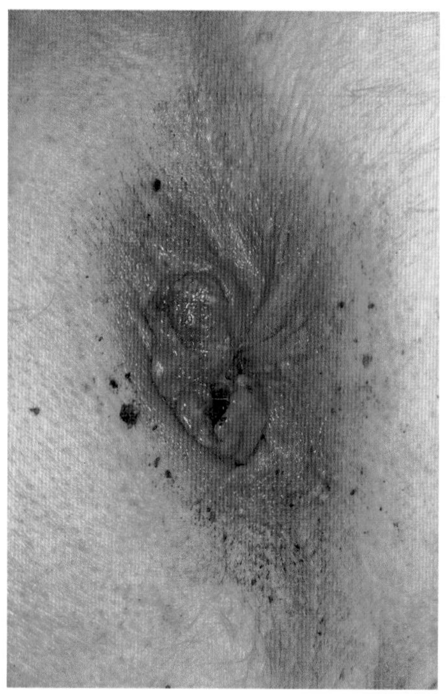

Figure 80.1

On the same day that the previous patient (Case 79, p. 158) attended the colorectal clinic, a patient with the lesion shown in Fig. 80.1 presented. He was a male nurse aged 55 years who had noticed a lump at his anal verge about 6 months previously, which bled on the toilet paper and onto his underpants. He thought he had piles and treated himself with various ointments he bought from the chemists. It was now getting bigger, bled more, was painful and was tender to touch. Examination revealed a healthy, middle-aged man. No abnormality was found on abdominal examination and careful examination revealed no inguinal lymphadenopathy. The anal ulcer was tender, had raised everted edges and was rubbery hard. Its upper border extended into the anal canal.

What would be your clinical diagnosis on these findings?

A malignant ulcerating tumour, probably an epithelioma of the anal verge.

What other malignant tumours may present at the anal verge?

Downward spread from an advanced adenocarcinoma of the lower rectum, malignant melanoma, basal cell carcinoma (rodent ulcer), carcinoid tumour and lymphoma. All of these are uncommon.

Under local anaesthetic, injected with a fine needle through the normal skin at the ulcer edge, a punch biopsy was taken. What would be the histology report, and why?

A squamous carcinoma arising from the stratified squamous epithelium that lines the lower half of the anal canal. This is in contrast to the columnar epithelial lining of the upper half.

Is the difference in the histology between these two situations of any importance in the management of the patient?

Very much so! Squamous cell carcinomas are usually radio-sensitive (e.g. skin, larynx, cervix of the uterus) and can be treated by radiotherapy. Indeed, this is how this patient was managed.

Adenocarcinomas, as a rule, are relatively radio-resistant, which is why the previous patient with a low rectal tumour required an abdomino-perineal excision of the rectum.

This patient's tumour was painful; he also required local anaesthetic for a biopsy to be taken. This contrasts with the previous case, whose large growth caused no pain and whose biopsy was performed without a need for an anaesthetic. Can you explain this?

The lower anal canal receives a somatic innervation from the pudendal nerve (S2, S3 and S4), which transmits normal cutaneous sensation of heat, cold, touch and pain. The upper anal canal, like the rest of the alimentary canal from the oesophago-gastric junction downwards, has an autonomic nerve supply, with sensation transmitted by sympathetic afferent nerves. These are insensitive to pricking, cutting and burning. Pain from a rectal carcinoma immediately suggests invasion of the surrounding pelvic tissues.

Why did the surgeon pay great attention to the patient's inguinal lymph nodes?

The lower anal canal, together with the anal verge, has its own lymphatic drainage to the inguinal lymph nodes. If these are implicated, a block dissection of the groin on one or both sides may be required. In contrast, the upper anal canal, like the rectum itself, drains along lymphatics that accompany the superior rectal veins to nodes lying alongside these vessels and then along the pedicle of the inferior mesenteric vessels.

Case 81 A large swelling in the groin

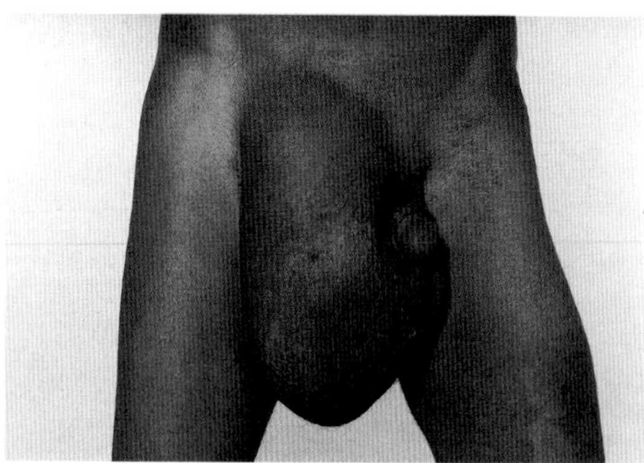

Figure 81.1

Figure 81.1 is a photograph of a 57-year-old vagrant, who had 'lived rough' for the past decade. He had noticed a lump in his right groin several years previously, which gradually enlarged until it reached its present size a couple of years ago. It was now getting to be uncomfortable but did not hurt. He found that the lump would disappear after he had lain down for a few minutes, but would return on standing up. Apart from the lump and a 'smoker's cough' (he smoked as many cigarette ends as he could collect), he was surprisingly fit.

Just on this brief history and on inspection of Fig. 81.1, what would be your working diagnosis?

An indirect, reducible, right inguino-scrotal hernia.

Describe the anatomical basis of this swelling

The sac of an indirect inguinal hernia, a protrusion of the parietal peritoneum, enters the inguinal canal at the internal (deep) ring. This orifice lies lateral to the inferior epigastric vessels. The sac then passes obliquely along the inguinal canal. This canal is about 4 cm in length. Its posterior wall is made up of the transversalis fascia, reinforced medially by the conjoint tendon, while its anterior wall comprises the aponeurosis of the external oblique reinforced laterally by fibres of the internal oblique. The canal terminates at the external (superficial) ring, which is a slit-like opening in the external oblique.

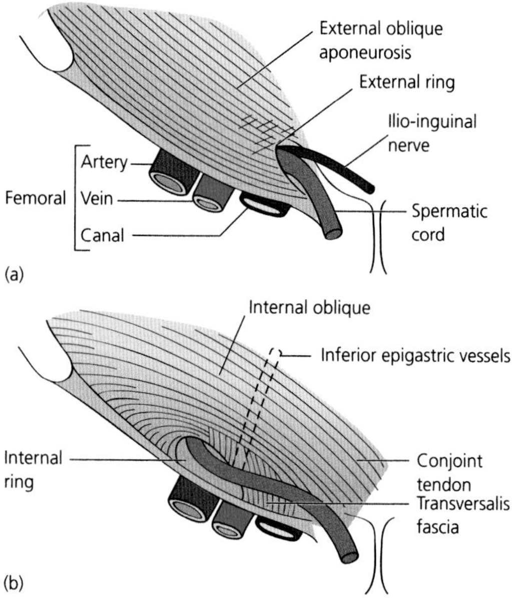

Figure 81.2 The right inguinal canal (a) with the external oblique aponeurosis intact and (b) with the aponeurosis laid open.

The canal transmits the spermatic cord in the male, together with the ilio-inguinal nerve (Fig. 81.2). In the female, the much narrower canal transmits the round ligament to the labium majus, together with the ilio-inguinal nerve.

Note that when the hernia is reduced, the peritoneal sac remains *in situ* but empty. When the subject coughs or strains, or in this case merely stands up, the hernia contents – which are usually small intestine but may also comprise large bowel, omentum or indeed any intraperitoneal viscus – descend into the sac.

What further tests would you perform in your clinical examination of this patient to confirm (or refute) your initial working diagnosis?

Lay the patient flat on the examination couch. In his case, the hernia contents reduced spontaneously. Sometimes gentle massage is required to reduce the hernia. This distinguishes a reducible from an irreducible hernia.

Now identify the position of the internal ring. This is done by palpating the femoral pulse at the groin, half way between the anterior superior iliac spine and the midline (the pubic symphysis), and sliding the index finger just above the line of the inguinal ligament above this point. Get the patient to cough – the hernia is controlled. Now release your finger, get the patient to cough again – the hernia appears and is seen to pass obliquely downwards into the scrotum. If visible and/or audible peristalsis is detected in the mass, this indicates small bowel contents.

What is the difference between a direct and an indirect inguinal hernia?

A direct inguinal hernia is a bulge of peritoneum through the posterior wall of the inguinal canal. Since this usually results from some progressive weakening of the transversalis fascia it is very rare in children and not common in young adults. It is also unusual in females, due to the small size of the inguinal canal. The hernia is seen to pass directly forward ('direct') on coughing, and does not descend towards or into the scrotum. Its neck lies medial to the inferior epigastric vessels and therefore the hernia is not controlled by finger pressure over the internal ring. Because it has a wide neck it immediately reduces on lying down. The wide neck also accounts for the fact that the direct hernia is at little risk of strangulation.

Often the differential diagnosis is suggested by careful inspection. Look at this photograph of a 67-year-old man with bilateral inguinal herniae (Fig. 81.3). The left is passing towards the top of the scrotum, while the right is bulging directly forward. The diagnosis of direct right and indirect left inguinal hernia was confirmed at operation later that day. (Note also the large sebaceous cyst with punctum to the right of his umbilicus, which was also removed.)

Not unusually at operation a patient is found to have an indirect sac descending into the spermatic cord through the internal ring and a direct bulge through the posterior wall of the canal medial to the inferior epigastric vessels. This is given the evocative name of a pantaloon hernia. Indeed, the standard technique of inguinal hernia repair involves removal of the indirect sac and reinforcement of the internal ring orifice and of the posterior wall of the canal.

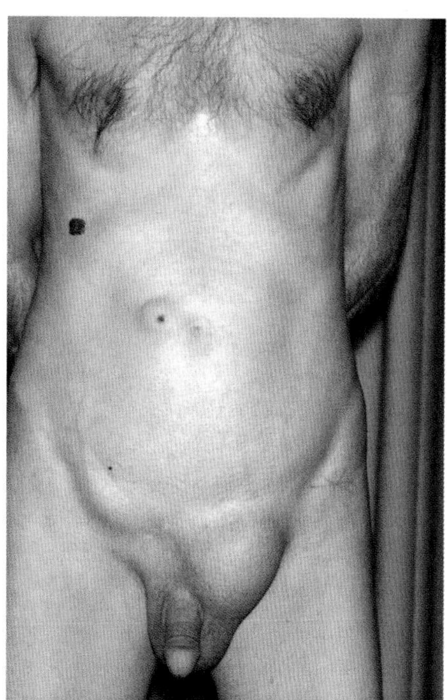

Figure 81.3 Bilateral inguinal herniae.

Which is the more common side for an inguinal hernia?

For some unknown reason, inguinal herniae are much commoner on the right side – 60% of unilateral herniae. Another 20% are on the left and 20% are bilateral.

What is the very real danger of leaving this man's hernia untreated?

Indirect inguinal herniae are likely to strangulate, and this especially so in large inguino-scrotal herniae such as this. Often, following a cough or straining, the contents of the sac are trapped – usually at the internal or the external ring – their blood supply cut off and gangrene of the trapped viscus will occur unless the hernia is operated upon urgently and the obstruction relieved.

Note that although large inguino-scrotal herniae such as this were common in the UK 40 or 50 years ago – and in consequence strangulated inguinal hernia headed the list of causes of small bowel obstruction – today the majority of patients report at a much earlier stage in the evolution of their herniae and are submitted to elective repair. In emerging countries, with poor medical facilities, giant inguinal herniae remain common and are a frequent cause of obstruction.

Case 82 A groin lump in an old woman

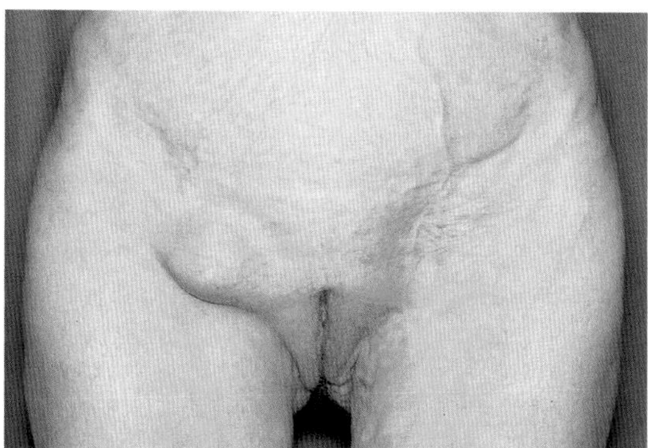

Figure 82.1

Figure 82.1 illustrates the groins of a woman aged 75 years, shaved in preparation for operation later that day. She noticed this lump on the right side 3 months previously. At first it was quite small and went away on lying down, but it is now larger, present all the time and, although not actually painful, is rather uncomfortable. She is otherwise remarkably well for her age.

On examination, the lump was smooth, slightly mobile from side to side and slightly tender. It could not be reduced by gentle pressure. It was definitely situated below and lateral to the pubic tubercle. Clinical examination was otherwise essentially normal.

What diagnosis would you make on these characteristic findings?

An irreducible right femoral hernia.

What is the sex distribution of this condition?

It is much commoner in females than males, probably because of the wide female pelvis. However, it is certainly found in men, as shown in Fig. 82.2 of this condition in a 60-year-old male. A femoral hernia is an acquired condition, extremely rare in children and unusual in young adults.

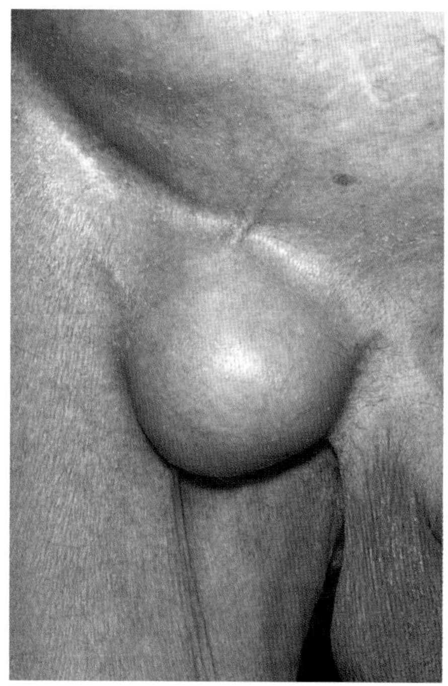

Figure 82.2 An irreducible right fermoral hernia in a male.

Describe the anatomy of the femoral canal

- Anteriorly – the inguinal ligament (Fig. 82.3).
- Medially – the sharp edge of the lacunar part of the inguinal ligament (Gimbernat's ligament).
- Laterally – the femoral vein.
- Posteriorly – the pectineal ligament of Astley Cooper,* which is the thickened periosteum along the superior pubic ramus.

---

*Sir Astley Paston Cooper (1768–1841), surgeon, Guy's Hospital, London.

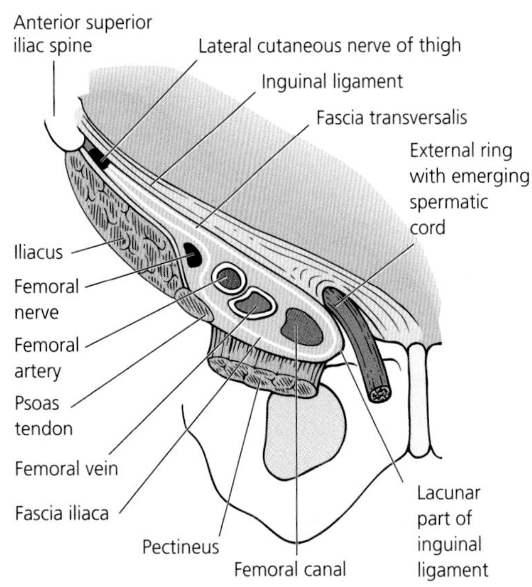

Figure 82.3 The anatomy of the femoral canal and its surrounds to show the relationships of a femoral hernia.

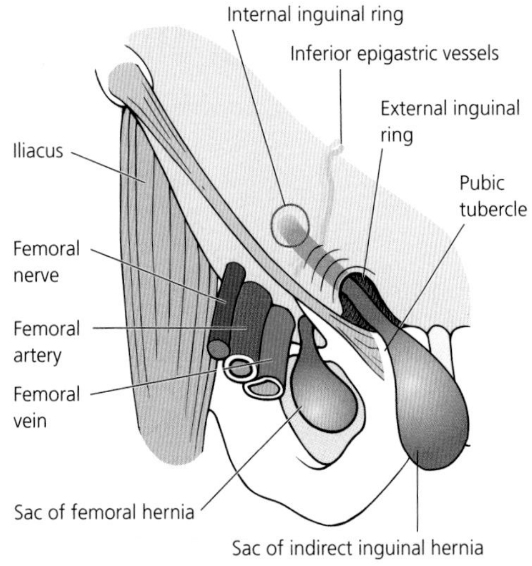

Figure 82.4 The relationships of an indirect inguinal and a femoral hernia compared: the inguinal hernia emerges above and medial to the public tubercule; the femoral hernia lies below and lateral to it.

• The canal normally contains a plug of fat and a lymph node – the node of Cloquet.†

Note that an inguinal hernia will lie above and medial to the pubic tubercle, whereas a femoral hernia lies below and lateral to this landmark (Fig. 82.4).

What is an irreducible hernia and how does this differ from a strangulated hernia?

A hernia becomes irreducible usually because its contents become adherent to the inner wall of the sac, or sometimes because adhesions within the contents become larger than the neck of the sac. In strangulation, the blood supply to the contents is cut off by the neck of the sac (Fig. 82.5). Unrelieved, gangrene of the contents is inevitable and, if gut is involved, perforation of the gangrenous loop will eventually take place.

What is the differential diagnosis of a lump in the groin?

Whenever you consider the differential diagnosis of a lump anywhere in the body, whether this is situated on the top of the skull, the right iliac fossa or, in this case, the groin, the process is the same. You must consider all the anatomical structures in that area, think of the pathologies that may affect those structures and then decide on the most likely cause of the mass in question.

So, in this case:

• Is the lump in the skin or subcutaneous tissues? It could be a sebaceous cyst or lipoma.

• Is it vascular? It could be a saphena varix or femoral aneurysm.

• Is it an enlarged lymph node? An enlarged Cloquet's node may be difficult to differentiate unless there is an obvious primary focus of infection or tumour in the lymphatic drainage area of the groin nodes, or a generalized lymphadenopathy.

• Is it an inguinal hernia? It would lie above and medial to the pubic tubercle.

What treatment would you advise this woman to have?

Femoral herniae are at great risk of strangulation. This is because they have a narrow neck and lie adjacent to the tough, sharp, reflected part of the inguinal ligament on the medial border. Indeed, many patients with this condition present as an emergency. Elective surgery is therefore

†Jules Germain Cloquet (1790–1883), Professor of surgery, Paris.

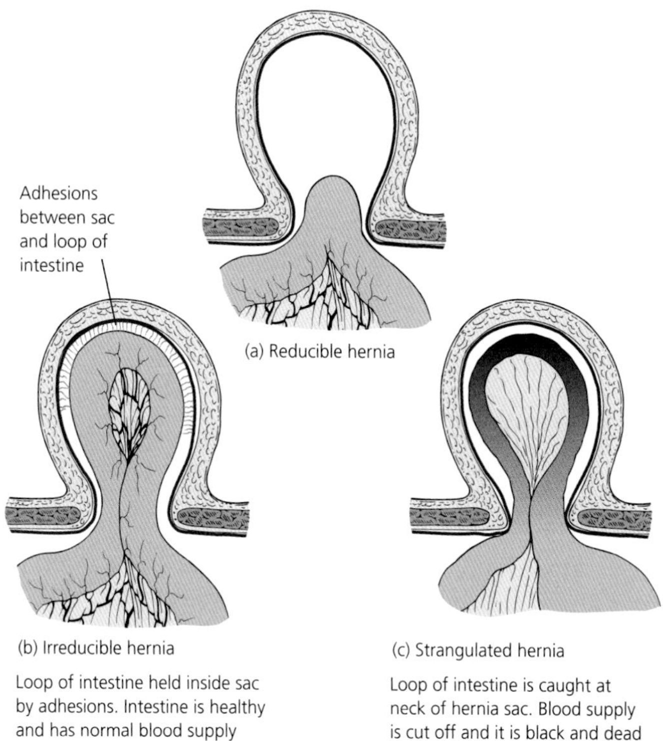

Figure 82.5 The differences between (a) a reducible, (b) an irreducible and (c) a strangulated hernia.

always advised in patients with a femoral hernia. Even in the unfit, the operation can be performed if necessary under local anaesthesia.

What is a Richter's hernia?‡

This is where only part of the wall of the intestine involved in a strangulated hernia is trapped by the neck of the sac. It is not a rare finding in a strangulated femoral hernia (or in the much less common obturator hernia), where the neck of the sac is small. The patient presents with a painful, tender, irreducible lump, but because the whole bowel lumen is not totally occluded, there may be no signs of intestinal obstruction.

‡August Gottlieb Richter (1742–1812), surgeon, Gottingen, Germany.

Case 83 A lump at the umbilicus

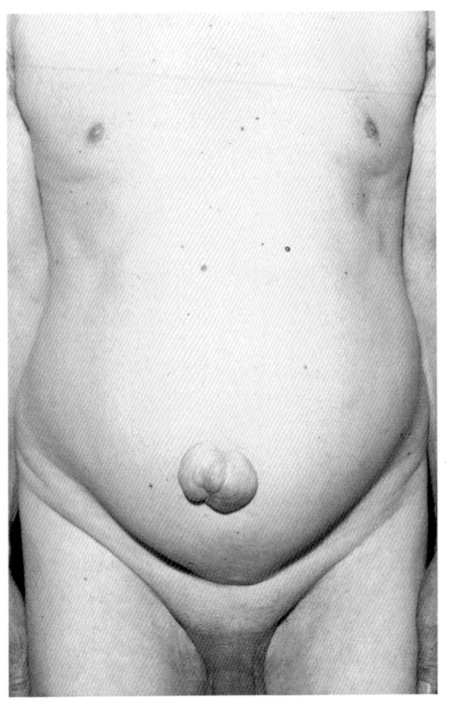

Figure 83.1

This 62-year-old, rather overweight man presented with a lump at the umbilicus. It was first noted 3 years previously and has slowly got larger. Initially it disappeared when he lay down and was only obvious to him after he got up and walked about. However, in the last few months he has noticed it is there all the time. It has remained painless.

What is this called? Full and correct title please!

The correct title for this is a paraumbilical hernia; these occur just above or just below the umbilicus and not through it. These herniae are commoner in females than males and they tend to occur in obese and multiparous women.

What, then, is an umbilical hernia?

This is quite a common finding in newborn babies, especially in Black children. It results from a defect in the umbilical scar, which bulges rather alarmingly when the baby cries. This looks frightening but in fact the great majority of these defects close spontaneously by the end of the first year. Surgery is only indicated in the rare cases when this does not occur.

To return to our adult patient, palpation of the lump revealed a rather soft nodular mass, which could not be reduced and did not enlarge on coughing. It was not tender to touch.

What further information do these findings give you about the hernia?

The hernia content is almost certainly greater omentum, hence its nodular feel. It is the commonest viscus to find its way into the sac of this type of hernia. Larger paraumbilical herniae often also contain transverse colon, with or without loops of small intestine. The hernia cannot be reduced; the contents have become adherent to the peritoneal lining of the sac. The absence of pain, tenderness or signs of bowel obstruction exclude strangulation.

Patients with this condition should be strongly advised to have the hernia repaired electively – why?

With its narrow neck, a paraumbilical hernia, like the femoral hernia of Case 82 (p. 167), is at considerable risk of strangulation, with danger, if unrelieved, of gangrene of its contents.

Case 84 A swelling in the abdominal wall

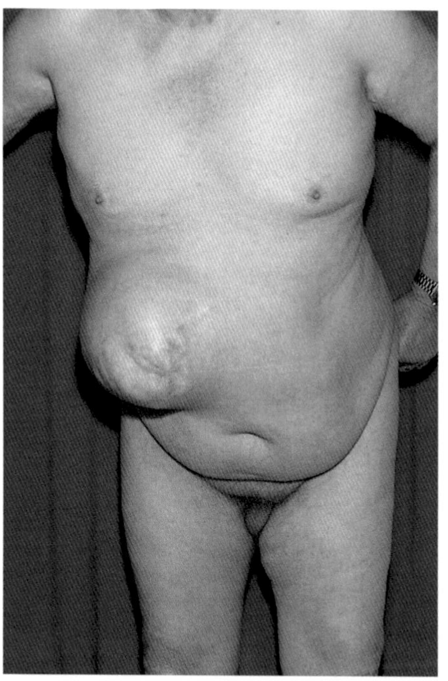

Figure 84.1

This patient, a store man aged 62 years, had had an appendicectomy performed as an emergency when he was 45. He remained well until 4 years ago when he was admitted to hospital as an emergency with a small bowel obstruction. He was operated on a few hours after admission and was told by the surgeon that his obstruction was caused by adhesions from his previous operation. Following surgery, he had a stormy time; the wound became seriously septic, discharged pus and broke down. He received prolonged courses of a variety of antibiotics and, after several weeks in hospital, was discharged home for daily dressings by the district nurse. Eventually, after about 3 months, the wound healed, leaving a rather ugly, wide scar. A few months later, an abscess appeared at the lateral end of the wound. He attended the hospital again, the abscess was drained and a long length of nylon suture, with a knot at its end, was removed. He was then well until a year ago, when he noticed a bulge in the scar, which gradually enlarged until it reached the size shown in Fig. 84.1. The lump disappeared as soon as he lay down, but bulged again as he stood up and enlarged when he coughed or strained. Apart from some discomfort, he was not particularly troubled by the lump, but on his holidays he was embarrassed by its appearance and avoided appearing in public in bathing trunks.

As can be seen, the patient is rather obese, but apart from the swelling, clinical examination was normal.

What is this lesion called?

An incisional hernia.

What was the abscess that appeared some months after he left hospital?

A stitch abscess. This was a collection of pus around the knot of the nylon suture that had been used to close the abdominal wall after his operation for intestinal obstruction. This is a common cause of a late wound abscess or discharging sinus.

Is this hernia dangerous? If not, why not?

The hernia has a wide neck and there is little danger here of obstruction. This is in contrast to the danger presented by a femoral hernia or an indirect inguinal hernia.

Classify the possible aetiological factors that might have resulted in the formation of this hernia

This is another exercise in the classification of causes of any postoperative complication. Consider the following:

- Possible factors present before the operation.
- Factors at the operation.
- Factors after the operation.

We have already gone through this exercise in Case 2 (p. 6), the patient with a postoperative burst abdomen; an incisional hernia might be regarded as a lesser degree of this. So consider:

• *Preoperative factors*: Anything that might affect wound healing, including vitamin C deficiency, uraemia, jaundice, protein deficiency or chronic cough.

• *Operative factors*: Poor technique.

• *Postoperative factors*: Cough, abdominal distension, wound infection or wound haematoma.

What is the treatment advised for this condition?

If the patient is troubled by the hernia and his general health is good, surgical repair of the hernia can be offered. If, however, the patient is not really bothered by the hernia, or he is in poor general condition, an abdominal corset can be prescribed.

Case 85 A jaundiced and very ill patient

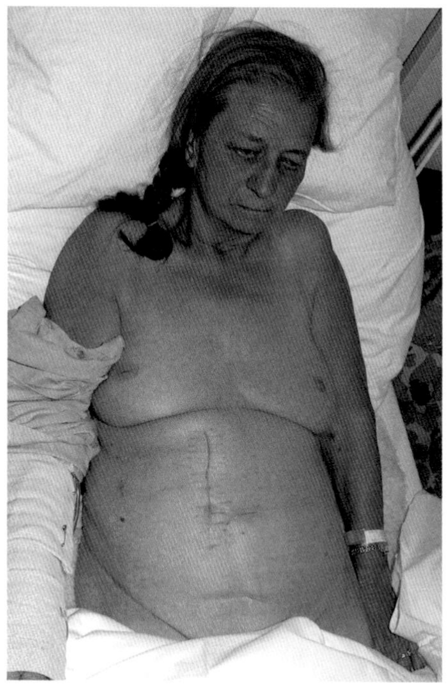

Figure 85.1

A housewife aged 64 years had been admitted to the surgical unit 6 months previously with a few weeks' history of vomiting after meals, anorexia and profound weight loss. The vomit contained pretty well unchanged food that she had just taken. There was almost continuous upper abdominal discomfort, rather than pain, and nothing seemed to relieve this. On her admission at that time, the notes stated that she was pale and looked unwell.

There was a rather ill defined tender mass in the upper abdomen; her haemoglobin was 9 g/dl and liver function tests were normal. An abdominal ultrasound showed several small lesions in the right lobe of the liver. An urgent gastroscopy was performed, which demonstrated an ulcerating tumour at the distal end of the stomach, biopsy of which showed a poorly differentiated adenocarcinoma. After a blood transfusion, she underwent a laparotomy. There was an obstructing mass occupying the antrum and pyloric end of the stomach, which was adherent posteriorly to the pancreas. Large firm lymph nodes could be felt along both curvatures of the stomach. Several hard nodules, up to 2 cm in diameter, could be felt in both the right and left lobes of the liver. Frozen section of one of the nodes and of a biopsy of a liver nodule showed adenocarcinoma. A palliative anterior gastro-jejunostomy was carried out to bypass the obstruction.

She had quite a stormy postoperative recovery – pulmonary collapse, treated with vigorous physiotherapy; bilateral deep vein thrombosis, in spite of prophylactic low molecular weight heparin and thromboembolic deterrent (TED) stockings, which required continuous intravenous heparin; and delayed opening of the gastro-jejunostomy stoma, which necessitated over a week of nasogastric aspiration and intravenous feeding. Eventually, 4 weeks after her admission, she was able to leave hospital and to tolerate a light diet.

She has now been readmitted as an emergency in a very sorry state, as shown in Fig. 85.1. She feels very weak and her husband had noted her colour change a few days before. She has completely lost her appetite and noticed that her stools have gone white and her urine a dark brown colour.

On admission, examination, apart from the obvious jaundice, showed that the surgical scar was well healed but that the abdomen was swollen, there was an obvious hepatomegaly, three to four finger-breadths below the right costal margin, and clinical evidence of marked ascites.

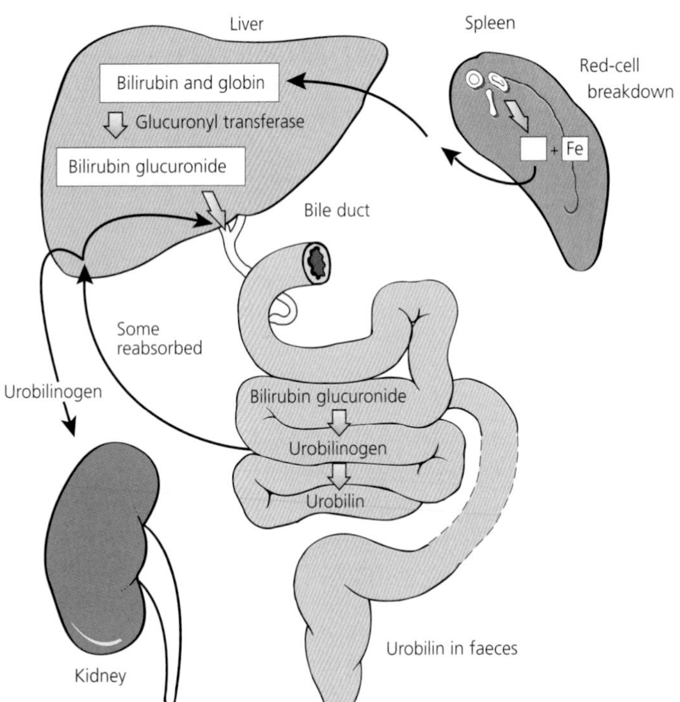

Figure 85.2 The metabolism of bilirubin.

What is the biochemical explanation of this patient's colour change?

Jaundice is due to staining of the tissues of the body with bilirubin (Fig. 85.2). This is detected clinically most easily in the conjunctivae. The normal serum bilirubin is under 17 µmol/L and jaundice becomes clinically detectable when the level rises to over 35 µmol/L.

Can you classify the three large subgroups of the causes of jaundice?

- *Prehepatic*: Due to excessive breakdown of haemoglobin, for example in haemolytic diseases and incompatible blood transfusion.
- *Hepatic*: Due to liver disease, for example hepatitis, cirrhosis or extensive destruction from tumour deposits – as in this case.
- *Posthepatic*: Due to bile duct obstruction. This can be further subdivided into:
  - Obstruction within the lumen of the bile duct, for example from calculi.
- Obstruction in the wall, e.g. congenital atresia, post-traumatic stricture or bile duct tumour.
- External compression of the ducts, e.g. pancreatic tumour or pancreatitis.

How do you make differential diagnoses of the cause of jaundice in a patient?

Of course, as in any diagnosis, this is made from a detailed history, careful clinical examination and then laboratory investigations. Table 85.1 lists the more important of the laboratory findings.

Which of the three aetiological groups usually only produces a tinge of jaundice?

Prehepatic jaundice, where the serum bilirubin is seldom raised above 100 µmol/L, and the colour change may often only be detected by careful inspection of the conjunctivae. An example of this is shown in Fig. 85.3, a woman with haemolytic jaundice. Since the bile ducts are not obstructed, large amounts of excess bilirubin are excreted into the gut.

Table 85.1 Laboratory tests useful in the diagnosis of the cause of jaundice.

Test	Prehepatic	Hepatic	Obstructive
Urine	Urobilinogen	Urobilinogen	No urobilinogen. Bilirubin present
Serum bilirubin	Unconjugated bilirubin	Conjugated and unconjugated	Conjugated bilirubin
ALT (SGPT) and AST (SGOT)	Normal	Raised	Normal or moderately raised
ALP	Normal	Normal or moderately raised	Raised
Blood glucose	Normal	Low if liver failure	Sometimes raised if pancreatic tumour
Reticulocyte count	Raised in haemolysis	Normal	Normal
Haptoglobins	Low due to haemolysis	Normal	Normal
Prothrombin time	Normal	Prolonged due to poor synthetic function	Prolonged due to vitamin K malabsorption; corrects with vitamin K
Ultrasound	Normal	May be abnormal liver texture, e.g. dilated bile ducts, cirrhosis	

ALP, alkaline phosphatase; ALT, alanine aminotransferase; SGOT, serum glutamic oxalo-acetic transaminase; SGPT, serum glutamic pyruvic transaminase.

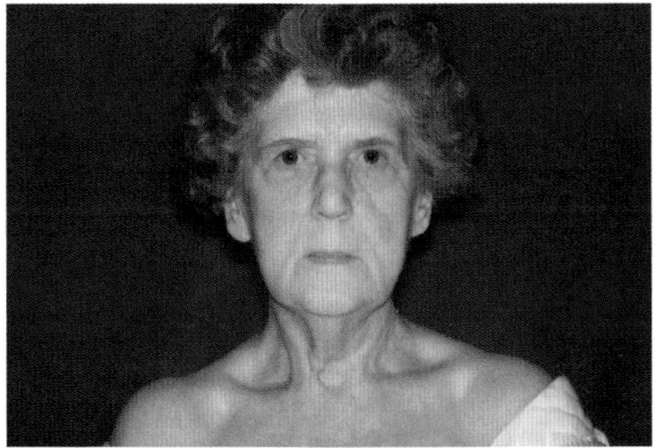

Figure 85.3 Haemolytic jaundice.

When our patient with jaundice and liver secondaries had her blood tests done, she was found to have a prolonged prothrombin time. Why was this?

Vitamin K, necessary for prothrombin synthesis in the liver, is fat-soluble and requires bile salts for its absorption from the gut. In addition, the extensive liver damage from her liver deposits may prevent the hepatic synthesis of prothrombin.

The important message from this is that jaundiced patients who are to undergo surgery require preoperative vitamin K by injection.

> *This poor lady was transferred a week later to the local hospice and died, fortunately peacefully, after 2 weeks. At the request both of the patient and her husband, an autopsy was performed because they both 'wished to help medical science and the doctors'. This forms the subject of Case 86.*

PART 2: CASES

Case 86 A postmortem finding

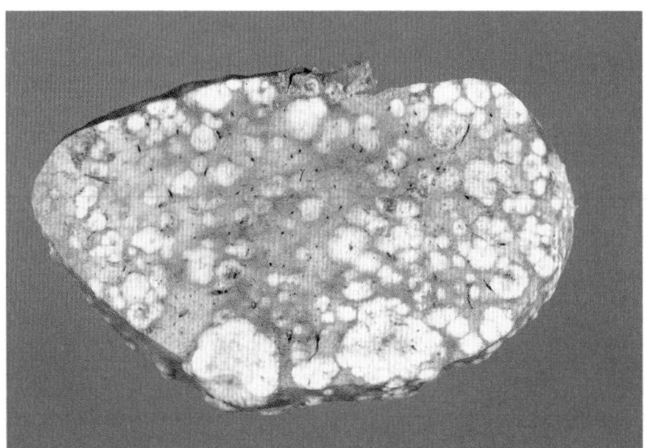

Figure 86.1

The patient described previously in Case 85 was submitted to postmortem examination 2 days after her death. The relevant findings were in the abdominal cavity. The omentum was adherent all along the previous abdominal incision, which was soundly healed. A large amount of ascitic fluid was present and was aspirated away. There was a large, fixed tumour mass that occupied the distal stomach, and was fixed to the posterior abdominal wall along the length of the pancreas. There were numerous enlarged, hard lymph nodes along both the gastric curvatures.

The striking finding was the liver, which was considerably enlarged and nodular. Figure 86.1 shows the appearance of a slice through it.

Describe what you can see in this specimen

The liver is almost replaced by widespread whitish deposits. Together with the clinical story, these are secondaries that have seeded to the liver from the primary gastric tumour via the portal vein.

What is the description of the characteristic cut surface of these lesions and what produces this appearance?

The cut surface has a depressed centre, described as an umbilicated surface. This is due to necrosis of the centre of the tumour, which has outgrown its blood supply from the adjacent blood vessels in the liver.

List the common primary sites for tumours that metastasize to the liver in the UK

Primary carcinomas of the lung, breast, large bowel and stomach account for the great majority of cases, although carcinomas at any site and malignant melanoma may metastasize to the liver. Malignant melanoma of the retina has a sinister reputation for this, hence the old surgical aphorism: 'Beware of the patient with a glass eye and a large liver'.

Approximately what proportion of patients dying of malignant disease will be found to have liver secondaries at autopsy?

About one-third of cases.

Case 87 A man with a grossly swollen abdomen

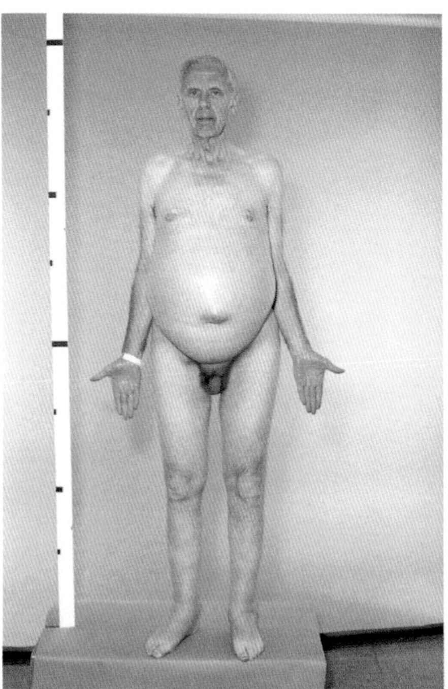

Figure 87.1

Figure 87.1 shows the appearance of a 68-year-old pensioner who used to work in a variety of public houses and bars as a barman. He has abused alcohol – beer and spirits – since his teens. He now presents with slight clinical jaundice – best seen on examining his conjunctivae – gross ascites, as demonstrated by shifting dullness in his flank, and marked pitting oedema of the legs almost to his knees. He has never vomited blood or passed black tarry stools.

What is the likely diagnosis that would fit this clinical picture?

Cirrhosis of the liver due to alcohol.

What are the factors responsible for the ascites in this case?

Transudation of fluid into the peritoneal cavity is here due to a combination of factors:

- Splanchnic vasodilatation secondary to the liver failure results in systemic hypotension, renal hypoperfusion and activation of the renin–angiotensin system, resulting in raised serum aldosterone, thus producing sodium and water retention.
- The portal venous pressure is raised due to compression of the portal venous radicles in the liver by the scarred surrounding hepatic tissue.
- The serum albumin, which is synthesized in the liver, is reduced, resulting in lowering of the serum osmotic pressure.

What do you notice about the patient's umbilicus?

There is a large paraumbilical hernia – a common finding in a grossly distended abdomen from any cause.

What CNS changes would you look for in this patient, and how are they explained?

Mental changes, manifesting as varying degrees of encephalopathy from lethargy and mild confusion to, in severe cases, hepatic coma, are secondary to a combination of factors. Principal among these are the inability of the diseased liver to detoxify various nitrogenous breakdown products of protein metabolism and the portosystemic shunting that diverts these products directly into the systemic circulation.

What treatment modalities can be offered to reduce the ascites in this patient?

- A low sodium diet and diuretics (spironolactone, occasionally combined with a loop diuretic).

- In intractable cases, repeated total volume paracentesis with albumin replacement provides symptomatic improvement.
- The formation of a portosystemic shunt, usually by means of a transjugular intrahepatic portosystemic shunt (TIPS), may be considered.
- Diuretic-resistant ascites is an indication for consideration of liver transplantation if the patient is otherwise suitable.

Case 88 A massive haematemesis

A married woman aged 50 years, who used to be a shop assistant but who is now out of work, was brought by ambulance to the accident and emergency department having vomited several basins full of bright red blood and clots. She complained of feeling very faint and dizzy, but was not in any pain. She had seen bright red blood in her stools several times in the previous couple of months but had done nothing about this.

Her husband explained that his wife had been an alcoholic for the past 10 years, drinking a bottle of gin – or any other spirits she could lay her hands on – each day. Efforts by her family and friends, her family doctor and the local psychiatric unit to control the habit had been completely ineffective. On several occasions she had attended Alcoholics Anonymous, but each time defected after the first session. She had been told by the doctors that 'she was poisoning her liver' and the psychiatrist told her husband that the liver tests they had carried out were 'very bad'. Over the last year she had eaten very little and had lost a great deal of weight.

On examination, the patient was thin, looked 10 years older than her chronological age, was deathly pale, covered in a cold sweat and with a definite icteric tinge to her skin and especially to her conjunctivae. Her pulse was 110/min and blood pressure 94/60 mmHg. The abdomen was distended and there was shifting dullness in the flanks. The spleen was palpable a couple of finger-breadths below the left costal margin but the liver could not be felt. There was pitting oedema of the ankles.

What is your clinical diagnosis in this sad case, and what is the anatomical basis of her massive haematemesis?

The whole clinical picture is that of severe cirrhosis of the liver resulting from her alcohol abuse – the jaundice, ascites and ankle oedema. Portal hypertension due to obstruction of the portal venous channels in her liver has resulted in her splenomegaly and the development of portosystemic anastomoses. The normal portal venous pressure is between 8 and 15 cm of water, this rises to 50 cm or more in portal hypertension.

Why do varices develop at the oesophago-gastric junction?

The lower oesophagus and the cardia of the stomach are the site of the most important of the anastomoses between the portal and systemic venous systems – here between the oesophageal branch of the left gastric vein (which drains into the portal vein) and the oesophageal veins draining into the azygos veins (systemic circulation).

Other anastomoses are between the superior (portal) and inferior (systemic) rectal veins in the anal canal, over the surface of the liver, and at the umbilicus, where the recanalized umbilical vein in the round ligament drains into the epigastric veins to form the caput medusae – dilated varices over the anterior abdominal wall. These anastomoses are shown in Fig. 88.1.

A blood transfusion was commenced in the A&E department, but she had another massive vomit of blood and her blood pressure became unrecordable. What emergency procedures would be used in an to effort to control the bleeding varices?

The patient was resuscitated aggressively with intravenous fluids, including blood to replace that lost, and her coagulation was corrected with fresh frozen plasma and platelets; she proceded to endoscopy once cardiovascularly stable. At fibreoptic endoscopy, bleeding oesophageal varices were identified and controlled by variceal band ligation, where a small elastic band is secured around the base of the varix. Injection of the varices with a sclerosant solution at endoscopy is sometimes required where banding is technically difficult. Intravenous vasopressin analogues, such as terlipressin or glypressin, or somatostatin analogues such as octreotide, are frequently

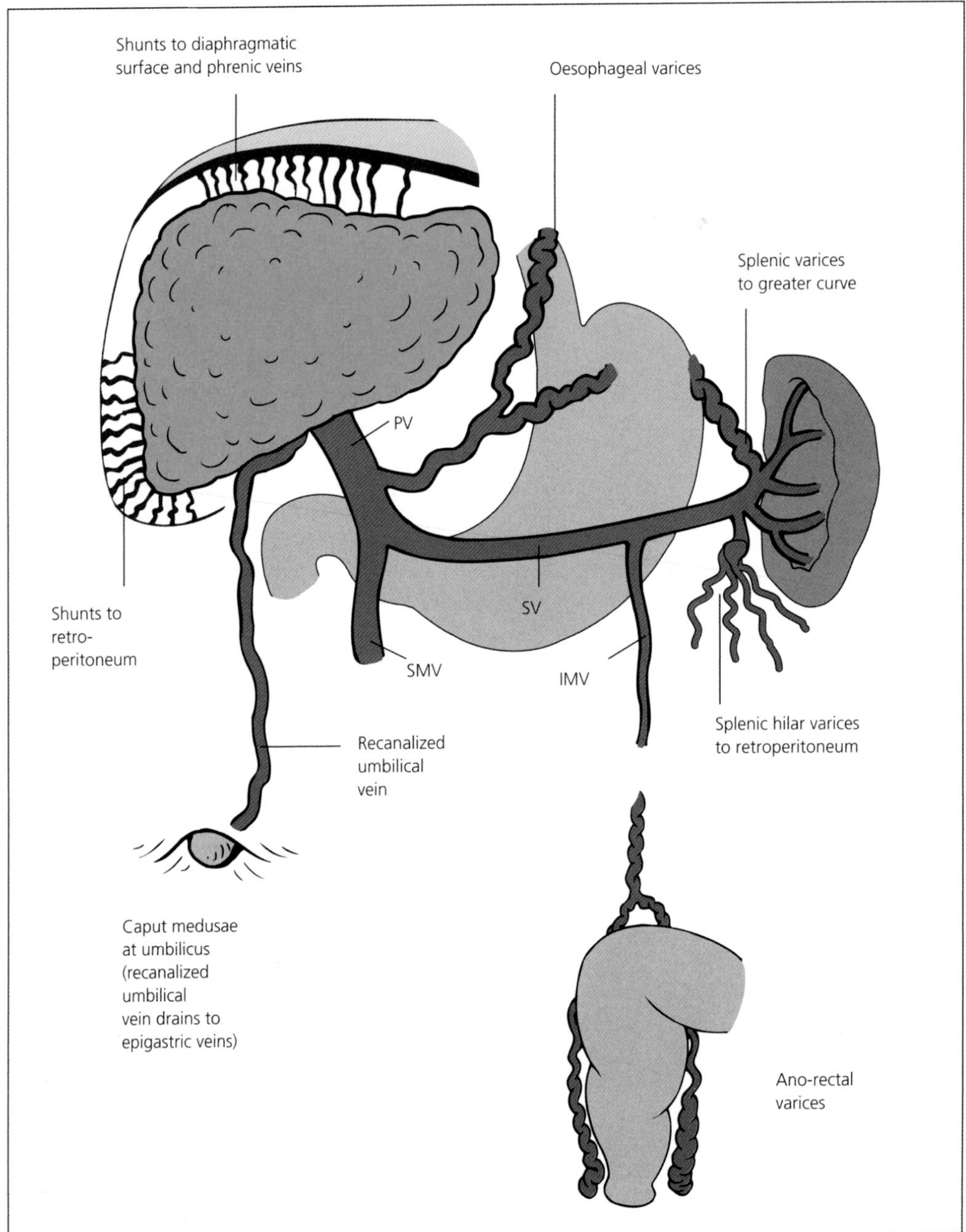

Figure 88.1 The sites of occurrence of portosystemic communications in patients with portal hypertension. IMV, inferior mesenteric vein; PV, portal vein; SMV, superior mesenteric vein; SV, splenic vein.

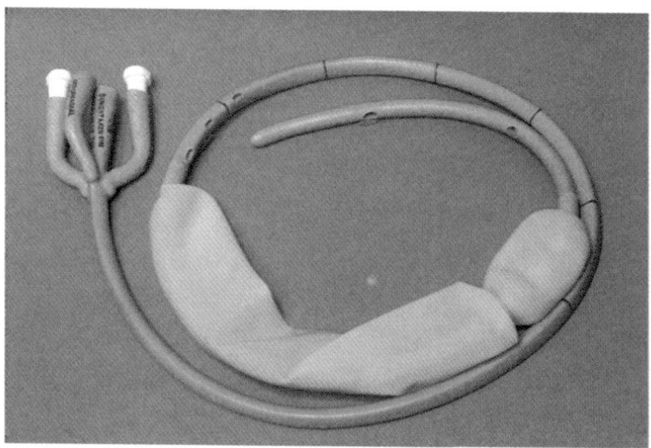

Figure 88.2 A Sengstaken–Blakemore double balloon catheter.

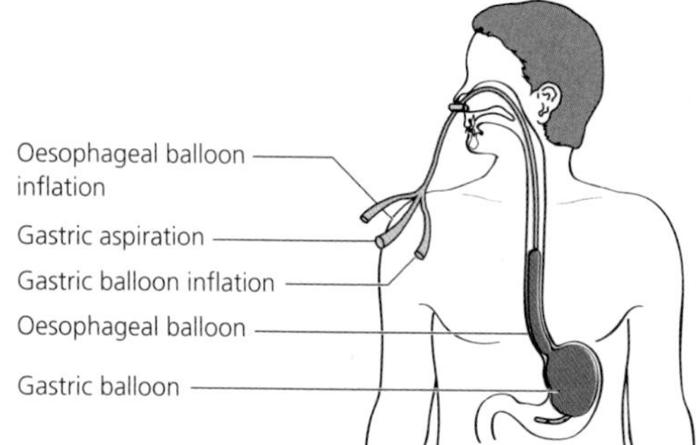

Figure 88.3 The double balloon catheter procedure.

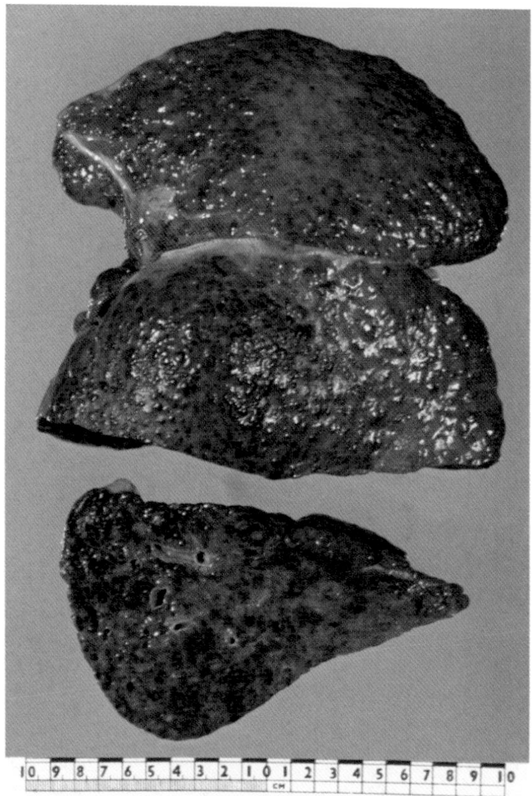

Figure 88.4 Slice of the patient's liver.

given in conjunction to produce a fall in portal venous pressure by mesenteric arteriolar constriction.

What other techniques are available to control the haemorrhage in these often desperate cases?

A Sengstaken–Blakemore* double balloon catheter (Fig. 88.2) was passed into the stomach and inflated. The lower balloon is inflated and the tube pulled back so that this balloon impacts at the oesophago-gastric junction (Fig. 88.3). Compressing the oesophago-gastric junction reduces portal blood flow into the oesophageal varices and in most cases arrests the bleeding. If bleeding continues the upper balloon is inflated to directly tamponade the oesophageal varices. The distal end of the tube is used to aspirate the stomach contents. Transjugular intrahepatic portosystemic shunt (TIPS) formation or surgical portosystemic shunt formation are occasionally required.

*Robert Sengstaken (b. 1923), neurosurgeon, New York; Arthur H. Blakemore (1897–1970), surgeon, Columbia Presbyterian Medical Center, New York.

Sadly, this patient died in spite of the attempts to stop the bleeding and replace her massive blood loss. The coroner was notified and an autopsy performed. Figure 88.4 shows a slice through her liver.

Describe the appearance of the liver in Fig. 88.4 and what would a section of it look like under the microscope?

The liver is coarsely nodular. The nodules are of varying size and comprise rounded areas of regenerating liver cells separated by fibrous septa.

This patient's spleen was palpable on clinical examination and her splenomegaly was confirmed at autopsy. How large must a spleen be before it is likely to be palpable?

The normal spleen 'fits into the palm of the hand'. It is tucked against the left leaf of the diaphragm in front of the 9th to 11th rib. A spleen must be at least three times its normal size before it can be detected clinically, so an easily palpable spleen represents considerable enlargement.

Case 89 A schoolmistress with attacks of abdominal pain

A single woman, an infant schoolteacher aged 45 years, was referred urgently to surgical outpatients by her family doctor. She gave a year's history of attacks of abdominal pain. These were always situated in the right upper abdomen and, on direct questioning, she said these went through to the lower end of her right shoulder blade. She might have two or three attacks of pain one week, then go several weeks in relative comfort. The attacks of pain would last up to several hours, were severe, continuous and made her double up. During these attacks she would be nauseated and would quite often be sick, bringing up recently ingested food. She thought that fatty foods brought on the pain and she was avoiding these. Ordinary painkillers did not help. The last attack, a week ago, was the worst ever, lasted all day and she had a temperature. She called her doctor who gave her an injection of pethidine, with great relief.

She had never noticed going yellow in these attacks, nor any changes in the colour of her urine or stools. Moreover, the doctor's referral letter stated that she was not jaundiced when he visited her in the last attack. She had lost about half a stone in the last year, which she said was due to the fact that she avoided eating large meals. There was nothing of note in her past history; she did not smoke and was a moderate 'social' drinker.

On examination in the clinic she was an intelligent, overweight woman. She was not clinically anaemic or jaundiced. The abdomen was very tender below the right costal margin and it was painful when she took a deep breath with the surgeon's fingers placed there. No masses could be felt and the rest of her examination was essentially normal.

This is a fairly classical story – what is your clinical impression?

The history suggests attacks of biliary colic over the past year, while her last attack suggests an episode of acute cholecystitis, which settled.

What are the typical features of biliary colic?

The pain is severe, often 'worse than having a baby' or 'the worst I have ever experienced'. It is usually situated in the right subcostal region but may be epigastric or spread as a band across the upper abdomen. Radiation to the lower pole of the right scapula (the gallbladder receives its autonomic afferent fibres from the T8 segment) is common, but often needs to be sought from the patient by direct questioning. Characteristically the pain is continuous. The patient is typically restless and rolls about seeking a comfortable position during the attack. There may be associated vomiting and sweating. Jaundice, with dark urine and clay-coloured stools, is suggestive of associated calculi in the biliary duct system, often impacted at the lower end of the common bile duct. This patient's most recent attack suggests an episode of acute cholecystitis.

What is a simple, safe and reliable investigation to confirm or refute the diagnosis of gallstones?

Abdominal ultrasound. Gallstones in the gallbladder show up as intensely echogenic foci, which cast a typical 'acoustic shadow'. It is much less sensitive in the detection of calculi in the biliary ducts. This woman's ultrasound is shown in Fig. 89.1.

The patient was admitted from the urgent waiting list after this. Her full assessment, including chest X-ray, blood count and liver function tests, was otherwise normal. She underwent a laparoscopic cholecystectomy. Figure 89.2 shows the operative specimen, which has been cut open.

What does the specimen in Fig. 89.2 demonstrate?

The gallbladder wall is considerably thickened and reddened – a typical appearance of cholecystitis. It also contains multiple stones (see also Case 90, p. 185).

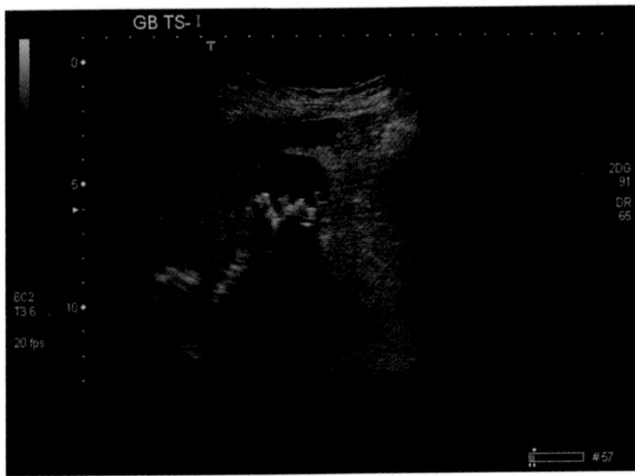

Figure 89.1 Ultrasound a gallbladder.

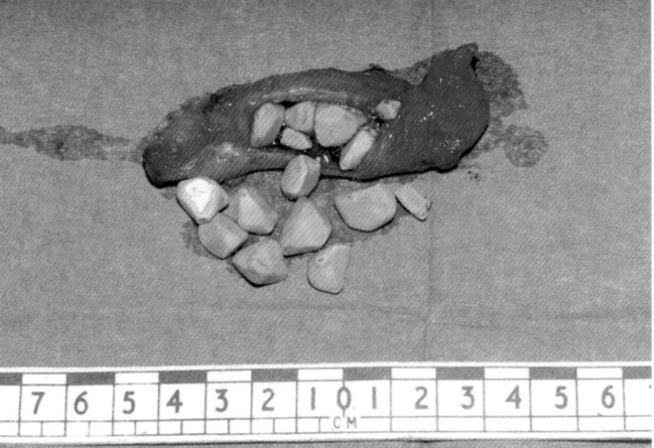

Figure 89.2 A gallbladder removed at cholecystectomy.

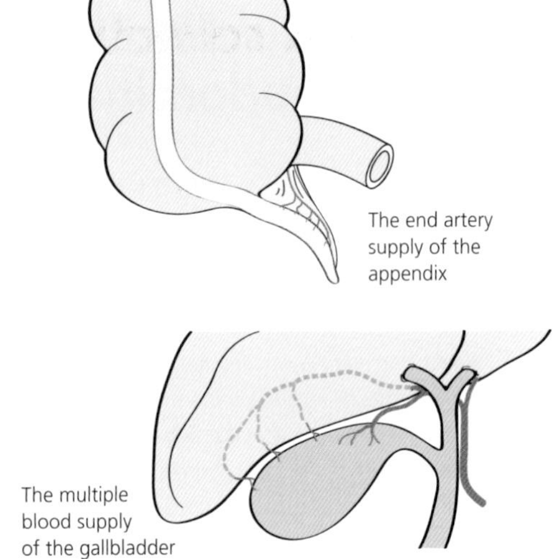

Figure 89.3 Blood supply of (a) the appendix and (b) the gallbladder.

Patients with acute cholecystitis are treated conservatively in the first instance (pethidine, bed rest, intravenous antibiotics and intravenous fluids if necessary), investigated and then have an elective cholecystectomy when things have settled down. In contrast, patients diagnosed with acute appendicitis are taken to theatre for urgent appendicectomy. Can you explain the anatomical reason for this?

The difference in treatment is a result of the difference between the blood supply of the two organs (Fig. 89.3).

The appendicular artery is an end artery – a branch of the ileocolic branch of the superior mesenteric artery, in fact. If this end artery thromboses in the inflammatory process, the entire blood supply to the appendix is lost, the dead tissues are invaded by bacteria within the lumen of the organ and gangrene must result. Untreated, the gangrenous organ will then perforate with either a resulting general peritonitis or with formation of a local appendix abscess.

In contrast, the gallbladder receives not only a blood supply from the cystic artery, derived from the hepatic artery – usually its right hepatic branch – but it also receives numerous small branches from the right hepatic artery that pass to it across its bed in the liver. Gangrene of the inflamed gallbladder is rare and resolution is the usual consequence.

Case 90 A collection of calculi

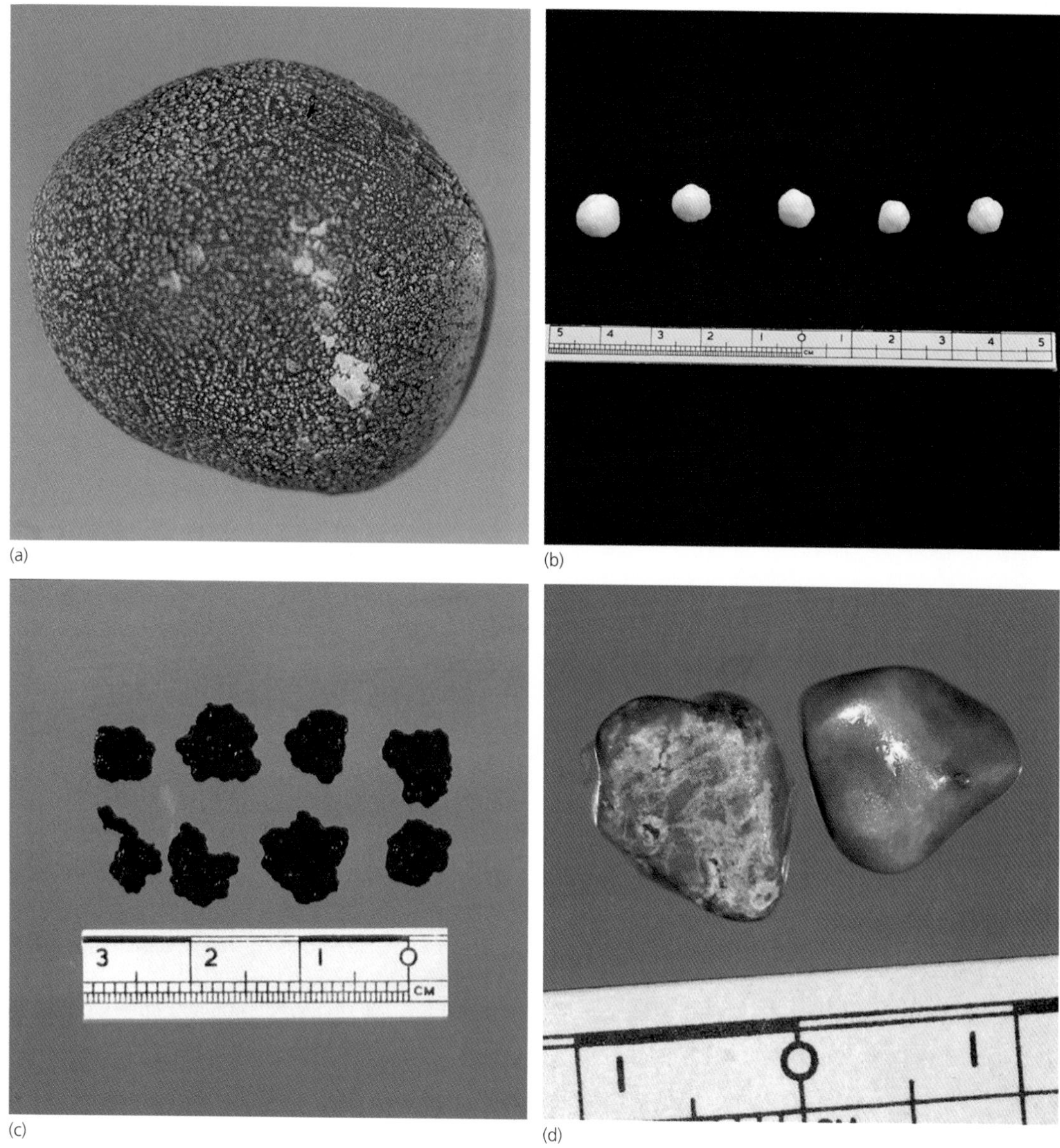

(a) (b) (c) (d)

Figure 90.1

> *Figure 90.1 shows examples of gallstones removed from four different patients at cholecystectomy. Look at them carefully!*

Name the principal constituents of the calculi in each example

- Specimen A – cholesterol.
- Specimen B – cholesterol.
- Specimen C – bile pigment.
- Specimen D – mixture of bile pigment and cholesterol.

What are the other names commonly given to the calculi shown in A, B and D?

- Specimen A – a cholesterol 'solitaire'.
- Specimen B – a collection of 'mulberry stones'.
- Specimen D – mixed faceted stones.

If the stones shown in A and D are cut open, what would be the appearances of their cut surfaces?

The cholesterol stone, A, would show radiating crystals of cholesterol. The mixed stone, D, would show concentric rings of cholesterol and pigment. Diagrams of the various stones are shown in Fig. 90.2.

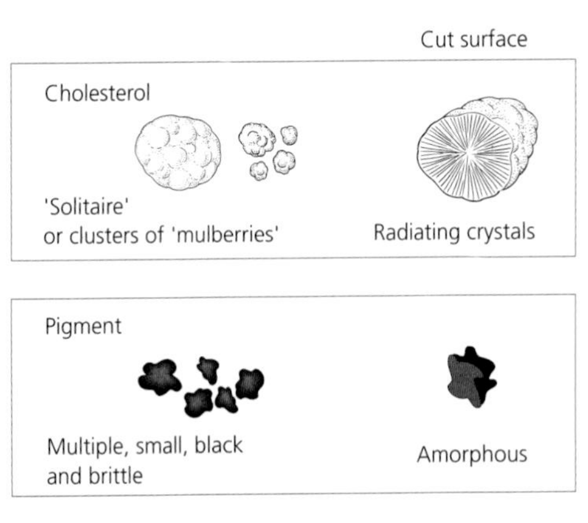

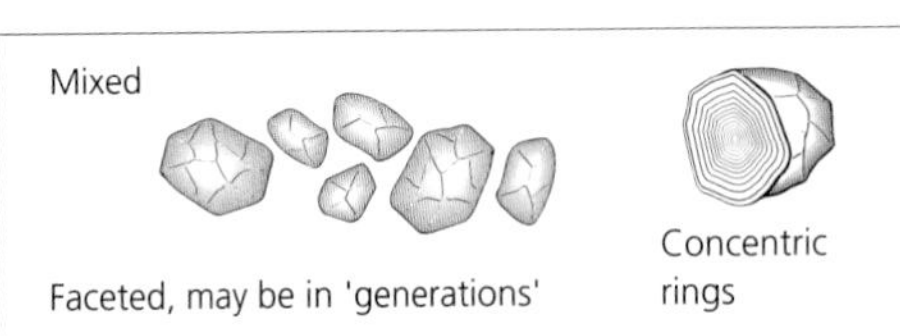

Figure 90.2 Varieties of gallstones.

Cholesterol is insoluble in water. What mechanism keeps it in solution in bile? What relationship has this with the aetiology of cholesterol-containing stones?

Cholesterol is held in solution in bile as a mixed micelle with bile salts and phospholipids. The bile of patients with cholesterol-containing calculi shows a reduction in the concentration of these substances in relation to the cholesterol content, which favours cholesterol deposition ('lithogenic' or stone-forming bile).

What associated diseases may be found in patients who develop pigment stones?

Pigment stones occur particularly in patients with the haemolytic anaemias, for example sickle cell disease, where an excess of bile pigments from extensive red cell breakdown are deposited in the biliary tract.

List the possible consequences of having a stone, or stones, in the gallbladder

These can be classified as follows:

- Gallstone(s) may be entirely symptomless – in fact, about 10% of the adult population of the UK have them, females more than males.
- Biliary colic: Caused by a stone lodging at the neck of the gallbladder or in the duct system.
- Acute cholecystitis: The gallbladder outlet is obstructed, and the contained bile is concentrated and sets up a chemical inflammatory reaction in the gallbladder wall. Secondary bacterial infection may occur. Repeated attacks of inflammation may result in the changes of chronic cholecystitis (see Case 89. p. 183).
- Mucocele of the gallbladder: Occasionally a calculus impacts at the neck of an empty gallbladder. The goblet cells in its wall continue to secrete mucus, which distend it to a considerable size.
- The stone (or stones) may migrate into the bile duct system, with attacks of biliary colic. If impaction occurs at the lower end of the common bile duct, obstructive jaundice results, with pale stools and dark urine. If infection follows, the patient becomes seriously ill with high fever and rigors – acute cholangitis.

• Carcinoma of the gallbladder: This is uncommon. When it does occur, it is nearly always associated with the presence of gallstones.
• Acute or chronic pancreatitis: Both have a strong association with gallstone disease.
• A large stone in the gallbladder may fistulate into the adjacent first part of the duodenum, travel along the intestine and impact at its narrowest part – about 0.6 m from the ileocaecal valve, to produce acute intestinal obstruction (gallstone ileus).

Case 91 A patient with jaundice and interesting physical signs

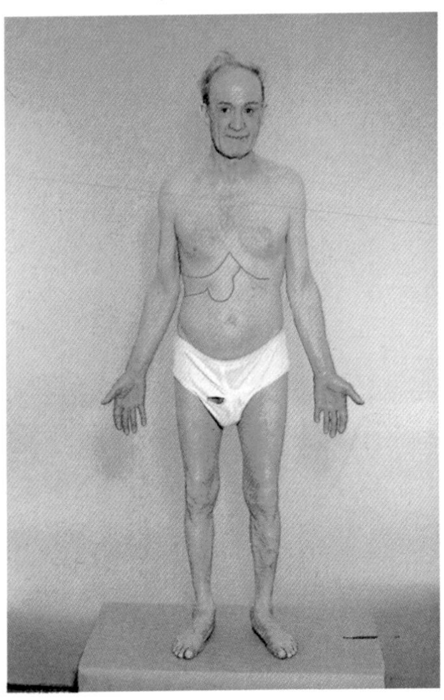

Figure 91.1

Figure 91.1 is a photograph of a lorry driver aged 60 years who was admitted to the surgical unit urgently from the outpatient clinic. About 6 weeks previously, his wife noticed that his eyes had turned yellow. His skin then became obviously discoloured and became itchy, his stools turned greyish white and his urine became dark brown. His appetite, normally excellent, became poor and he thought he had lost a few pounds in weight. However, he had experienced no abdominal pain or discomfort during this time. There was nothing relevant in the rest of his functional enquiry, past or family history. He was a non-smoker and a life-time teetotaller.

On examination he was a cheerful, well built man, but obviously deeply jaundiced. The abdominal signs were striking, and have been outlined with a marker pen. There was a firm, smooth mass extending 5 cm below the right costal margin, which was dull to percussion, and this dull note extended up to the fifth rib in the mid-clavicular line. From its lower border, a globular mass projected towards the umbilicus. There was no clinical evidence of ascites and the supraclavicular nodes were not palpable. Rectal examination revealed a moderate smooth enlargement of the prostate and clay-coloured stool was seen on the examining finger. Apart from a Dupuytren's contracture of his left little finger and varicose veins of both legs, general examination was otherwise normal.

A ward test of his dark brown urine specimen was strongly positive for bile pigment.

What physical signs are demonstrated in this jaundiced patient's abdomen?

The liver is enlarged and the gallbladder is grossly distended.

What is the name of the law based on these signs and what conclusion can you draw from these?

Courvoisier's law,* which states that, in the presence of jaundice, if the gallbladder is palpable, the jaundice is unlikely to be due to a stone, or stones, impacted in the bile duct system and, therefore, is probably due to a tumour at the head of the pancreas which is obstructing the common bile duct.

Can you explain this phenomenon, which, in clinical practice, is found to be pretty reliable?

The law, and its exceptions, are explained in Fig. 91.2. Obstructive jaundice due to stones is usually associated

*Ludwig Courvoisier (1843–1918), Professor of surgery, Basle, Switzerland.

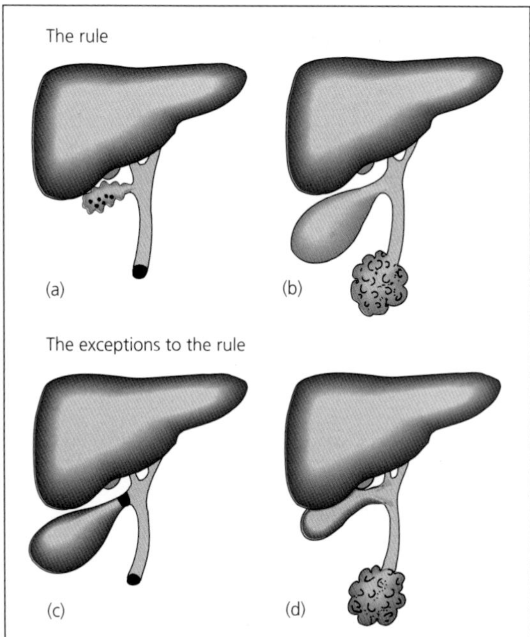

Figure 91.2 Obstructive jaundice due to stone is usually associated with a thickened contracted gallbladder (a). Therefore, in the presence of jaundice, a palpable gallbladder indicates that the obstruction is probably due to some other cause – the commonest being carcinoma of the pancreas (b). Exceptions to the rule are a palpable gallbladder produced by one stone impacted in Hartmann's pouch resulting in a mucocele, another in the common duct causing the obstruction (c), which is a rare occurrence. Much more often, the gallbladder is indeed distended but is clinically impalpable (d).

with a thickened, contracted gallbladder (Fig. 91.2a; see Case 89, p. 183), which is incapable of becoming distended. Therefore, in the presence of jaundice, a palpable gallbladder is probably due to some other cause of the obstruction, the commonest by far being a tumour at the head of the pancreas (Fig. 91.2b).

Exceptions to the rule are a stone impacted at the neck of the gallbladder producing a mucocele and another in the common duct causing obstructive jaundice (Fig. 91.2c), which is a rare occurrence. Much more often, the gallbladder is indeed distended but is clinically impalpable (Fig. 91.2d). This occurs in about half the cases of obstructive jaundice in pancreatic cancer.

In view of this patient's complete absence of pain, what sort of pancreatic tumour may this patient have?

The absence of pain suggests that the patient has a periampullary tumour, arising in pancreatic tissue immediately adjacent to the termination of the common bile duct at the ampulla of Vater,† or in the duct itself, or, rarely, in the second part of the duodenum. This will result in early obstruction of the duct – with all the features of obstructive jaundice – before invasion of adjacent tissues produces pain. The majority of carcinomas of the pancreatic head present with upper lumbar and/or upper abdominal pain before jaundice becomes clinically obvious.

What physical sign, which you probably did not spot before, can you see on this patient's underpants?

He has dribbled some urine onto his pants; this has evaporated, leaving a brown stain. Obviously he has bilirubinuria! It is a common sign to find in the ward on the jaundiced patient's bed sheets, where there has been spillage from the urinal or bed pain. (This patient is further discussed in Case 92, p. 190.)

†Abraham Vater (1684–1751), Professor of anatomy, Wittenberg, Germany.

Case 92 The patient in Case 91 has surgery

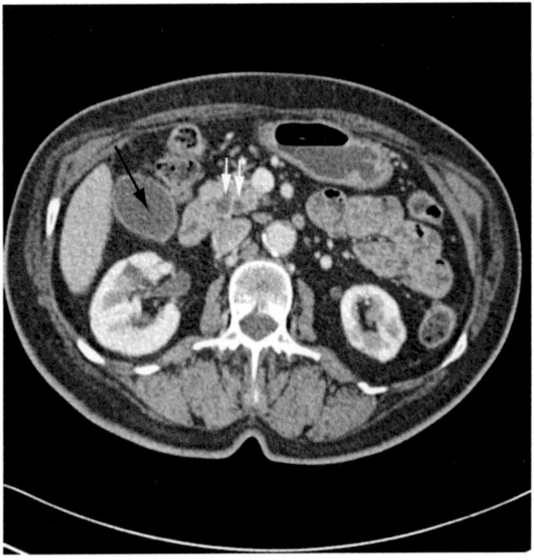

Figure 92.1 CT of the patient described in Case 91. There is a mass involving the second part of the duodenum (two white arrows) and the gall bladder is diotended (black arrow).

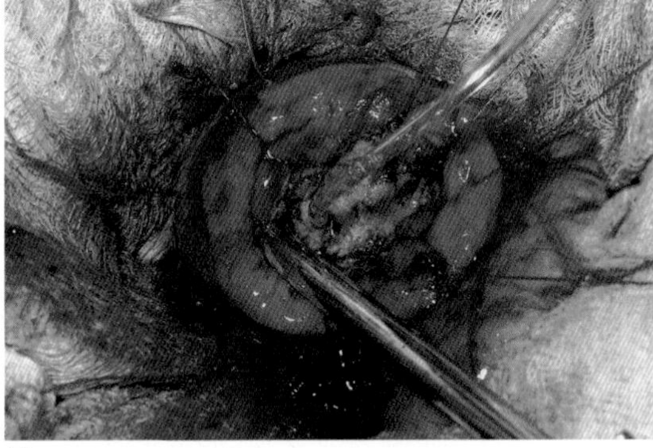

(a)

(b)

Figure 92.2 (a) Operative appearance of the tumour in the duodenum. (b) The resected specimen.

The patient described previously (Case 91) was intensively investigated. The most important finding, which established the diagnosis, was an upper gastroduodenal fibreoptic endoscopy. This revealed an ulcerating tumour in the second part of the duodenum, from which biopsy specimens were taken. A CT scan showed no evidence of metastases, and also revealed a typical 'double duct' sign where both bile and pancreatic ducts are visibly dilated (Fig. 92.1, arrowed).

After being given vitamin K by injection, he was submitted to laparotomy via an upper midline incision. The liver was smoothly enlarged but free from deposits; the gallbladder was tensely distended (also visible on the CT scan). A small mass could be felt within the second part of the duodenum. This was exposed by opening the second part of the duodenum longitudinally and is shown in Fig. 92.2a. The tumour was excised with diathermy and the specimen is shown in Fig. 92.2b. The duodenum was sutured and he made a satisfactory recovery. The jaundice faded completely over the subsequent 3 weeks.

What is this tumour and from which structures may it have originated?

This is a periampullary papiliferous and ulcerating carcinoma. It may have originated in the ampulla of Vater, the lower end of the common bile duct or, rarely, from the duodenal mucosa. The histological report on the specimen stated that it was a well differentiated adenocarcinoma and that excision was complete.

Fine catheters have been passed into two structures through the duodenal papilla. What is the upper one and what is the lower?

The upper catheter is in the orifice of the common bile duct, the lower in the opening of the main pancreatic duct as these come together at the ampulla of Vater (Fig. 92.2a).

What is the distribution of carcinoma of the pancreas through the head, body and tail of the pancreas?

Carcinoma of the pancreas occurs most commonly in the head, then in the body and then, least, in the tail. The proportions are approximately 60%, 25% and 15%, respectively.

What is the age and sex distribution of carcinoma of the pancreas and what is apparently happening to its incidence?

The disease occurs particularly in middle-aged and elderly subjects. Although it used to have a male predominance, it is now equally distributed between the sexes. It is commoner in smokers. The incidence of the tumour is increasing in the Western world. This may be because of the increasing longevity of the population and perhaps also because of more sophisticated techniques of diagnosis.

Why was the patient given vitamin K by intramuscular injection before his operation?

Vitamin K is essential for the hepatic synthesis of prothrombin. Vitamin K is fat-soluble and bile salts are essential for its absorption from the small gut. In obstructive jaundice, bile salts cannot reach the intestine through the blocked common bile duct, the serum prothrombin level falls and any surgery will be complicated by bleeding due to defective blood clotting.

Note that patients with severe hepatic disease – e.g. hepatitis or extensive tumour destruction – are unable to synthesize prothrombin. This accounts for the serious bleeding problems that are associated with operations on these patients, who require replacement by transfusion of essential components of the clotting cascade.

Case 93 A giant abdominal mass

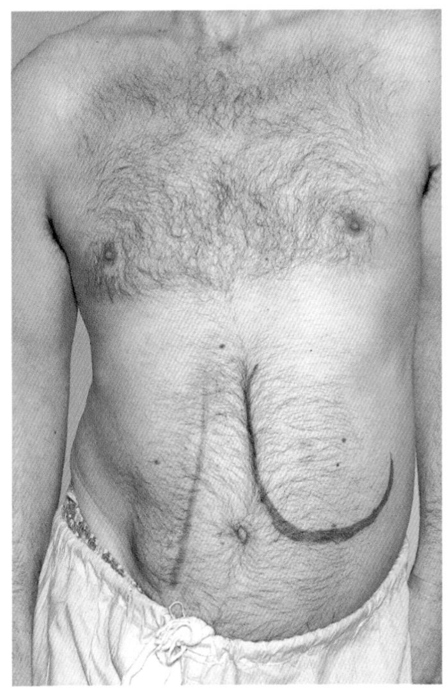

Figure 93.1

A 30-year-old English oil engineer was air evacuated to hospital in London from the Middle East, where he had been working. His accompanying medical notes (supplemented by his own history) stated that he had been admitted to a private clinic as an emergency 10 months previously with a 2-day history of acute abdominal pain. He admitted that this seemed to have followed an alcoholic 'binge' at a party, where he drank a large amount of home-brewed spirit. The pain was extremely severe, generalized and radiated to his dorsolumbar spine. Shortly after arriving at the clinic he was explored through a long right paramedian incision. This revealed copious amounts of turbid, slightly blood-stained free fluid. There were large numbers of white spots scattered over the exposed peritoneal surfaces, especially the greater omentum. There was a mass to be felt through the wall of the stomach, presumably the swollen pancreas, although this was not further explored. The peritoneal cavity was lavaged with warm saline and the abdomen closed.

Next day a blood specimen was sent to the government laboratory and his serum amylase was reported to be grossly elevated to 1000 Somogyi units. From the notes it was obvious that he had a stormy postoperative recovery, complicated by pulmonary collapse (he was a heavy smoker) and a prolonged paralytic ileus, which required nasogastric aspiration and parenteral nutrition for over a week. However, he slowly recovered and, following 6 weeks of sick leave in England, he returned to office work.

He remained well until about a month ago, when he noticed his belly was getting swollen. This was painless and he felt quite well. However, when the swelling became much greater and when he could now feel a large lump there, he reported back to his local surgeon, who arranged for him to be sent home.

On examination, he was a muscular, somewhat overweight young man, who looked very well. General examination was normal apart from the striking physical signs demonstrated in Fig. 93.1. There was a well healed, fairly recent (i.e. still red), long right paramedian scar. The abdomen looked distended, but palpation showed that this was due to a large mass, outlined with a marker pen, which descended from below the left costal margin to the level of the umbilicus. It was smooth, not tender, did not move with respiration and was distinctly dull to percussion. There was no clinical evidence of free fluid.

What is your clinical diagnosis and what has produced this large mass?

A pancreatic pseudocyst. Following the attack of acute pancreatitis, fluid accumulated in the lesser peritoneal sac. Presumably the foramen of Winslow* (the epiploic foramen), which is the orifice of the lesser sac into the general peritoneal cavity, became sealed off with inflammatory adhesions so that the lesser sac distended to its present size.

The pancreas is a retroperitoneal organ with the gas-filled stomach lying in front of it. Why, then, was this pancreatic pseudocyst dull to percussion?

When small, the cyst is indeed retroperitoneal and is apparently resonant to percussion because of the gas-filled stomach and loops of intestine that lie anterior to it. As it increases in size, the intestine is pushed away and the stomach is tautly stretched over the front of the cyst so that it becomes dull to percussion, as in this instance (Fig. 93.2).

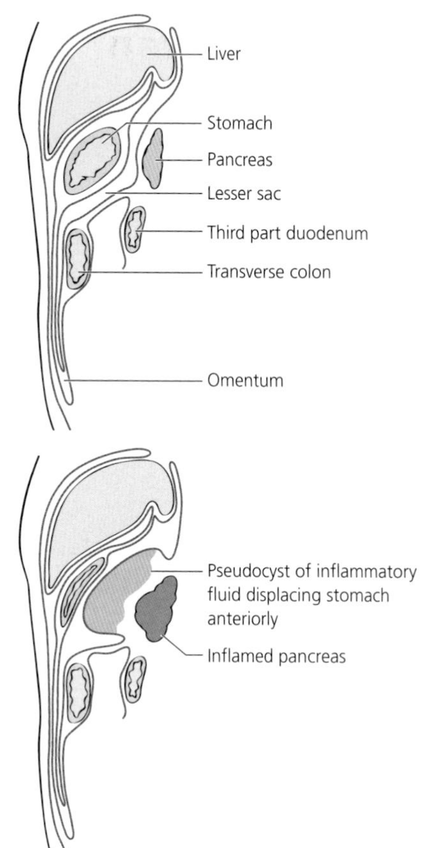

Figure 93.2 (a) A small cyst in the lesser sac does not disturb the other organs around it. (b) As it enlarges it, it displaces the stomach.

What special investigations are useful in delineating this mass?

It may be demonstrated by abdominal ultrasonography, but the cyst may be obscured by gas within the upper gastrointestinal tract – air is the great bugbear in ultrasonographic examinations. Computerized tomography is the investigation of choice and may be enhanced by giving oral contrast so that the stomach outline is clearly delineated. Figure 93.3 is a CT scan showing a transverse section through the abdomen illustrating a large pancreatic pseudocyst (single large arrow) filling the lesser sac and displacing the stomach anteriorly (double arrow).

What is the treatment of this condition?

Follow-up CT scans on patients with acute pancreatitis have shown that small fluid collections in the lesser sac – clinically undetectable – are quite common and absorb spontaneously. It is often possible to drain an obvious pseudocyst percutaneously under ultrasound or CT control. This was carried out in this patient but the cyst filled up again to the same size within a couple of days.

He was therefore submitted to laparotomy. The stomach was found to be tensely stretched over a massive cyst and cystgastrostomy was performed (Fig. 93.4). In this, the anterior wall of the stomach was incised, a trocar passed through the posterior wall of the stomach into the cyst mass, several litres of turbid, whitish fluid aspirated and an anastomosis made between a 5 cm incision through the posterior wall of the stomach and the underlying cyst wall. The incision in the anterior wall of the stomach was then closed.

In the original operation notes mention was made of white spots scattered over the peritoneal cavity. What were these? How are the three digestive enzymes produced by the exogenous secretion of the pancreas correlated with three features of acute pancreatitis?

• The spots are areas of fat necrosis.

*Jacob Winsløw (1669–1760), Danish, Professor of surgery and anatomy, Jardin du Roi, Paris.

PART 2: CASES

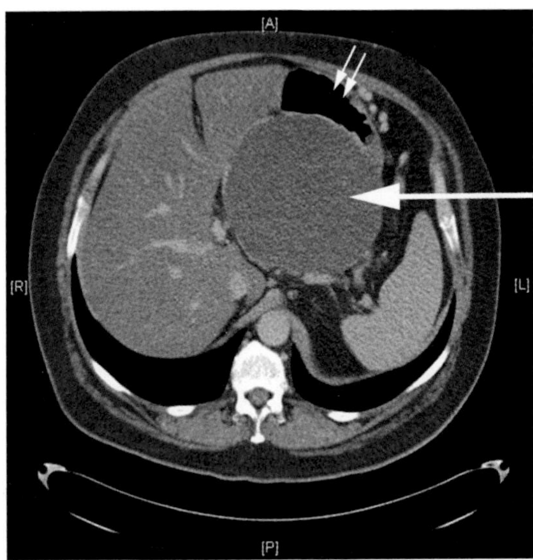

Figure 93.3 CT scan of a transverse section through the abdomen showing a large pancreatic pseudocyst (single large arrow) displacing the stomach (double arrow).

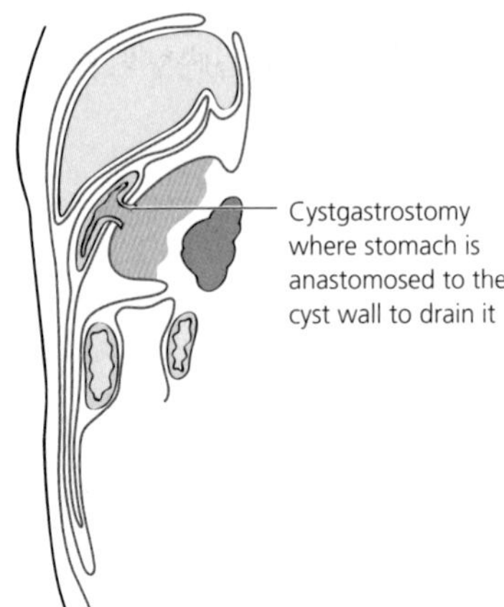

Figure 93.4 Cystgastrostomy.

• Liberated lipase breaks down intra-abdominal fat into fatty acids. These react with serum calcium to produce these little spots, which represent deposits of calcium soaps.

• The liberated pancreatic amylase in the peritoneal cavity is absorbed and accounts for the very considerable rise in the serum amylase – a useful aid to diagnosis of this condition. This patient had a massive increase in his serum amylase level, even though the test was carried out after the event.

• The liberated and activated pancreatic trypsin accounts for the autodigestion of the pancreas, which is the basic pathology of acute pancreatitis.

Case 94 A severe abdominal injury

A 28-year-old builder's labourer was brought by ambulance to the A&E department within 30 min of his injury. He was driving his motor cycle, coming home from work, along a wet and slippery road at some speed, when he skidded and crashed head on into a lorry on the other side of the road. He was aware of going head over heels over the handle bars of his bike, striking his upper belly against them, then landing on the road. He was wearing his crash helmet and, although he hit his forehead on the road, he did not lose consciousness. He now had a great deal of abdominal pain and felt faint and dizzy.

Examination after his motor cycling gear had been removed completely revealed a muscular, thin young man – pale, sweating and in obvious great pain. His blood pressure was 100/60 and pulse 110. He was fully conscious, had no neck pain or tenderness. His chest was clear. There was no bruising to see over the abdominal wall, but there was marked generalized guarding of the abdomen and generalized tenderness, especially marked over the left upper abdomen. A striking finding was that, on pressing the left upper abdomen, he complained that this produced severe pain in his left shoulder tip. On percussion, there was dullness in the left flank and the abdomen was silent on auscultation. Full examination was otherwise negative, apart from some superficial abrasions to the face and hands.

Intravenous morphine was given, and an i.v. line set up with Hartmann's solution. Blood sent for urgent grouping and cross-match of 4 units of blood. The bladder was catheterized and clear urine obtained; it tested negative for blood. A portable anteroposterior chest X-ray was clear.

What would be your working diagnosis at this stage if you were managing this patient?

He is obviously bleeding – and seriously – into the abdominal cavity, hence the classical features of shock associated with his obvious abdominal trauma. Clinical assessment and the simple investigations that have been carried out exclude other injuries to the CNS, spine, chest and urinary tract.

A splenic tear or rupture is the commonest cause of a haemoperitoneum after closed abdominal injury. Other viscera that may be injured and cause intraperitoneal bleeding are the liver, small bowel mesentery and diaphragm. Indeed, more than one organ may be involved.

The left upper quadrant pain and tenderness, the dullness to percussion in the left flank and the shoulder tip pain all strongly suggest splenic injury.

What is the explanation of the left shoulder tip pain?

The diaphragm is supplied with sensory as well as motor innervation by the phrenic nerve, which derives from cervical nerve roots 3, 4 and 5. Irritation of the diaphragm, in this instance by blood from the spleen under its left dome, produces referred pain to the cutaneous distribution of these nerves – the shoulder tip. Occasionally, remarkably, the patient's only complaint of pain is to the shoulder. Often it is necessary to enquire specifically for this symptom – the patient knows that he has been injured in the abdomen and disregards the fact that the left shoulder is also hurting unless directly questioned about this.

Over the next 30 min, the patient's condition deteriorated. His blood pressure fell to 90, his pulse rose to 120 and he was cold and clammy. He was taken directly to theatre, with a second intravenous line running and cross-matched blood, now available, was given in the transfusion. Laparotomy was carried on under general anaesthesia via an upper midline incision, which allowed access to the peritoneal cavity in under a minute. Blood and clots poured out. The spleen was palpated and felt to be severely damaged, and was rapidly mobilized and removed. No other abdominal injury was found. He received all 4 units of blood and his condition was stable by the end of the operation.

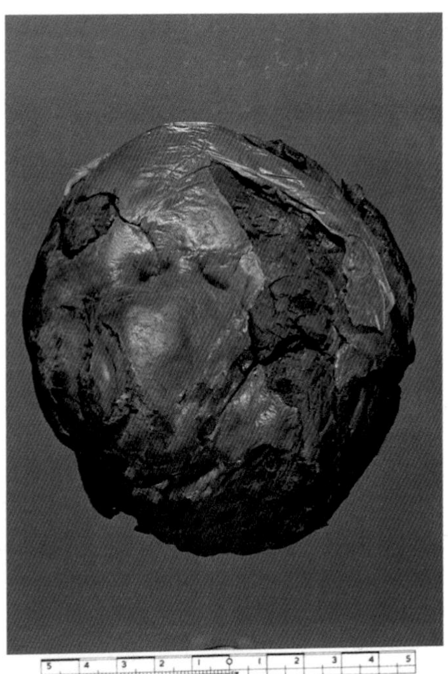

Figure 94.1 Shattered spleen.

Figure 94.1 shows the specimen of shattered spleen that was removed.

This is an example of massive immediate bleeding from a shattered spleen, which calls for immediate splenectomy. What other clinical types of splenic rupture may occur?

• There may be progressive blood loss over several hours from a relatively small tear in the splenic capsule.
• Delayed rupture of the spleen may occur many hours, or even days, after the abdominal injury. There is an initial history of an abdominal injury, with pain resulting from the local blow. This may partly or entirely settle down, but then symptoms and signs of splenic rupture, as described above, become manifest. This is explained by the fact that the initial trauma has produced a subcapsular haematoma. As oozing of blood continues, the thin splenic capsule ruptures, with resultant brisk bleeding into the peritoneal cavity.
• Spontaneous rupture may occur in a diseased and enlarged spleen, for example in malaria, glandular fever or leukaemia, after quite trivial injury.

Are there any special investigations that may help confirm the diagnosis of splenic rupture in a less acute situation than with this patient?

In a relatively stable patient, the investigation of choice is a CT scan of the abdomen. This will usually demonstrate the splenic tear, the presence of fluid in the peritoneal cavity and possible injury to other viscera.

Are there any late dangers to the patient following splenectomy?

Splenectomy predisposes the patient, especially if a child, to infection, particularly from pneumococci, with shock and collapse – a condition termed 'overwhelming post-splenectomy sepsis.' For this reason, if a minor laceration of the spleen is found at laparotomy, attempts are made to preserve it by using fine sutures to repair the tear or by wrapping the organ in haemostatic absorbable gauze.

Following splenectomy, immunization with pneumococcal, meningococcal and *Haemophilus influenzae* vaccines should be administered. In addition, children should receive prophylactic low dose penicillin daily until adulthood. Adults should receive daily penicillin for a year – for longer if they are immunosuppressed.

Case 95 A painless lump in the neck

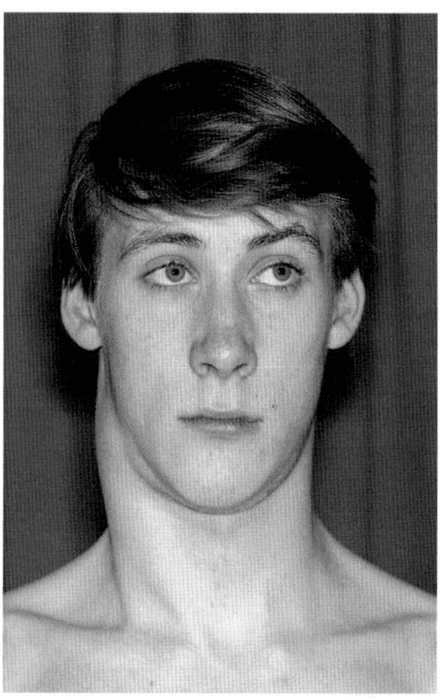

Figure 95.1

This 18-year-old student noticed a small, painless lump in the right side of his neck 3 months previously. He thought nothing about it at first, but it then enlarged quite rapidly to its present size. This brought him to the students' medical officer and then to the surgical outpatient clinic.

On examination, he was a very fit, thin, muscular young man. There was a non-tender mass of discrete rubbery lymph nodes to feel in the right anterior triangle of the neck (Fig. 95.1).

What steps would you now take in your clinical examination of this young man to try to establish the cause of his lymphadenopathy?

• Search the area drained by the involved lymph nodes for a possible primary source of infection or malignant disease. In this instance, this requires a careful examination of the head, neck and throat.

• Examine the other lymph node areas – the opposite side of the neck, both axillae and both groins – to determine if this is part of a generalized lymphadenopathy.

• Examine the abdomen for splenomegaly and/or hepatomegaly. Their enlargement would suggest lymphoma, lymphatic leukaemia, sarcoid or glandular fever as possible clinical diagnoses.

You have done all this with great care; everything apart from these enlarged, non-tender, rubbery, discrete nodes is entirely negative. Are you in the position to make a provisional clinical diagnosis?

These findings are suspicious of Hodgkin's disease or non-Hodgkin's lymphoma.*

The time has now come to order laboratory and imaging special investigations. What should these be, and how will they assist in establishing the cause of this patient's lymphadenopathy?

• Order a blood film examination and a full blood count. This may show a leucocytosis in the region of 11.0×10^9/L with a predominance of atypical monocytes, strongly suggesting glandular fever (infectious mononucleosis), which can be confirmed by the 'monospot' test. A leucocytosis of 100×10^9/L, with atypical lymphocytes, indicates lymphatic leukaemia.

• Arrange a chest X-ray, which may reveal unsuspected enlarged mediastinal nodes or an unsuspected primary lung tumour. This will require further investigation – a CT scan and biopsy.

---

*Thomas Hodgkin (1798–1866), curator of pathology, Guy's Hospital, London.

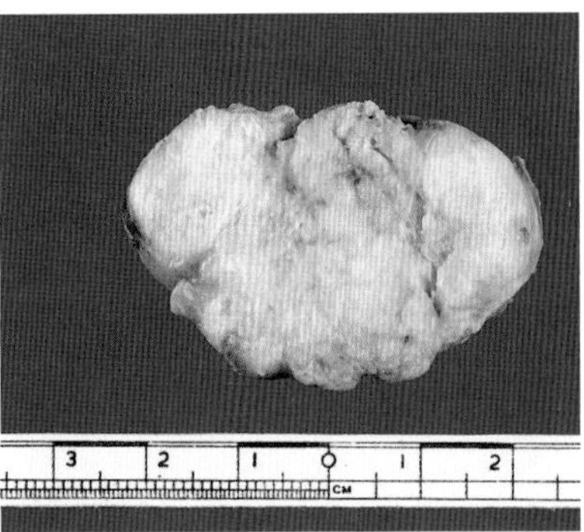

Figure 95.2 Excised lymph node.

• The diagnosis will be established beyond doubt by removing one of the nodes for histological examination.

A lymph node was excised under local anaesthetic. It shelled out easily and its cut surface is shown in Fig. 95.2. Describe its macroscopic appearance

The lymph node appears discrete and enclosed in its own capsule. Its cut surface is lobulated and has a diffuse appearance.

Histological examination showed this to be Hodgkin's disease. What are the characteristic cells seen under the microscope in this condition?

Dorothy Reed giant cells,† also known as Reed–Sternberg cells (Fig. 95.3).‡

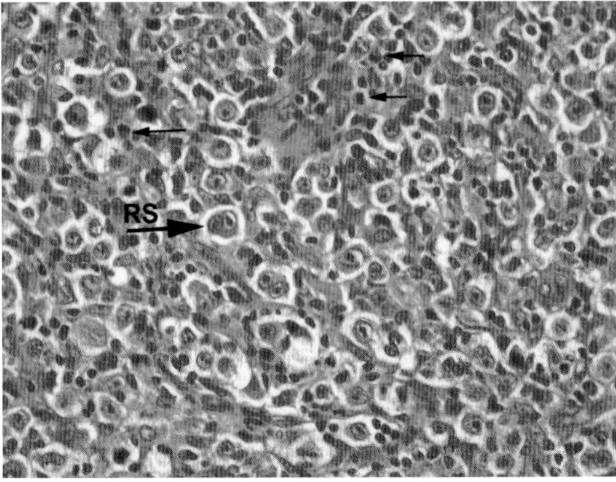

(a)

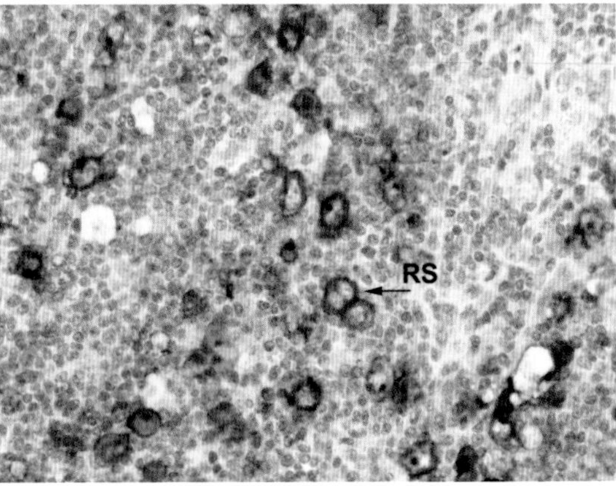

(b)

Figure 95.3 Photomicrographs of Hodgkin's disease: (a) stained with haematoxylin and eosin and (b) an immunohistochemistry slide stained with a CD30 antibody. CD30 is expressed on Reed giant cells (RS) and the stain is used as a confirmatory test of Hodgkin's disease. Numerous eosinophils are also shown on (a), some of which are arrowed.

†Dorothy Reed (1874–1964), paediatrician, Foundling Hospital, New York. She described the giant cells of Hodgkin's disease in 1902 when assistant to William Welch, pathologist at Johns Hopkins Hospital, Baltimore, and clearly distinguished Hodgkin's disease from tuberculosis, both diseases being present in some patients.

‡Carl Sternberg (1872–1935), pathologist, Vienna. He described the cells in 1898, but failed to distinguish Hodgkin's disease from tuberculosis. The cells were actually first described by William Greenfield (1846–1915), an English pathologist, in 1878.

Case 96 Swollen legs in a young woman

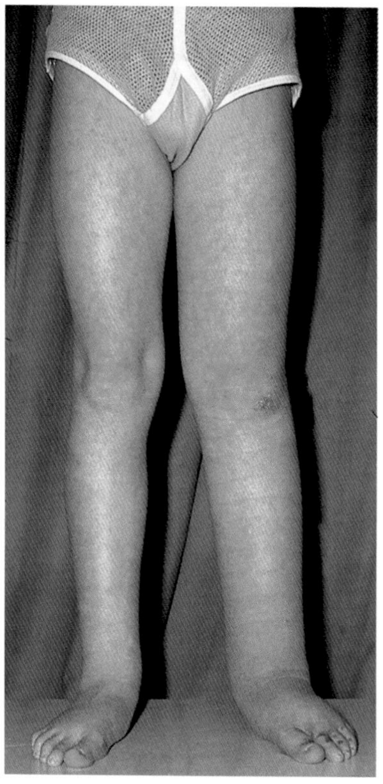

Figure 96.1

Figure 96.1 shows the legs of a 21-year-old shop assistant. Her legs have been swollen since she was 14 years old and have slowly become slightly worse, although entirely painless, until they have reached their present size. She is otherwise very fit, but is now very bothered by the appearance of her legs, especially the more swollen left one. She usually wears trousers or jeans and feels too embarrassed to wear a bathing costume on holiday. Her periods are normal and regular; they commenced just about the time that her leg swelling first appeared.

She has never been ill. Her parents and her two sisters are well and have no problems with their legs – nor, as far as her mother knows, have any of her other relations.

What is this condition called, and how is it classified?

She has lymphoedema of the legs. Lymphoedema can be classified into:

• *Primary lymphoedema*: There is some congenital defect of the lymphatic drainage of the limb.

• *Secondary lymphoedema*: There is some extrinsic cause producing lymphatic obstruction.

Secondary lymphoedema is not uncommonly seen, affecting the upper or lower limb(s); can you list the causes of this?

A wide range of conditions may result in this phenomenon. They include:

• Blockage of the lymphatics and lymph nodes by metastatic tumour deposits, or following radiotherapy to, or block dissection of, involved nodes. This is not uncommonly seen in the arm of patients with advanced breast cancer, for example.

• Secondary to severe bacterial or parasitic infection. Filariasis, caused by *Wuchereria bancrofti** infestation of the lymphatics, is the cause of gross lymphoedema of the legs, and often the scrotum, in the tropics.

How is primary lymphoedema further subdivided?

• *Lymphoedema congenital*: As the name suggests, the congenital form. The child presents with swollen legs at about the first year of life. The leg, or legs, may be affected right up to the groin. It is rather more common in males

---

*Joseph Bancroft (1836–1894), physician and public health officer, Brisbane, Australia.

and in about 10% there is a family history. This familial form is known as Milroy's disease.†

• *Lymphoedema praecox*: This first appears in children or in adults up to the early thirties, with a 3 : 1 predominance in females. The onset peaks at about the menarche, as in our present case, and usually only affects the leg up to the knee, again as occurs here. When a family history is positive, the condition is termed Meig's disease.‡

• *Lymphoedema tarda*: This commences after the age of 35. It is important to exclude the secondary causes of lymphoedema, listed above, in these cases, and also to consider whether the cause may be a previous deep vein thrombosis leading to chronic venous oedema.

Methylene blue was injected subcutaneously into the dorsum of the patient's left foot 24 h previously. What do you notice now on Fig. 96.1?

The dye has persisted. This confirms the virtual absence of lymphatic drainage from the foot. In the normal subject the dye would rapidly disappear over a few hours.

What is the aetiology of primary lymphoedema?

Lymphangiographic studies – performed in the 1950s by placing a very fine cannula into a foot lymphatic and visualized by methylene blue injection – defined the congenital anomalies that might affect the lymphatics of the lower limb. These might show aplasia (almost total absence), hypoplasia or varicose dilatation of the lymphatic channels (megalymphatics).

How can this condition be treated?

• The great majority of patients are treated conservatively. This includes elevation of the legs when the subject is sitting down or in bed (heels higher than the knees, knees higher than the hips) and graduated compression stockings. Many respond to this, which may be supplemented with ingenious intermittent pneumatic compression machines in the physiotherapy department.

• The patient is warned to be careful about scratches and abrasions to the legs. The absence of lymphatic drainage renders the limb susceptible to cellulitis, which may damage residual lymphatics. This might well be the aetiology of cases of lymphoedema tarda. Cellulitis of the limb therefore calls for urgent antibiotic treatment.

• Radical surgical excision of the lymphoedematous subcutaneous tissue, down to the deep fascia, is a major procedure and is only indicated in very advanced and disabling cases.

†Wiliam Forsyth Milroy (1855–1942), Professor of medicine, Omaha, Nebraska.

‡Henri Meig (1866–1940), Professor of medicine, Hôpital Salpêtrière, Paris.

Case 97 A frightened girl with a breast lump

A 17-year-old schoolgirl, about to take her 'A' level examinations, was seen in the breast clinic. She was crying and very upset. Her mother explained that the girl had found a lump in her left breast while showering a week ago and was convinced that she had cancer. This girl's grandmother, on her mother's side, had had a mastectomy 10 years ago. She remains very well and the girl is much attached to her. The patient was otherwise very well, an athlete and school prefect. Her periods had commenced when she was 13 and were regular. There was no other family history of breast cancer apart from her grandmother.

On examination, she was a healthy, but very upset, nervous and crying young woman. There was a highly mobile, rubbery, well defined 2 cm lump in the upper outer quadrant of her left breast. The right breast and the axillae were clear and no abnormalities were found elsewhere.

What would be your clinical diagnosis at this stage?

The age of the patient and the physical signs make the diagnosis of a fibroadenoma of the breast a very near certainty. The nickname of 'breast mouse' fits well with this mobile little firm lump.

What are the pathological features of this condition, and what is its age distribution and natural history?

The fibroadenoma arises from a breast lobule. It is encapsulated and is made up of fibrous tissue surrounding epithelial duct proliferation (Fig. 97.1). It was formerly classified as a benign neoplasm, but it is now regarded as an aberration of normal development. Quite often bilateral or multiple fibroadenomas may occur. There is no increased risk of malignant change and the majority will disappear over a number of years. It is commonly found in teenagers, but it is seen rarely in middle-aged or even elderly women.

What would be your management of this very frightened girl?

She requires reassurance, but, as with every breast lump, the diagnosis must first be established without doubt. Although mammography is a standard investigation in older women (35 years plus), it is less valuable in young people, where the breast stroma is dense, and was therefore not ordered in this case. Instead she underwent an ultrasound and core biopsy.

The diagnosis confirmed – what now?

The patient was told that she had an entirely benign lump that would not be of any danger to her and which would probably disappear if left alone. However, the girl was terrified by her lump and wanted to get rid of it. She was therefore admitted shortly afterwards to the day surgery unit and the lump removed under a general anaesthetic. It shelled out easily through a small circumareolar incision, which leaves a near invisible scar. Figure 97.2 shows the exercised specimen.

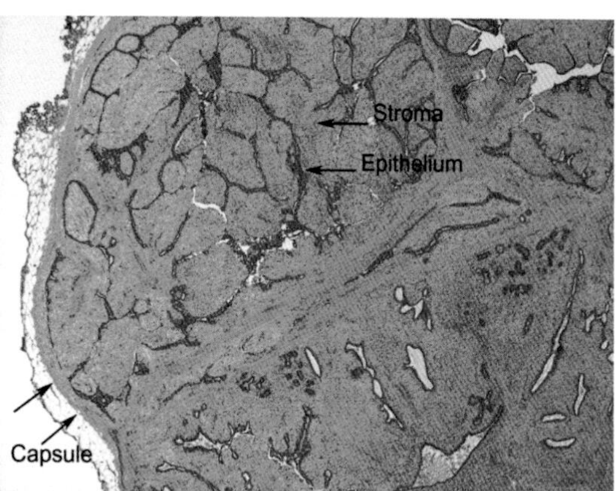

Figure 97.1 A well demarcated lesion with proliferating interlobular stroma surrounding and distorting the epithelium.

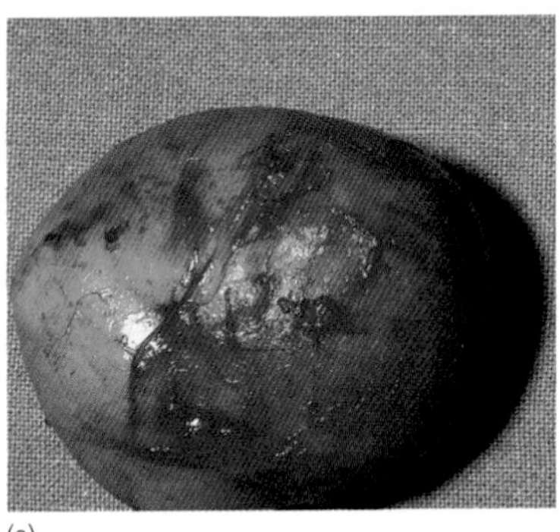
(a)

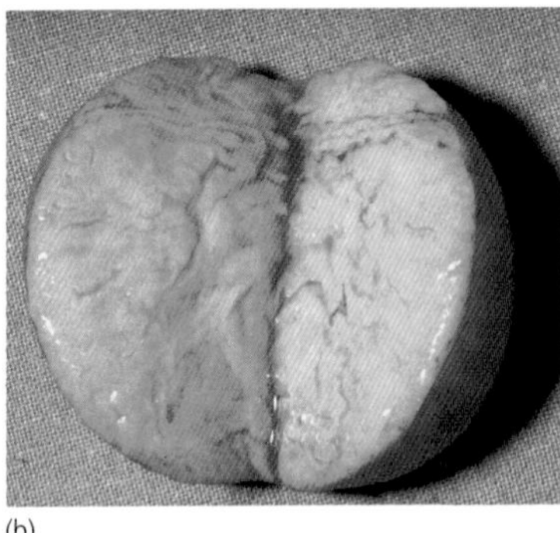
(b)

Figure 97.2 (a) The intact appearance and (b) the cut surface of the excised specimen.

Describe the naked eye appearance of the specimen

An encapsulated tumour with a characteristic whorled appearance of its cut surface.

Case 98 Breast screening

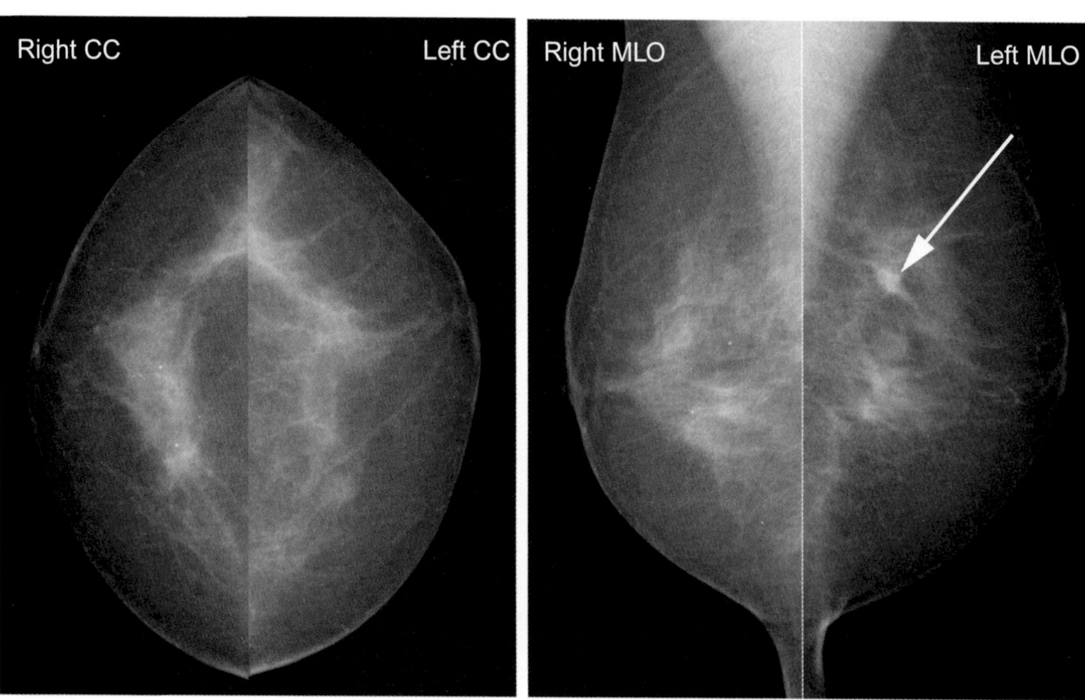

Figure 98.1

A 55-year-old woman who worked as a ward clerk on a surgical ward attended her second routine screening mammogram. She was otherwise asymptomatic, with no family history of breast disease. Her only past history was of a cholecystectomy following an episode of acute cholecystitis 5 years ago.

She was recalled a week later for further investigation, at which time she was told that there was an abnormality in the left breast on the mammogram. The mammogram shows a spiculated lesion with microcalcification in the upper outer quadrant of the left breast best seen on the mediolateral oblique (MLO) view (white arrow) (Fig. 98.1).

The MLO view images the breast obliquely with the pectoralis major visible obliquely from above; the craniocaudal (CC) view images the breast from above.

What further investigation is required to prove the diagnosis?

Any breast lump requires a triple assessment comprising clinical examination, radiological imaging and biopsy. On this occasion there was no palpable lesion and no palpable lymphadenopathy. Needle core biopsy was performed using ultrasound guidance and confirmed carcinoma.

Outline the surgical management

The tumour is excised, either by wide local excision or, if the tumour is large and central, by mastectomy. In this case the tumour was impalpable and a decision was made to perform wide local excision. The tumour position was identified radiologically and a guide wire placed in the centre under ultrasound or mammographic control. Blue dye and radoisotope were injected into the tumour at the same time. A wide excision of the tissue at the tip of the guide wire was then performed with minimal delay. Through a separate axillary incision, the sentinel lymph nodes were identified by virtue of taking up the blue dye and radioisotope, and excised. In this case the axillary nodes were found to be free of tumour; the primary itself was a 1.5 cm diameter, well differentiated, invasive duct carcinoma.

How would you determine what adjuvant therapy is appropriate for this patient?

The tumour needs to be formally staged to exclude distant metastatic spread. This involves excluding lung, liver (CT scans of the chest and abdomen) and bone (isotope bone scan) metastases. A full blood count may indicate marrow involvement and abnormal liver function tests (particularly raised alkaline phosphatase) may indicate early liver involvement.

Staging investigations failed to detect evidence of distant metastases. What is the TNM stage of the tumour and what adjuvant treatment is appropriate?

The tumour was 1.5 cm in diameter (T1), without nodal (N0) or distant metastatic (M0) spread, hence stage T1N0M0. In the absence of distant spread, local radiotherapy is the only adjuvant therapy required, and this will reduce the risk of local recurrence.

What is the prognosis of such a screen-detected tumour?

Tumours that are asymptomatic when detected by screening generally have a better prognosis than tumours that present with symptoms, possibly because they represent a slower growing lesion. In addition small tumours, well differentiated tumours and tumours without axillary or distant spread all have better prognosis. This woman has a 95% 10-year survival likelihood.

Breast cancer, like cervical cancer, is the subject of a national screening programme. What are the requirements for an effective screening programme for a given condition?

Effective screening for a condition like breast cancer using a specific test, such as mammography, has the following prerequisites:

- The condition, if untreated, is sufficiently serious to warrant its prevention.
- The natural history of the condition should be understood.
- The condition has a recognizable early stage.
- Effective treatment is available.
- Treatment at an early stage could improve the prognosis, and is of more benefit than treatment started later in the disease.
- The screening test is simple, reliable and acceptable to the patient.
- The screening test should have minimal false-positive and false-negative outcomes (i.e. it should be both sensitive and specific).

Case 99 An ulcerating breast lesion

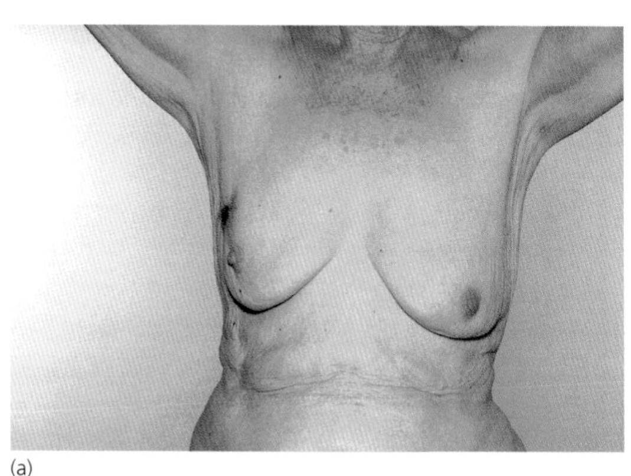
(a)

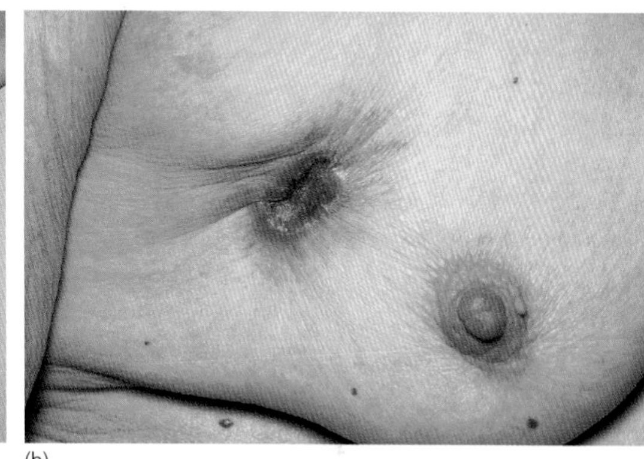
(b)

Figure 99.1

Figure 99.1 shows a general and close-up view of an ulcerating lesion of the right breast in a widow aged 75 years, who was referred urgently by her family doctor to the breast clinic of the local hospital. She explained that she had found a lump in the right breast 'about the size of a grape' about 2 years before. This gave her a terrible fright so she ignored it completely and did not consciously examine her breasts again. However, a few months ago this ulcer appeared and began to discharge and to bleed. She finally got enough courage to show it to her doctor. It was quite painless and she was otherwise well.

The patient had never had children and there was no one in the family, as far as she knew, who had had breast cancer. Her periods ceased when she was 45. She lived on her own in a two-roomed flat.

What is the diagnosis?

She has, without much doubt, an ulcerating carcinoma of the right breast. In the Western world it is unusual to see patients presenting at such a late stage of the disease – although they still sometimes do. However, older clinicians will have seen many such cases decades ago and such examples are still common in the developing world.

Enumerate the signs of advanced breast cancer that you can see in Fig. 99.1

There is an ulcerating lesion in the upper outer quadrant of the right breast. It has raised everted edges and there is puckering of the adjacent skin. The nipple is indrawn and the breast is somewhat shrunken and also elevated.

How common is carcinoma of the breast in the UK?

It is the commonest killing cancer of women in the UK and indeed in the Western world. In the UK there are 44 000 new cases annually, and it accounts for some 12 500 deaths.

Is it ever found in male subjects?

There is breast ductal tissue beneath the male nipple, which extends just outside the areolar margin – hence there are cases of gynaecomastia in the male at puberty or in response to stilboestrol. Carcinoma of the male breast accounts for roughly 1% of all cases. Because the male patient often thinks little of a painless lump in the region of the nipple, many cases in the male present at a fairly advanced stage.

Where would you examine this woman for evidence of dissemination of her tumour?

- *Lymphatic spread*: Examine the axillary and supraclavicular nodes on the affected side.
- *Blood spread*: Examine the liver, lungs, skeleton and CNS.
- *Transcoelomic spread*: Examine for the presence of ascites and pleural effusion.

Is anything known about the aetiology or predisposing factors of this common cancer?

In spite of much study, surprisingly little is known.

- There is a family tendency – a premenopausal first-degree relative, mother or sister, with breast cancer confers a lifetime risk of 25%, which reduces to 14% if the relative is postmenopausal at the time of her diagnosis. If both the mother and sister have developed breast cancer premenopausally, the risk rises to 33%.
- The disease is rare in the Far East.
- An early age of commencement of periods (11 years or under) and a late menopause (51 years or over) are associated with higher risk – and both these factors are becoming more common.
- Nulliparous women have a higher risk than parous, and early age at first pregnancy appears to play a protective role, as does breastfeeding.
- Hormone replacement therapy may slightly increase the risk, and this is proportionate to the length of time of treatment.
- Carriage of the *BRCA1* and *BRCA2* genes are significant risk factors.

The chest X-ray, bone scan, abdominal ultrasound (for hepatic involvement or evidence of free fluid) and full blood count were normal. A biopsy of the ulcer edge, performed under local anaesthetic, showed a moderately well differentiated, invasive ductal carcinoma, oestrogen receptor positive. The patient was treated as an outpatient with radiotherapy and tamoxifen and the ulcer slowly healed.

Case 100 A sinister break

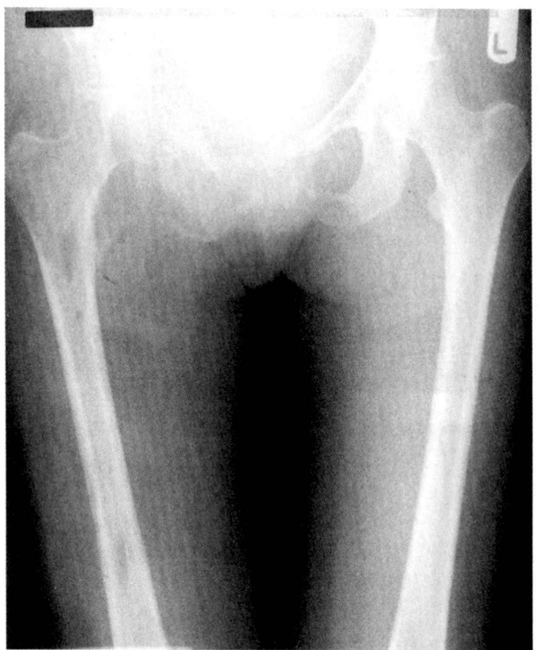

Figure 100.1

The woman described in Case 99 continued to be followed up by the oncologists and she remained well. However, 18 months after first being seen in the breast clinic, she suddenly developed severe pain in her right hip while out walking, her hip gave way and she fell down in the street. She was brought to hospital by ambulance. The X-ray taken in the accident and emergency department is shown in Fig. 100.1.

Describe the lesion you can see on this X-ray

There are extensive lytic lesions seen in the right femoral neck, the trochanters and the femoral shaft. Further lytic areas are seen in the right pubis, where there is a pathological fracture of its upper ramus. Smaller areas of lysis are seen in the pubic bone on the left side.

What would be your diagnosis?

Osteolytic secondary bone deposits from the initial carcinoma of the left breast, with a pathological fracture.

Where else are bone secondary deposits found – and why is this?

Bony deposits occur at the sites of red bone marrow, which is highly vascular. These sites are the vault of the skull, the vertebral bodies, the ribs, sternum and upper end of the humerus as well as the pelvis and upper end of the femur, as has occurred in this patient.

What other primary tumours commonly spread by the blood stream to bone?

In the male, lung carcinoma is the commonest tumour to spread by the blood stream, followed by prostate (see Case 116, p. 241). In the female, breast carcinoma is commonest, followed by lung. These are the cause of the majority of cases of bone secondaries in practice. Secondary deposits to bone may occasionally be found in patients with carcinoma of the kidney and thyroid. Apart from these five tumours, bone deposits from other cancers are rare.

As part of her further investigation, a chest X-ray was performed (Fig. 100.2); there were no chest symptoms but clinically there was dullness at the right lung base. What does the X-ray show ?

There is an obvious effusion at the right lung base, with the typical appearance of a pleural fluid collection. Numerous opacities are seen in both lung fields, suggesting lung secondary deposits.

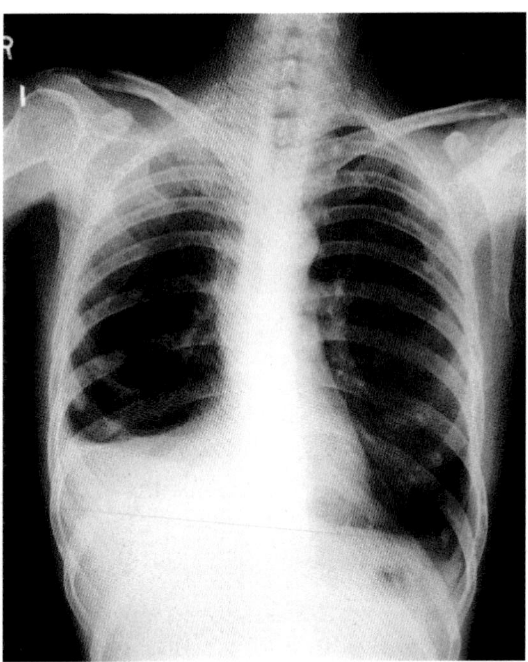

Figure 100.2 Chest X-ray.

Aspiration of the right pleural effusion produced yellow fluid. Malignant cells were identified on its cytological examination. Cytotoxic therapy was commenced but the patient showed no response to this; indeed, the treatment was discontinued because of severe toxicity. She was transferred to the local hospice and died peacefully 2 months after her fall.

Case 101 A woman with a sore nipple

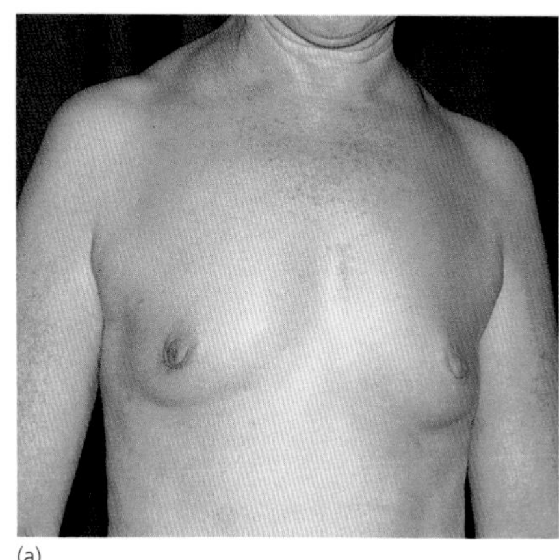

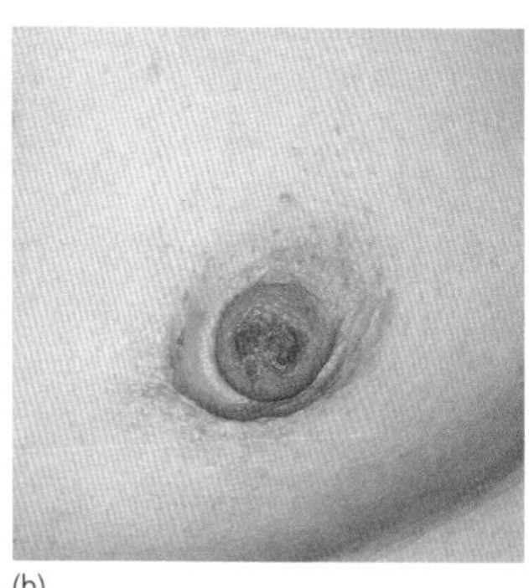

Figure 101.1 (a) (b)

PART 2: CASES

Figure 101.1a shows the chest wall and breasts of a 66-year-old housewife, who was referred urgently to the breast clinic by her family practitioner. She stated that her right nipple had become discoloured and thickened over the past year and recently she had noticed some slight blood staining of her brassiere and nightdress. The lesion was slightly sore but not really painful. Figure 101.1b shows a close-up of the affected nipple. She was otherwise well. She had had two children, both girls and both breastfed. Her periods had stopped when she was about 50 and she had not had any hormonal replacement therapy. As far as she knew, there was no history of breast disease in any of the female members of her family.

On examination, the right nipple had the appearance shown in Fig. 101.1b. It was thickened and slightly tender to touch, but no masses could be felt in either breast and the axillae were clear. There were no other relevant findings.

What is your clinical diagnosis?

This has the typical appearance of Paget's disease of the nipple.

Describe the typical features of this condition

A unilateral, red, bleeding eczematous condition of the nipple, which is eventually destroyed by the disease. There may or may not be an underlying carcinoma to feel.

There are two other diseases that bear this surgeon's name; what are they?

Sir James Paget* also described Paget's disease of bone (osteitis deformans), which is common and still of unknown aetiology, and Paget's disease of the glans penis, a rare condition but similar in appearance to the nipple disease and which may also develop into a frank carcinoma.

---

*Sir James Paget (1814–1899), surgeon, St Bartholomew's Hospital, London.

A biopsy was taken of this lesion. What are the typical microscopic findings?

The deep layers of the epithelium contain multiple clear large Paget cells with small dark nuclei (Fig. 101.2, arrowed in the inset). The underlying dermis contains an inflammatory cellular infiltrate. As is usually the case, the specimen in Fig. 101.2 also shows an associated invasive ductal carcinoma.

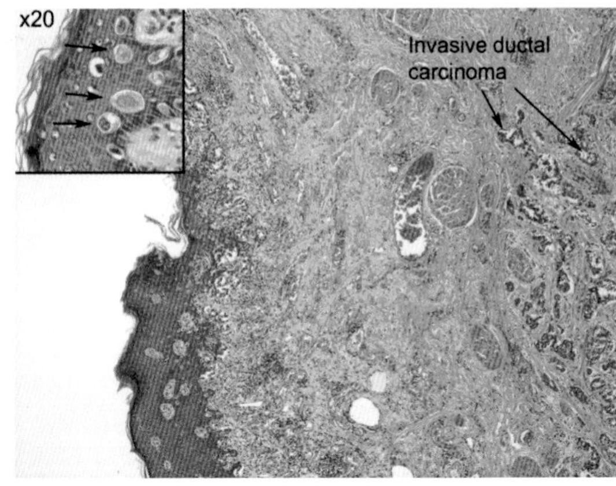

Figure 101.2 Invasive ductal carcinoma (magnification × 4 (inset × 20), haematoxylin and eosin stain).

What is the commonly held theory of the aetiology of this disease?

Paget's disease probably represents invasion of the nipple by malignant cells that arise in a mammary duct and that also give rise to the associated solid breast tumour when this develops.

Case 102 A painless lump in the neck

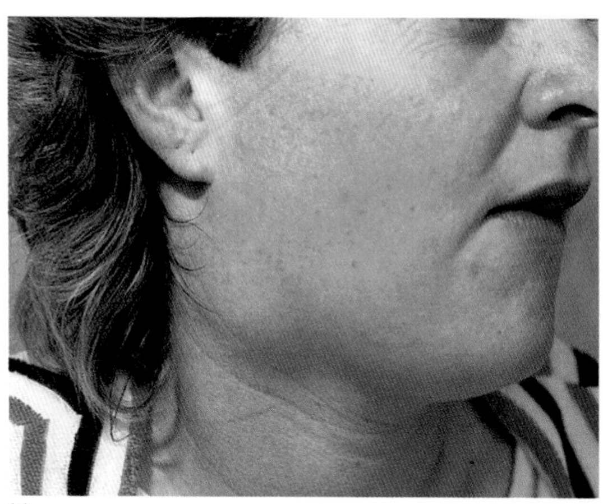

(a)

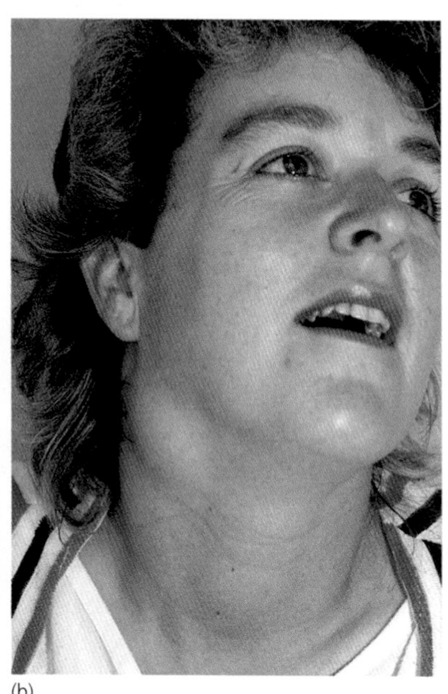

(b)

Figure 102.1

Figure 102.1 shows two photographs of a 45-year-old office worker who noticed a lump in the right side of her neck 3 months ago. At first it was small, and she thought it was 'just a swollen gland'. However, she had a mild throat infection a month ago and the lump, although still quite painless, got larger. Now she was getting concerned. She consulted her own doctor, who referred her to the surgical outpatients clinic.

On examination, the lump was smooth, round and not attached to the overlying skin. Its anterior part emerged from under the anterior border of sternocleidomastoid. It fluctuated and transilluminated brilliantly to torchlight.

What is the likely diagnosis?

This has the typical features of a branchial cyst.

There is some controversy about the aetiology of this condition. Can you give an account of the two 'popular' theories of its aetiology?

1 *The embryological hypothesis.* In the development of the side of the neck, the second branchial arch of the fetus grows down over the third and fourth arches to form the cervical sinus. Normally, this sinus disappears before birth. It is postulated that its persistence leads to the formation of a branchial cyst. There is little doubt that this accounts for the rather uncommon branchial fistula – a track that is present at birth, opens in front of the origin of sternocleidomastoid above the sternoclavicular joint, and tracks upwards almost to the level of the palatine tonsil. Figure 102.2 shows an example of this in a young man.

2 *The cervical lymph node theory*. The cervical lymph nodes, on histological examination, are often found to contain rests of stratified squamous epithelium. One of these rests is postulated to break down into a cystic space – hence the squamous lining of the cyst. The fact that the cyst may enlarge after a throat infection – as happened in this case – supports this theory.

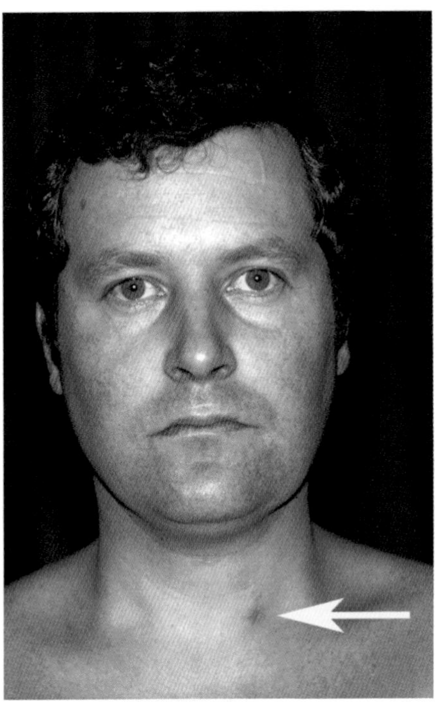

Figure 102.2 Branchial fistula (arrowed).

What does the fluid inside the cyst look like to the naked eye and what is its microscopic appearance?

The fluid is thick, turbid, yellowish white and looks just like pus. However, under the microscope, it is seen to contain typical cholesterol crystals. This woman's cyst was indeed aspirated in the clinic, to confirm the diagnosis, and Fig. 102.3 demonstrates the macroscopic and microscopic findings.

What may complicate this condition?

The cyst may become infected, producing an abscess, which requires surgical drainage followed by a rather difficult removal of the now adherent cyst wall to prevent further infections.

Are there any other diagnoses you might have to consider?

A tuberculous lymph node (see Case 103, p. 214) or, if infected, an acute cervical lymphadenitis.

What treatment do you think was advised in this case?

Elective surgical excision of the cyst, first to obviate the risk of infection and second because the patient was now anxious to get rid of her rather unsightly lump. This was duly carried out as a day case. Figure 102.4 shows the cyst exposed at operation and the excised specimen.

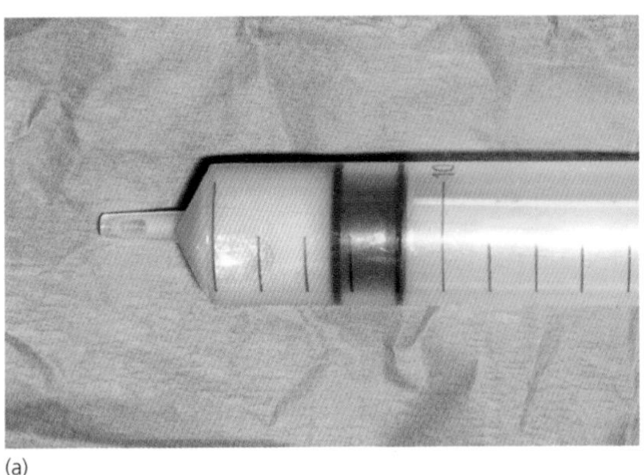

(a)

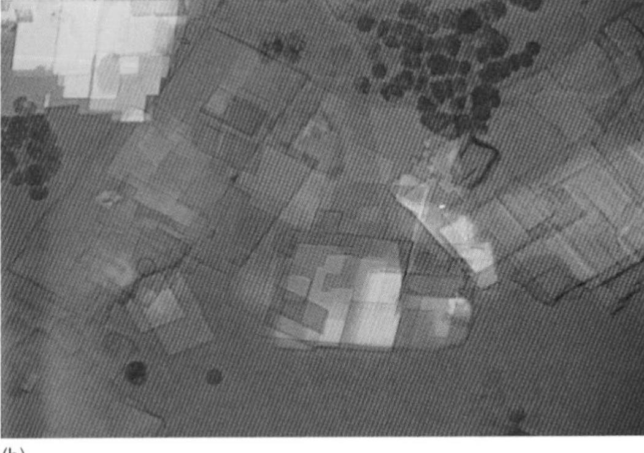

(b)

Figure 102.3 Branchial cyst aspirate: (a) macroscopic and (b) microscopic findings.

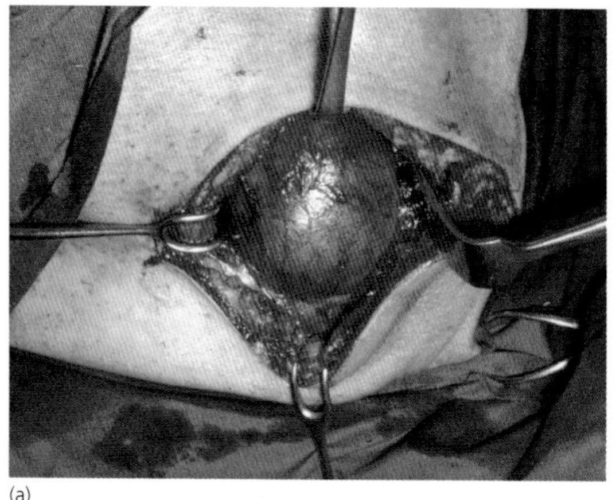
(a)

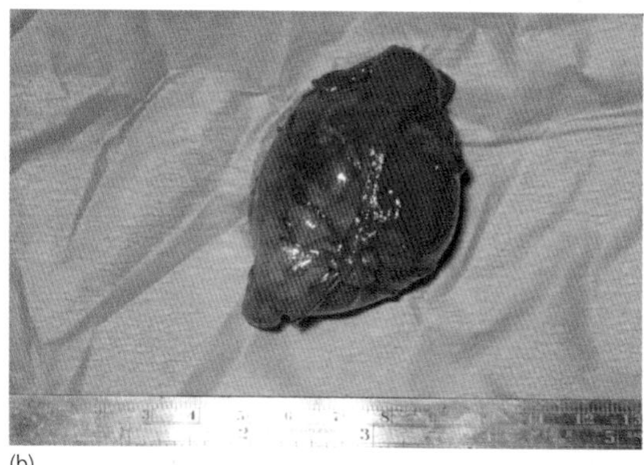
(b)

Figure 102.4 (a) The cyst as exposed at operation. (b) The excised specimen.

Case 103 A young immigrant with a lump in the neck

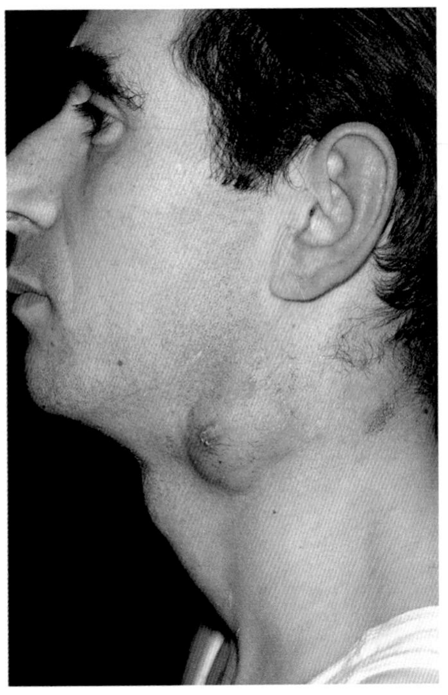

Figure 103.1

Figure 103.1 is of a 26-year-old catering worker, a recent immigrant from the Middle East. He had noticed a lump in the left anterior triangle of his neck about 6 months previously. It had gradually enlarged, and then, in the last couple of weeks, it became considerably bigger. It was uncomfortable rather than painful and he was now worried about its appearance. Apart from this, he was well and was still at work.

On examination, the lump was soft, smooth, not tender and definitely fluctuated, although it did not transilluminate. At the centre of the mass, the overlying skin was adherent to the lump and, as can be seen, was slightly reddened. However, the skin did not feel warmer than its surrounds.

He was afebrile. There was no other lymphadenopathy, no local focus of infection on full clinical examination, and the spleen and liver could not be felt.

Taking all these features into consideration, what would be the probable diagnosis?

This patient presents the clinical features of a tuberculous 'cold' abscess.

What is the origin and the natural history of tuberculosis of the cervical lymph nodes?

This condition is now rare in children and young adults born in the Western world, where milk comes from tuberculosis-free herds of cows or, at the least, is pasteurized. It is still quite commonly encountered in patients coming to the UK from developing countries, especially the Middle East and the Indian subcontinent. Tuberculous mycobacteria in infected milk are taken up by the lymphoid tissue in the palatine tonsils, passes to the tonsillar lymph node and may spread to the other nodes in the deep cervical chain. The nodes enlarge, and then break down to form a tuberculous abscess. This is demonstrated in Fig. 103.2 showing a mass of tuberculous cervical nodes excised from a girl of 14 who had recently arrived from the Indian subcontinent.

Left untreated, the pus from the infected nodes breaks through the deep fascia to lie in the subcutaneous tissue – a 'collar stud abscess'. This is what has happened in this young man. There is an abscess in the superficial tissues of his neck that leads down through a track through the deep fascia down into the breaking down mass of deep cervical lymph nodes. If treatment is still further delayed, the abscess discharges spontaneously through the overlying skin, resulting in a chronic tuberculous sinus.

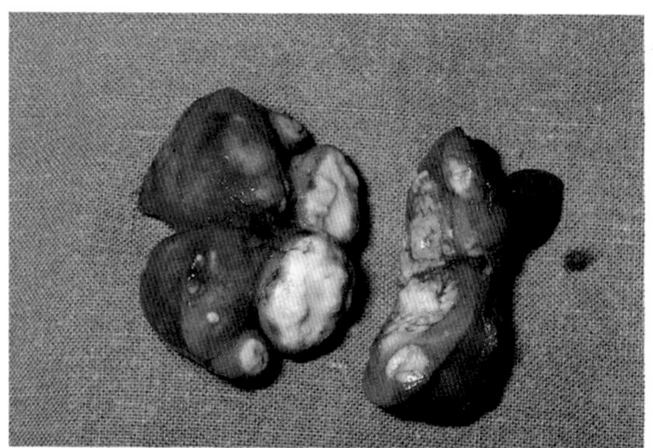

Figure 103.2 Tuberculous cervical nodes.

What is your differential diagnosis in this patient?

- Acute lymphadenitis, but this is very painful and tender and the inflamed skin feels hot to the touch (unlike this 'cold' abscess).
- An infected branchial cyst (see Case 102, p. 211).

An X-ray of the neck may be helpful as chronically infected tuberculous nodes usually show flecks of calcification.

What is the name given to tuberculous pus?

'Caseous' pus – the word caseous means 'cheesy', because of its resemblance to cream cheese.

Discuss the treatment of tuberculous cervical lymph nodes

Enlarged nodes should be excised; this was performed in the young girl whose specimen is shown in Fig. 103.2. If the patient presents with a 'collar stud abscess', as in our catering worker, the pus is evacuated, a search made for the hole penetrating through the deep fascia, and the underlying caseating node evacuated by curettage. The operative treatment is combined with antituberculous chemotherapy.

Case 104 A lump in the neck that moves on swallowing

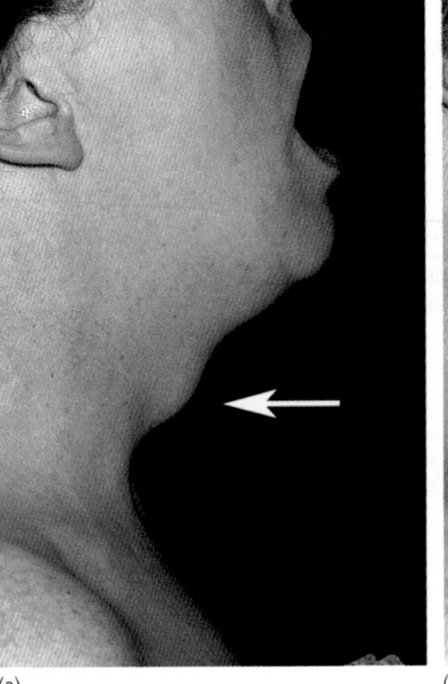
(a)

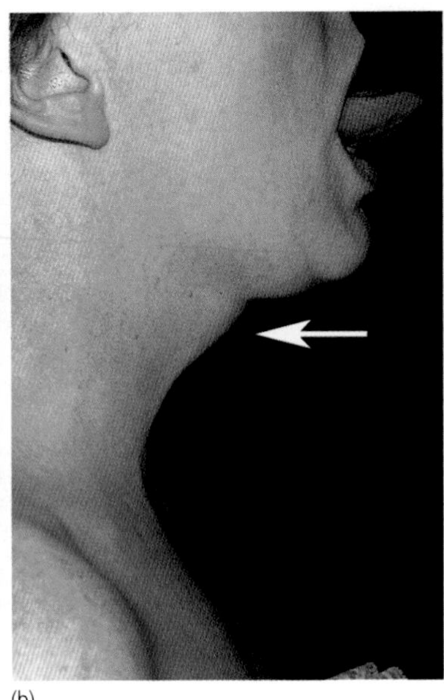
(b)

Figure 104.1

A hairdresser aged 29 years noticed a lump in her neck 3 months before being seen in the outpatient clinic. It was quite painless and not tender, but both she and her friends noticed that it 'bobbed up and down' when she swallowed. It seemed to her that it was getting bigger and she was worried about its appearance. Apart from this, she was perfectly well.

On examination, she was a healthy young woman, although rather overweight. There was a lump just to the right of the midline to the lamina of the thyroid cartilage, which moved upwards on swallowing. Figure 104.1 shows a side view of her neck, with her mouth open (a), and what happened when she was asked to put out her tongue (b).

The lump in this woman's neck (arrowed) moves on swallowing. What does this imply, and why?

In clinical practice, the only lumps you will see that move on swallowing have something to do with the thyroid gland. The gland is attached to the sides of the larynx and the larynx moves upwards on swallowing.

This lump also moves upwards when she protrudes her tongue. What is the undoubted diagnosis here?

She has a thyroglossal cyst.

What is the embryological explanation of this lesion and of its physical signs?

The thyroid gland develops as a diverticulum of the tongue at the junction of its anterior two-thirds and posterior one-third. This leaves a pit, the foramen caecum, which can be seen on the dorsum of the back of the tongue. This diverticulum descends along the front of the neck, passes in close relationship to the body of the hyoid bone, and takes up its definitive position on either side of the larynx and trachea, with its isthmus crossing the front of the trachea. The thyroglossal cyst develops in the

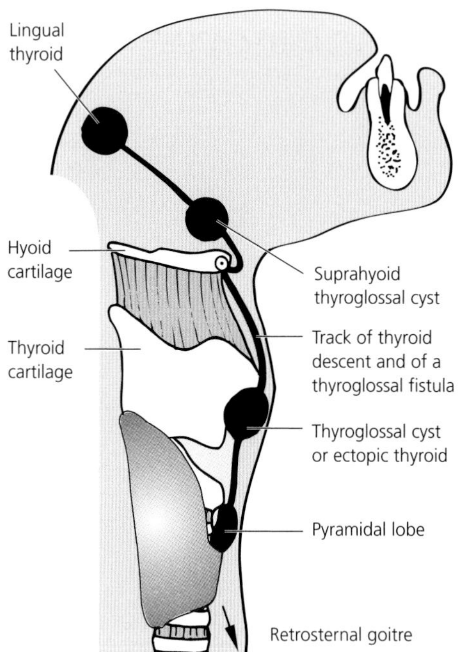

Figure 104.2 The descent of the thyroid, showing possible sites of ectopic thyroid tissue or thyroglossal cysts, and also the course of a thyroglossal fistula. The arrow shows the further descent of the thyroid that may take place retrosternally into the superior mediastinum.

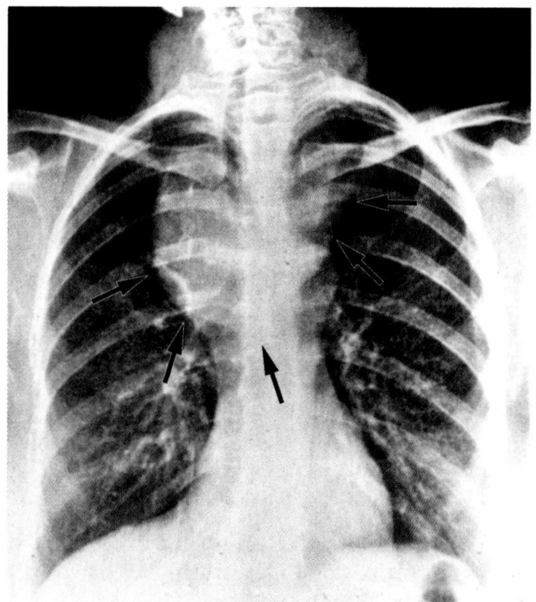

Figure 104.3 Retrosternal thyroid (arrowed) shown on a chest X-ray.

remnants of this thyroglossal track and retains its attachment to the base of the tongue, so that it moves upwards when the tongue is protruded. It also moves upwards on swallowing because of its attachment to the larynx.

What other congenital anomalies, apart from thyroglossal cysts, may result from this embryological process?

These are shown in Fig. 104.2:

• *Lingual thyroid*: All or, more usually, a part of the gland persists at the tongue base.

• *Thyroglossal fistula*: This may result if the cyst becomes infected and ruptures, or if incomplete excision of the tract is performed.

• *Pyramidal lobe*: This a common finding, attached to the isthmus of the thyroid gland.

• *Retrosternal thyroid*: The thyroid descends beyond its station into the superior mediastinum. Indeed, this is the commonest cause of a superior mediastinal mass, and an example is shown in Fig. 104.3.

How was this woman's thyroglossal cyst treated?

A radioactive thyroid scan was performed to ensure the presence of normal thyroid tissue in the correct place. Following this, the neck was explored through a transverse skin crease (Kocher*) incision. The cyst was excised together with the track, which led upwards behind the cyst and was in intimate contact with the back of the body of the hyoid bone, the central piece of which was also excised; the track was removed up to the base of the tongue. Inferiorly, the cyst was attached to a pyramidal lobe, which was also resected. It is important to remove the whole of the track as well as the cyst in order to prevent the development of a thyroglossal fistula from the duct remnant. The excised specimen is shown in Fig. 104.4.

The patient made a smooth recovery from her operation.

*Theodor Kocher (1841–1917), Professor of surgery, Berne. He was the first of the seven surgeons to have gained the Nobel Prize.

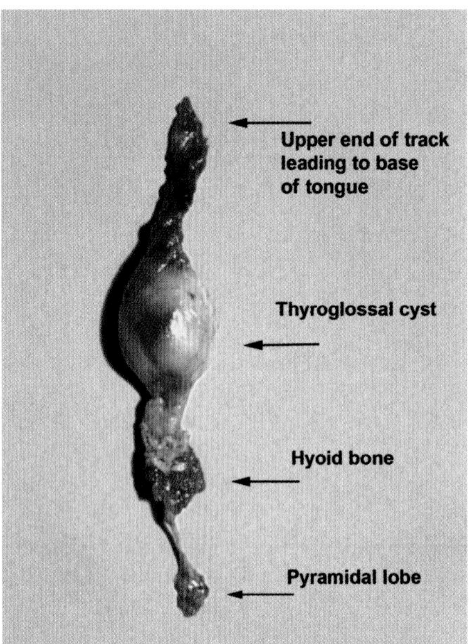

Figure 104.4 Thyroglossal cyst.

Case 105 A woman with an obvious endocrine disease

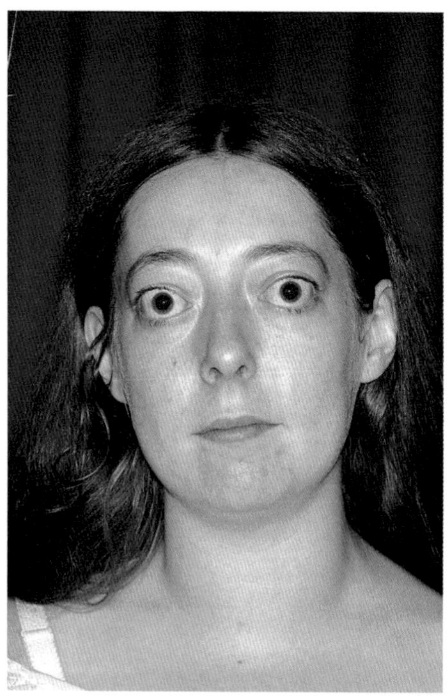

Figure 105.1

The young woman in Fig. 105.1 has an endocrine disease that can be diagnosed at a glance. When her history was taken in the clinic it was briefly as follows. She was a 26-year-old married dressmaker, with no children. Previously quite healthy, she had become nervous, irritable and trembly over the past 6 months, and for no apparent reason – no family or work problems were out of the usual. Then she noticed that her neck was getting swollen, she was experiencing palpitations on slight exertion, she was losing weight and, the thing that worried her the most, her eyes were becoming increasingly prominent and 'starey'.

What disease is it?

She has primary hyperthyroidism (Graves' disease*), with marked exophthalmos.

Can you classify the possible clinical manifestations of hyperthyroidism?

The features of hyperthyroidism are widespread. However, it is important to remember that not all of them may be present in a particular patient, and so the diagnosis may be overlooked. They can be classified as follows:

- The thyroid gland is usually – but not always – enlarged.
- The eyes may show exophthalmos.
- Cardiovascular: Tachycardia and palpitations with a rapid pulse even when asleep. The patient may develop atrial fibrillation and progress to heart failure.
- CNS: Nervousness, irritability and tremor of the hands.
- Alimentary: Increased appetite (due to the raised basal metabolic rate, BMR) but loss of weight, which may be profound. There may be diarrhoea.
- Skin: Because of the raised BMR, the patient feels hot and sweats profusely – they will open the windows and switch off the central heating when everyone else feels cold.
- Genitourinary: Female patients may have irregular, scanty periods and are subfertile. However, pregnancy may occur and treatment of the hyperthyroidism then presents a serious problem since the drugs used will also affect the fetus.

Classical cases of hyperthyroidism, with every feature listed above, are quite common, but the clinician must be on guard for less typical examples. Thus, a patient may be admitted in congestive heart failure with atrial fibrillation but the diagnosis of hyperthyroidism is

*Robert Graves (1796–1853), physician, Meath Hospital, Dublin.

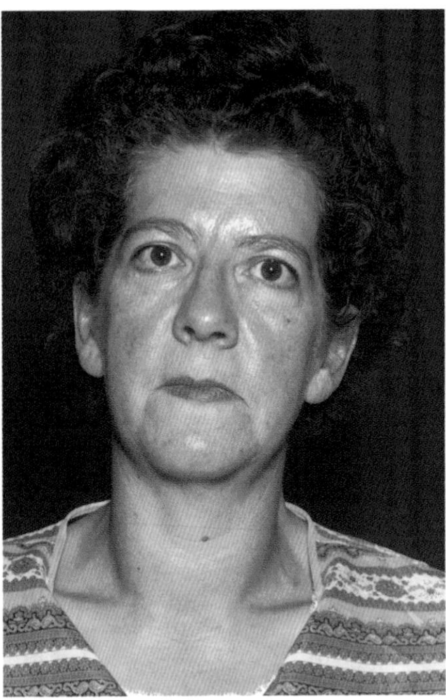

Figure 105.2 Hyperthyroidism presenting with heart failure and atrial fibrillation, and no goitre.

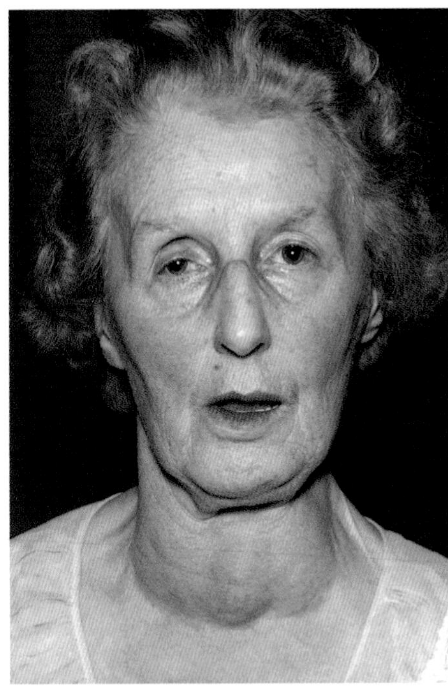

Figure 105.3 Nodular thyroid enlargement.

missed because the thyroid gland is not palpably enlarged and there is no exophthalmos. Figure 105.2 shows just such an example. This lady, aged 65, admitted as an emergency in heart failure and atrial fibrillation, was picked up as a case of hyperthyroidism by the astute and careful clinician dealing with her.

What changes within the orbit produce the eye signs?

Exophthalmos in Graves' disease is the result of an autoimune inflammatory process, with fibroblast proliferation, deposition of extracellular matrix and adipocyte differentiation and proliferation. The result is interstitial oedema, an increase in the volume of the orbital pad of fat and enlargement of the extrinsic muscles of the eye.

What may happen in very advanced exophthalmos?

If the exophthalmos is severe, the swollen and oedematous extrinsic muscles may be so damaged that incoordination or paralysis of eye movements may occur (exophthalmic ophthalmoplegia). If the patient cannot close the eyelids, corneal ulceration may develop. The patient may require partial suture of the eyelids together (tarsorrhaphy) or even surgical decompression of the bony orbit.

Clinically we distinguish between primary and secondary hyperthyroidism – can you discuss this?

- *Primary hyperthyroidism*: Often called Graves' disease in the UK and Basedow's disease† in continental Europe, this occurs usually in young women with no previous history of thyroid enlargement. The gland is usually smoothly enlarged and exophthalmos is common. Symptoms, apart from the eye changes, are primarily those of nervousness and tremor. The condition is due to the action of autoantibodies that bind to, and stimulate, the thyroid-stimulating hormone (TSH) receptor. These thyroid-stimulating antibodies have a prolonged stimulatory effect compared to TSH, hence the name of long-acting thyroid stimulators (LATS).

†Carl Adolph von Basedow (1799–1854), physician, Meresburg, Germany.

• *Secondary hyperthyroidism*: This is overactivity that develops in an already hyperplastic gland. It is a disease of the middle age and occurs in patients with a pre-existing euthyroid enlarged nodular gland. Symptoms fall more on the cardiovascular system, although CNS signs may also be present. Figure 105.3 shows a typical example. This woman of 74 presented with mild heart failure and atrial fibrillation. She had had this nodular thyroid enlargement for many years.

Case 106 A mass of cervical lymph nodes

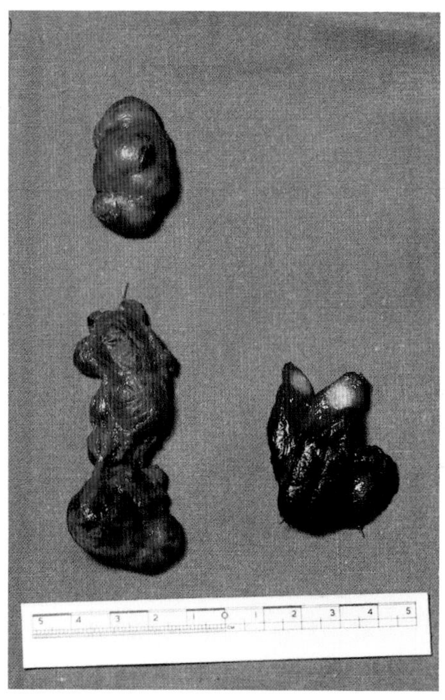

Figure 106.1

A 36-year-old divorcee, working as a clerk in the local tax office, noticed a lump in the right side of her neck about 2 months previously. The lump was painless and not tender to touch, but it gradually enlarged. In her past history, she had been treated 2 years ago for in situ carcinoma of the cervix after a positive smear test. She had never had children. There were no other relevant features in her history.

On examination, she was a healthy woman with no anomalies to find apart from an obvious collection of enlarged, rubbery-firm, non-tender lymph nodes in the right anterior triangle of the neck, which extended forward from deep to the sternocleidomastoid muscle.

A chest X-ray was normal. After biopsy of one of the nodes, she was submitted to a block dissection of the right cervical lymph nodes, together with the internal jugular vein, and removal of the right lobe of the thyroid gland. The right recurrent laryngeal nerve was identified and carefully preserved. Figure 106.1 shows the lymph nodes, together with the opened right lobe of the thyroid gland.

What does this specimen demonstrate?

There is a small white nodule of tumour in the upper pole of the thyroid gland. The chain of lymph nodes are greatly enlarged and must obviously have been invaded by secondary deposits.

What is the likely pathology of the white nodule of tumour in the upper pole of the thyroid gland?

A papillary carcinoma of the thyroid may typically metastasize to the cervical lymph nodes. Occasionally the primary tumour may be small and indeed impalpable – only a careful search of the specimen will reveal what usually proves to be a well differentiated tumour. The typical appearances are shown in Fig. 106.2.

In the past, these deposits in the chain of cervical lymph nodes were mistakenly thought to arise in 'lateral aberrant thyroid tissue'. However, a careful search will reveal, as in this case, a small focus of primary tumour in the ipsilateral lobe of the thyroid gland.

This woman had a papillary carcinoma, the commonest type of thyroid cancer. It accounts for about 60% of cases and occurs in young adults, adolescents and even children. It is usually slow growing and has a good prognosis. What are the other types of primary carcinomas of the thyroid?

• *Follicular*: Usually in young and middle-aged adults. It is particularly found in areas where goitre is endemic.

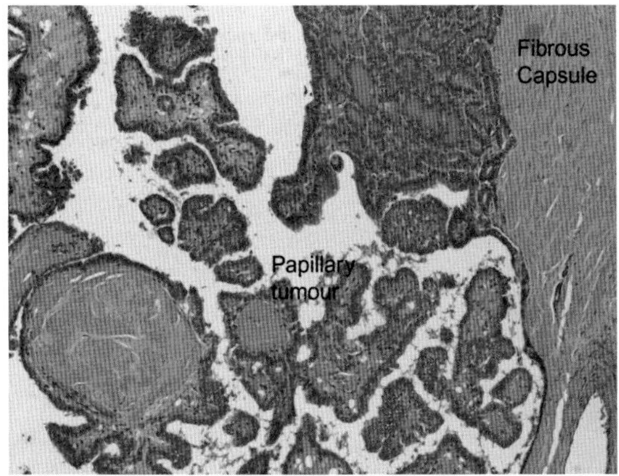

Figure 106.2 A papillary carcinoma of the thyroid (magnification × 20, haematoxylin and eosin stain).

It tends to spread by the blood stream rather than the lymphatics, so its prognosis is worse than the papillary type.

• *Medullary*: This arises from the parafollicular C-cells and may secrete calcitonin. It may occur at any age, be familial and be associated with the multiple endocrine neoplasia type 2 (MEN-2) syndrome, associated with phaeochromocytoma and either parathyroid tumour or multiple neurofibromas. The characteristic histological finding is of deposits of amyloid between the nests of tumour cells.

• *Anaplastic*: Usually found in elderly patients (see Case 107, p. 224).

• *Thyroid*: Lymphoma sometimes arises within the thyroid.

What is the sex distribution of thyroid carcinomas?

Medullary carcinoma has a roughly equal sex distribution, whereas the other tumours affect females twice as often as males.

What is the blood stream spread of thyroid cancers?

When haematogenous spread occurs, this is typically to the lungs and the brain. It is one of the tumours that may metastasize to bone (see Cases 100 and 116, pp. 207 and 241).

Case 107 A rapidly enlarging mass in the neck

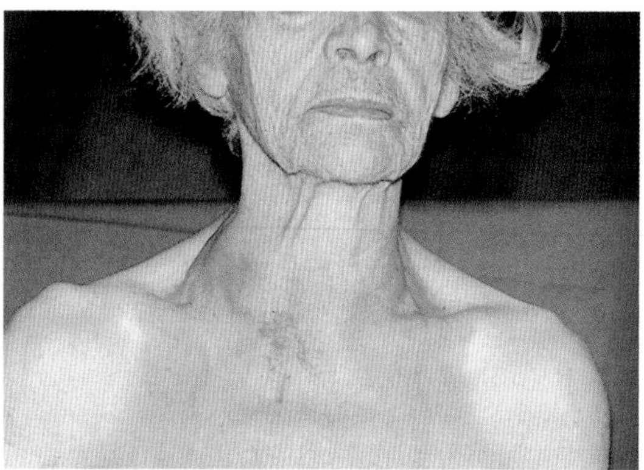

Figure 107.1

Figure 107.1 is of an 80-year-old woman who presented with a rapidly enlarging mass in the neck. She had only noticed this a couple of months ago, but she confessed that she was not a very good witness. For the last 2 weeks her voice had become weak, so that she could now only whisper. She was now having difficulty swallowing solid food, which seemed to stick in her throat, although liquids went down fairly well.

On examination she was a thin, frail old woman. There was a hard, tender, nodular mass, which definitely moved on swallowing. It occupied the front and lateral aspects of the neck, more on the right than the left. There was a mass of enlarged, hard nodes to feel in the right posterior triangle. There were no other relevant findings apart from what might be expected in a woman of this age – varicose veins, arthritic knees and fingers and a blood pressure of 180/100.

The clinical diagnosis is pretty obvious; what is it?

This is a malignant mass in the neck with lymph node metastases. It moves on swallowing, so it is a carcinoma of the thyroid gland.

Why has she recently lost her voice?

This must have been due to involvement of the recurrent laryngeal nerve, probably on the right side.

How would you confirm this?

The vocal cords should be inspected by laryngoscopy. This can be done easily and painlessly using a local anaesthetic spray and a fibreoptic laryngoscope. The paralysed cord will be immobile when the patient attempts to phonate.

What is the likely histological appearance of this thyroid tumour, and why is this anomalous when compared with tumours at other sites?

Rapidly enlarging thyroid tumours in the elderly are usually anaplastic carcinomas. This is the reversal of the state of affairs in other organs, in that the more malignant tumours of the thyroid gland occur in older age groups.

What treatment might be possible in the case of this old person?

This extensive tumour is already invading the recurrent laryngeal nerve (hence the loss of voice) and is beyond treatment by radical thyroidectomy. Radiotherapy to the neck may give temporary relief and a tracheostomy may eventually be required for obstruction of the airway.

Case 108 A patient with colic, and its endocrine underlying cause

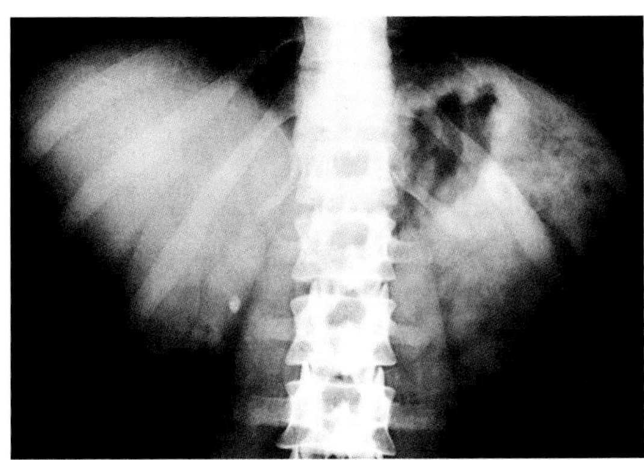

Figure 108.1

A married 33-year-old schoolteacher was admitted as an emergency on surgical take. She gave a history of being previously well before experiencing an attack of violent pain that had commenced 8 h before admission. The pain was situated in the right flank and spread around her side into her right iliac fossa and even down into her right groin. The pain was continuous, with sharp exacerbations, and made her double up and roll about in agony. She had had three children and said that the pain was rather like labour pain, except it was not intermittent and was 'much, much worse' – in fact, the worst pain she had ever experienced. She vomited several times – the food she had eaten and then just clear green fluid – and noticed that her urine had gone red in colour. She had had a normal period a week previously.

Her family doctor had come round to the house to see her, and had given her an injection of 100 mg of pethidine intramuscularly, which had helped ease the pain a good deal, and had arranged her urgent admission.

On examination, she was a healthy looking, slim young woman, but she was obviously in great pain. Her temperature was 37°C, pulse 86 and blood pressure 130/78. She was lying on her right side, doubled up and only reluctantly turned onto her back to be examined. The abdomen was soft but there was some tenderness in the right loin. No masses could be felt. She passed a specimen of urine, which looked blood stained and, indeed, when a drop was placed under the microscope, it was teeming with red cells.

Her haemoglobin and white cell count were normal, and a pregnancy test was negative. A chest X-ray was performed and was clear, a plain X-ray of the abdomen is shown in Fig. 108.1.

What does this X-ray of the patient's abdomen show, and what is now your working diagnosis?

The X-ray (Fig. 108.1) demonstrates a small, densely calcified shadow just to the right and slightly above the tip of the transverse process of the second lumbar vertebra. Putting all the information together, the patient is experiencing a violent attack of right renal colic with associated haematuria. The X-ray strongly suggests a calcified urinary stone at the level of the right pelviureteric junction – a common site for a stone to impact.

She was admitted under the urology team. That night she had two more violent attacks of the same pain, for which she received intravenous pethidine, and next morning passed a stone in her urine. This is shown in Fig. 108.2.

Can you identify this calculus?

This is a typical 'spiky' calcium oxalate stone – the commonest type of urinary calculus.

The much relieved patient was discharged from hospital and subjected to a series of further investigations as an outpatient. The relevant results of these were as follows:

- *Corrected serum calcium: 2.71 mmol/L (normal range 2.20–2.60 mmol/L).*
- *Parathyroid hormone level: 69 ng/L (normal range 9–54 ng/L).*

- *Repeated urine studies: sterile on culture, microscopy – occasional red blood cells and no white blood cells in unspun samples.*

What underlying cause of her stone are you thinking of now?

The raised serum calcium and raised serum parathyroid hormone level strongly indicate the presence of a functioning parathyroid adenoma. Excessive secretion of calcium in the urine has resulted in the formation of a calcium oxalate stone. Unless the tumour is located and removed, she will certainly have further problems from this.

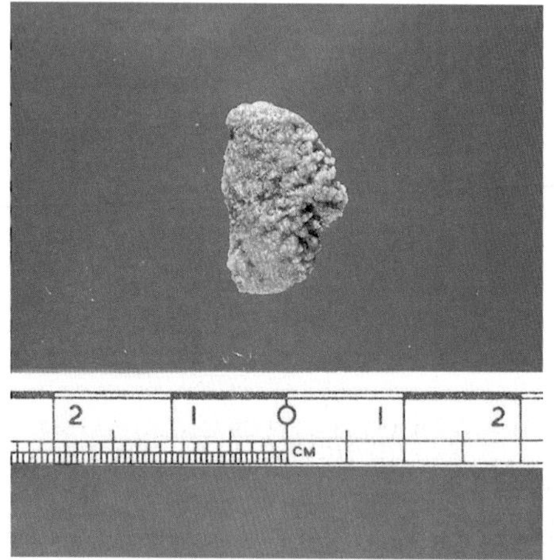

Figure 108.2 Urinary stone.

Is there a special investigation that is very useful in confirming the diagnosis of a parathyroid tumour and of locating which of the parathyroid glands contains it?

Yes, a sestamibi scan. This was carried out in our patient and is shown in Fig 108.3. The sestamibi scan involves injecting technetium-99m-labelled sestamibi intravenously. It is taken up both by the thyroid gland and parathyroid adenoma; uptake in the thyroid washes out quickly, but persists in the parathyroid adenoma and is detected by placing the patient on a gamma camera. Sestamibi (also known as MIBI, or methoxyisobutylisonitrile) is the same radiopharmaceutical used in cardiac imaging.

The patient was readmitted to hospital and the neck explored. The parathyroid adenoma was found below the lower pole of the right lobe of the thyroid gland. The operative findings are shown in Fig 108.4 and the adenoma in Fig. 108.5.

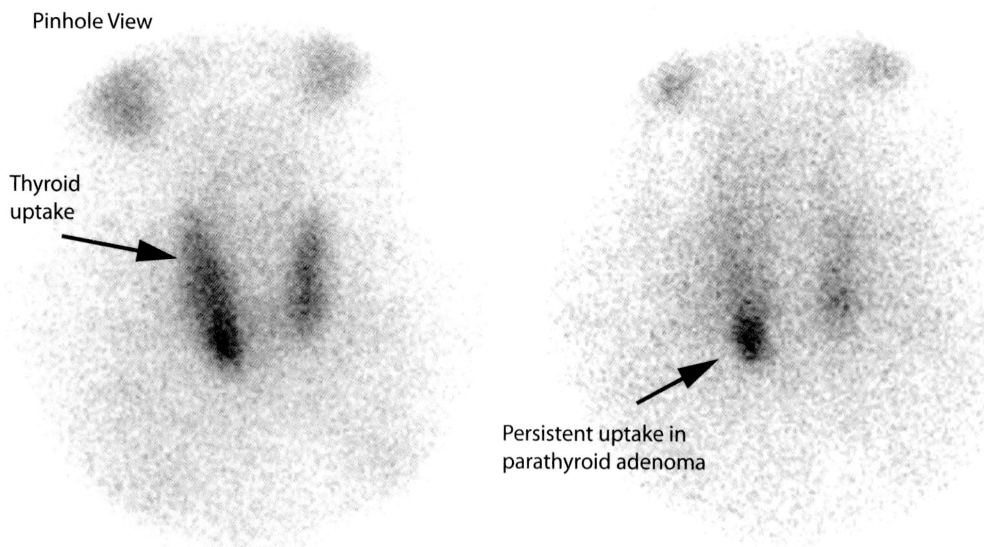

Figure 108.3 A sestamibi scan, (a) 15 min and (b) 135 min post-injection.

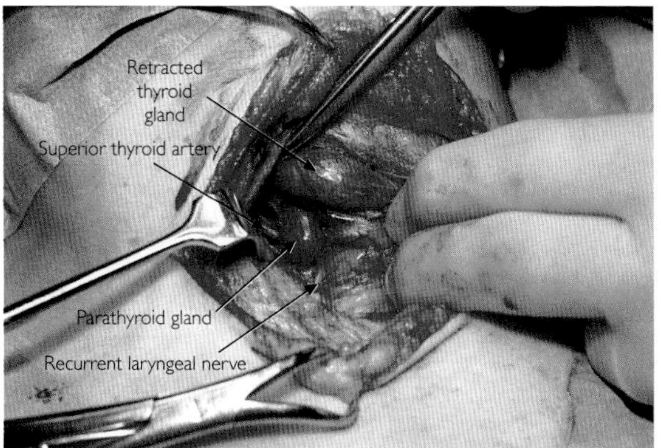

Figure 108.4 Operative findings.

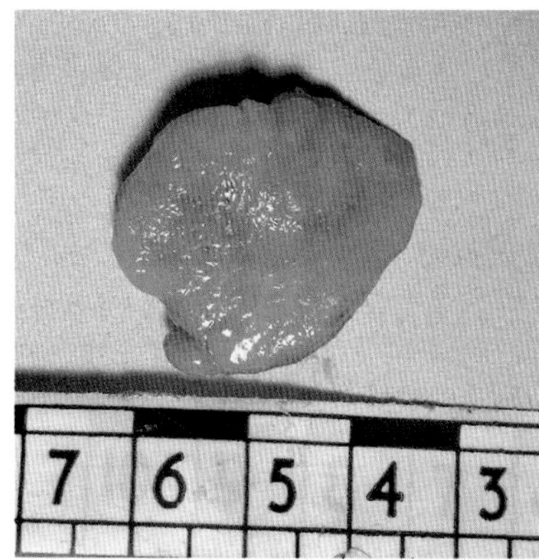

Figure 108.5 Parathyroid adenoma.

What other endocrine tumours may occasionally coexist with a parathyroid adenoma, and what is this syndrome called?

These are the multiple endocrine neoplasia (MEN) syndromes:

- MEN type 1 syndrome:
  - Parathyroid tumour.
  - Pancreatic tumour – islet cell, with the exception of the β cell (insulinoma).
  - Pituitary tumour, e.g. prolactinoma.
  - Adrenocortical tumour.
- MEN type 2 syndrome:
  - Parathyroid tumour (only in type 2A).
  - Medullary carcinoma of the thyroid.
  - Phaeochromocytoma of suprarenal medulla.
  - Neurofibromas of the tongue, lips and eyelids (only in type 2B).

Case 109 A girl with hirsutes

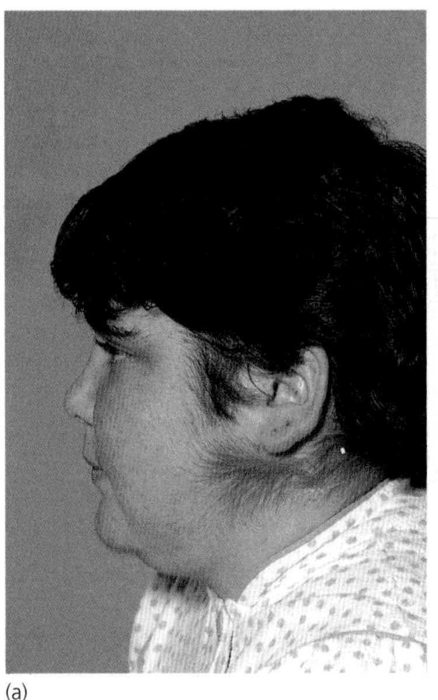
(a)

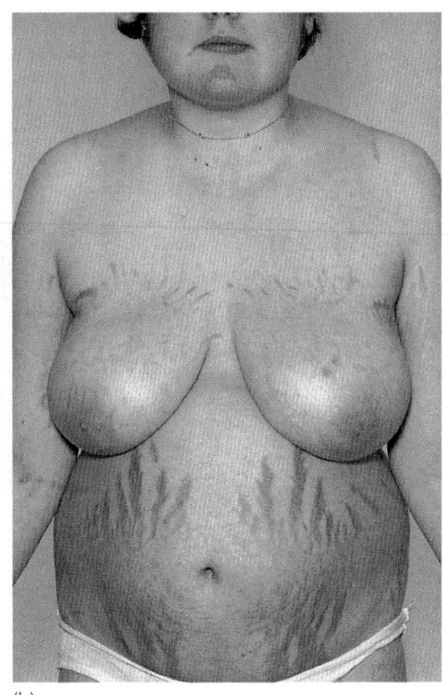
(b)

Figure 109.1

Figure 109.1a shows the side view of the face of a 17-year-old school girl who was brought by her mother to the family doctor. She was seriously worried by the growth of hair on her face. When the doctor examined her fully, there were also striking findings on inspection of the abdomen (Fig. 109.1b).

What is the eponymous name of the endocrine disease from which she is suffering?

Cushing's syndrome.*

What are the possible causes of this condition?

Cushing's syndrome occurs when there is prolonged exposure to supraphysiological levels of circulating glucocorticoids. The aetiology of Cushing's syndrome is most easily considered in terms of whether it is adrenocorticotrophic hormone (ACTH) dependent or independent:

1 *ACTH-dependent Cushing's syndrome*:
- Pituitary adenoma (so-called Cushing's disease).
- Ectopic ACTH secretion (e.g. from a small cell carcinoma of the lung).

2 *ACTH-independent Cushing's syndrome*:
- Exogenous steroids.
- Suprarenal adenoma or carcinoma.

The effects of oversecretion of suprarenal corticosteroids are widespread. Can you list the most important of these?

- Obesity: Principally involving the trunk and neck – so-called centripetal.

*Harvey Cushing (1869–1939), neurosurgeon, Peter Bent Brigham Hospital, Boston.

- Skin changes: Hirsutism, abdominal striae, excessive bruising, thin skin.
- Raised blood pressure.
- Proximal muscle weakness/wasting: Especially of the shoulder and pelvic girdles.
- Glucose intolerance/diabetes mellitus.
- Mental disturbance: Depression or psychosis.
- Growth retardation in childhood.

What laboratory and imaging investigations are useful in such cases?

The investigation of Cushing's syndrome should be considered in two stages.

1 *Confirmation of hypercortisolism*: Typically two or more of the following tests are used to confirm the diagnosis:

- Elevated 24 h urinary free cortisol (UFC) excretion – a minimum of three collections are required to ensure that mild cases are not missed.
- Failure of cortisol to suppress in response to dexamethasone. An overnight test administering 1 mg dexamethasone is often used for screening purposes, but has a significant false-positive rate, hence the conventional low dose 48 h test (0.5 mg 6-hourly for 48 h) should be used to confirm the diagnosis.
- Loss of circadian rhythm, with elevated midnight cortisol levels.

2 *Identification of source*: Measurement of the plasma ACTH helps to differentiate ACTH-dependent from ACTH-independent Cushing's syndrome.

- For ACTH-dependent cases, inferior petrosal venous sinus sampling (IPSS) reliably distinguishes pituitary from ectopic ACTH secretion. Pituitary MR imaging identifies approximately 60% of microadenomas. CT imaging, octreotide scintigraphy and positron emission tomography can be used to help localize ectopic tumours.
- For ACTH-independent cases (low/undetectable levels), a CT scan of the suprarenal glands is the next appropriate investigation.

What treatment is available for patients with Cushing's syndrome?

In those patients where a suprarenal tumour is found, adrenalectomy is performed. Trans-sphenoidal microsurgery is used to remove a pituitary adenoma. Medical pre-treatment with drugs such as metyrapone and ketoconazole can help to control hypercortisolaemia prior to surgery.

Case 110 Congenital disease of both kidneys

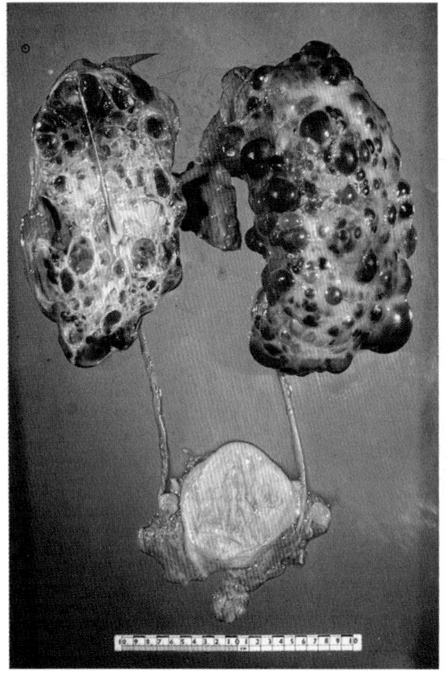

Figure 110.1

The specimen shown in Fig. 110.1 of both kidneys, ureters, bladder and adjacent aorta was obtained at postmortem on a 40-year-old man in the days before much could be done for patients with this congenital condition.

What is this abnormality called, and what is its embryological explanation?

Polycystic disease of the kidneys. It is believed to be due to failure of many of the tubules of the metanephros, which later develops into the kidney, to join with the metanephric duct, which gives rise to the calyces, the pelvis of the ureter and the ureter itself (Fig. 110.2).

There may be associated cysts in other viscera, particularly the liver (30%), lungs, spleen and pancreas. In addition, there is a strong association with intracranial berry aneurysms and the danger of subarachnoid haemorrhage.

Is it an inherited disease?

The condition is inherited as an autosomal dominant form, which presents usually in middle age. A less common autosomal recessive type presents in childhood, with renal failure. Genetically, the dominant form may result from a number of different gene mutations, the commonest being in the *PKD1* gene (chromosome 16p13.3).

How may this condition present clinically?

To some extent, this may be classified according to the age of the patient. It is surprising that patients with this gross bilateral renal disease may sometimes live on, untreated, into their sixties or more:

• *Antenatal*: The renal masses may be detected on routine ultrasound.

• *At birth*: There may be obstructed labour due to the abdominal masses.

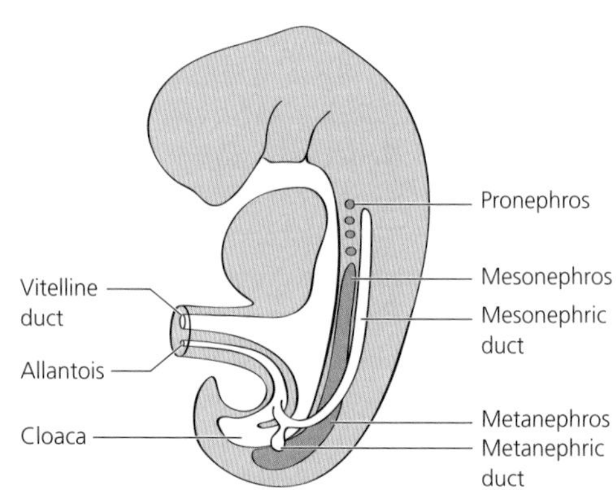

Figure 110.2 Development of the pro-, meso- and metanephric systems.

• *Infancy*: The baby may die from multiple congenital anomalies and renal failure.
• *Young adults*: Large bilateral symptomless masses may be found on a routine medical examination.

The patient, often a young adult, may present with hypertension. There may be urinary tract symptoms of loin pain, haematuria and renal infection. Eventually renal failure supervenes.

What are the two common forms of death from this condition, if untreated?

The patient either dies from renal failure or from the complications of hypertension – cardiac failure or a cerebrovascular catastrophe (cerebral haemorrhage or rupture of an associated berry aneurysm).

How is this condition treated?

Dialysis is commenced when the patient develops renal failure, followed by renal transplantation if he or she is fit enough.

Occasionally bilateral nephrectomy may be required, either to make room for the transplant, or to treat the otherwise uncontrolled hypertension, or for recurrent pain, infection or haematuria.

Case 111 Haematuria of sinister origin

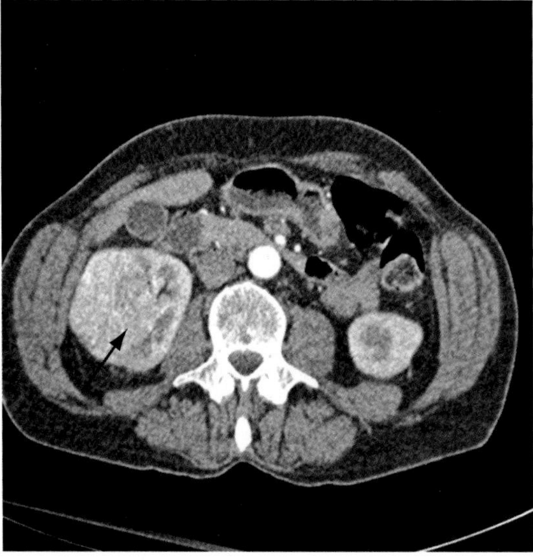

Figure 111.1

An electrician aged 60 years reported to his family practitioner with a 3-week history of passing blood in his urine, together with some clots. The practice nurse confirmed this by a dipstick test on a specimen of his urine and the patient was referred urgently to the urological clinic.

A detailed history and examination at the clinic gave little more information. The blood was noticed in every specimen of urine and some clots were seen in the outpatient specimen. He denied any abdominal or loin pain or, indeed, any other symptom. His appetite was good and, if anything, he had gained a few pounds in weight. Examination revealed a muscular, obese man.

Abdominal examination was normal, apart from an old appendicectomy scar. There was a moderate, smooth, rubbery enlargement of the prostate on rectal examination. Microscopy of the urine showed numerous red blood corpuscles. A full blood count and biochemistry profile were within normal limits and an outpatient flexible cystoscopy showed no abnormality in the urethra or bladder.

An urgent chest X-ray and abdominal CT were ordered. The chest film was clear. A typical film from the CT is shown in Fig. 111.1.

What does the CT demonstrate and what diagnosis does this suggest?

There is a solid mass in the right kidney (arrowed) and a normal left kidney. This is suggestive of a renal tumour as the cause of the patient's haematuria. As a result of this investigation a transabdominal right nephrectomy was performed.

Figure 111.2 is of a coronal section through the right kidney. What is the name given to this tumour, and what is its microscopic appearance?

This is an adenocarcinoma of the kidney. To the naked eye it has a golden yellow colour, together with haemorrhagic areas. 'Hypernephroma' is now an archaic term still occasionally used, dating back to the theory of its origin from suprarenal 'rests' postulated by Grawitz,* whose name is also eponymously applied to this tumour. Microscopically, the tumour cells are typically large with abundant foamy cytoplasm and with a small, central, densely staining nucleus – the so-called 'clear cell tumour'. The histology shows a typical example (Fig. 111.3), with a high power inset demonstrating the typical clear cells (arrowed).

What are the local symptoms that may draw attention to this tumour?

About 40% present with haematuria, as in the present case. This may be accompanied by the passage of clots. The clots may cause severe ureteric colic as they pass, or they may impact at the bladder outlet, with clot retention

*Paul Albert Grawitz (1850–1932), pathologist who worked with Virchow in Berlin.

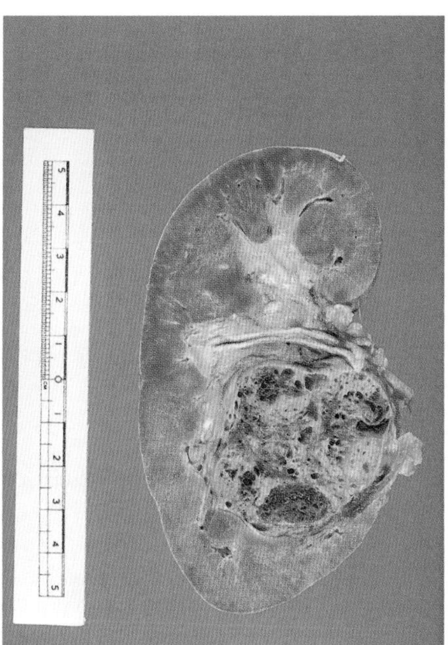
Figure 111.2 Coronal section through a right renal tumour.

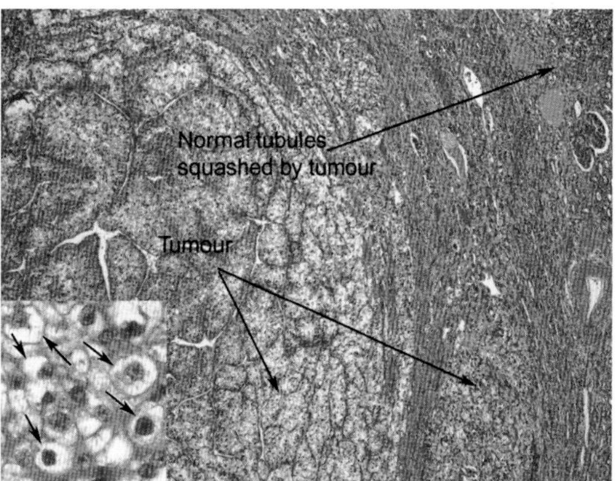

Figure 111.3 Histology picture of a renal carcinoma demonstrating the typical clear cells (arrowed) (magnification × 4 (inset × 20)).

of urine – either of these may bring the patient to hospital as an acute emergency. Another 40% present with an aching pain and/or a mass in the loin.

In what other ways may this tumour present?

The remaining 20% of patients manifest either with the effects of secondary deposits – typically to the lungs or bones (perhaps presenting with a pathological fracture, for example) – or with the general features of malignant disease, such as anaemia or loss of weight. Occasionally, the tumour presents with a pyrexia of unknown origin.

Describe how the tumour may metastasize

- By lymphatic spread to the para-aortic lymph nodes and thence by the thoracic duct to the supraclavicular nodes.
- By haematogenous spread via the renal vein into the inferior vena cava and thence to the lungs, skeleton, brain and elsewhere.

Case 112 A gross congenital abnormality

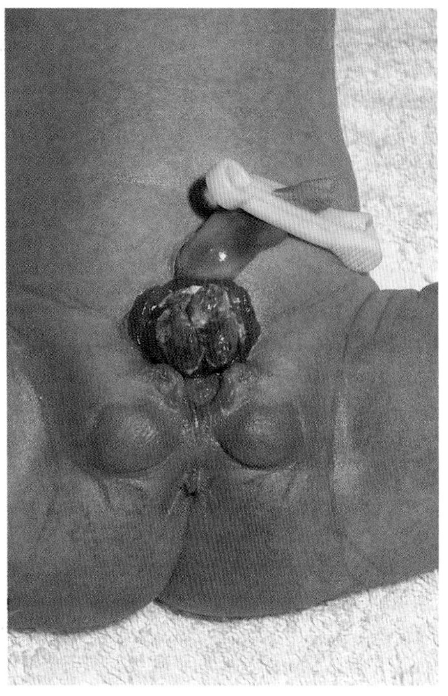

Figure 112.1

Figure 112.1 shows the appearance of the abdomen of a newly delivered baby girl. As well as the gross abnormality seen in the suprapubic area, it was also noted that urine was trickling continuously from below the protruding mass immediately distal of the clamped stump of the umbilical cord. Full examination of the baby revealed no other anomalies.

What is the name of this condition?

Ectopia vesicae – which means literally that the bladder is abnormally placed.

What is the nature of this condition?

The bladder fails to develop normally and the ureters, together with the trigone of the bladder (the triangle between the ureteric orifices and the bladder outlet), open directly onto the anterior abdominal wall. In the male there is associated epispadias of the penis.

This child has a commonly associated abnormality of the pelvic girdle; the visible nodule on each side of the exposed bladder mucosa is the corresponding pubic ramus. What does this comprise?

Frequently, as in this child, there is a failure of the pubic bones to meet in the midline at the symphysis. This results in a widened pelvis and the child eventually walks with a waddling gait.

Left untreated, what is the natural history of this condition?

The child may die of pyelonephritis due to ascending urinary tract infection. Carcinoma of the bladder rudiment may take place after initial metaplastic change. Note that this tumour is therefore a stratified squamous carcinoma, not a transitional cell tumour, which is the usual carcinoma of the uroepithelium.

What surgical treatment is usually carried out in this condition?

Attempts to reconstruct the bladder have been made, but are usually unsuccessful. Standard treatment usually comprises reimplantation of the ureters into an ileal conduit, which drains into a plastic bag attached around the ileostomy spout stoma. The bladder remnant is excised as a prophylaxis against malignant change.

Case 113 A bladder stone found at autopsy

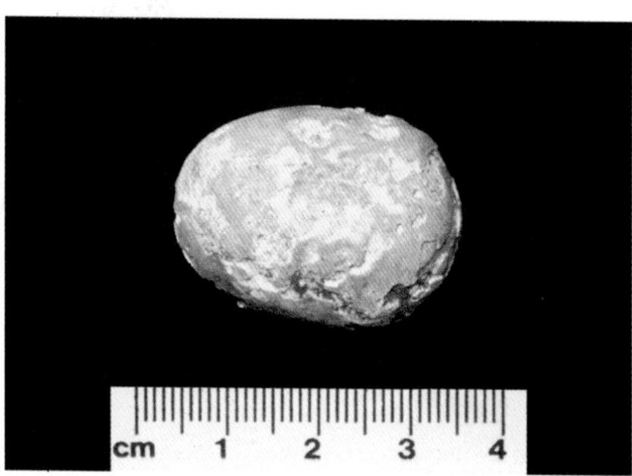

Figure 113.1

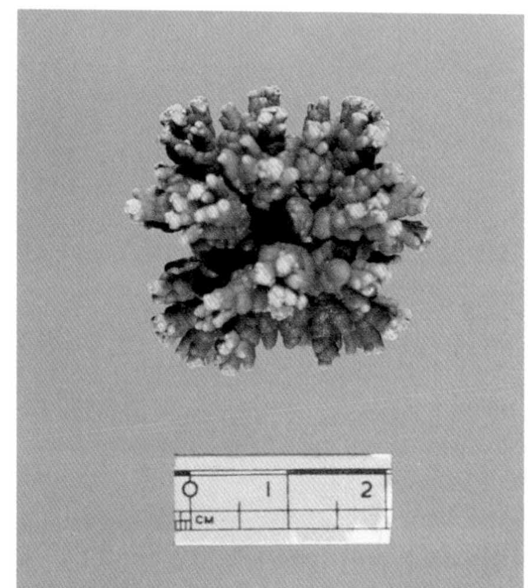

Figure 113.2 Oxalate stone.

Figure 113.1 shows a calculus removed from the bladder at the postmortem performed on an old gentleman of 92 years. He had contracted gonorrhoea while serving as a soldier in France in World War I at the age of 22. This had been treated with irrigations of antiseptic fluid. By the 1930s, when he was working as an agricultural labourer, he had developed a urethral stricture and attended hospital as an outpatient for regular dilatations of the urethra with metal bougies at the 'stricture clinic'. Over subsequent years he had repeated episodes of urinary tract infection and also of retention of urine, on one occasion requiring a temporary suprapubic cystotomy. He eventually died in an old people's home from bronchopneumonia (which complicated his smoker's chronic bronchitis) as well as congestive heart failure and urinary infection. He had requested that his body should be used 'to assist medical science'.

At autopsy the bladder was thick walled, heavily trabeculated and chronically inflamed. The urine in the bladder was full of debris, had a strong fishy smell and contained the large calculus shown in Fig. 113.1.

What is the likely chemical composition of this bladder stone?

It has the typical appearance of a calcium ammonium and magnesium phosphate ('triple phosphate') stone. It is greyish-white in colour.

Name the three other types of urinary calculi

- *Oxalate stones*: These are the most common, comprising about 60%. They are hard, with a sharp spiky surface, which traumatizes the urinary epithelium. The resultant bleeding often colours the stone a dark brown or black (see Case 108, p. 225). A typical example, removed from the bladder, is shown in Fig. 113.2.
- *Uric acid and urate stones* (5%): These are moderately hard, brown in colour and with a smooth surface. Pure uric acid stones are radiolucent but, fortunately, from the diagnosis point of view, usually contain enough calcium to show up on plain X-ray.

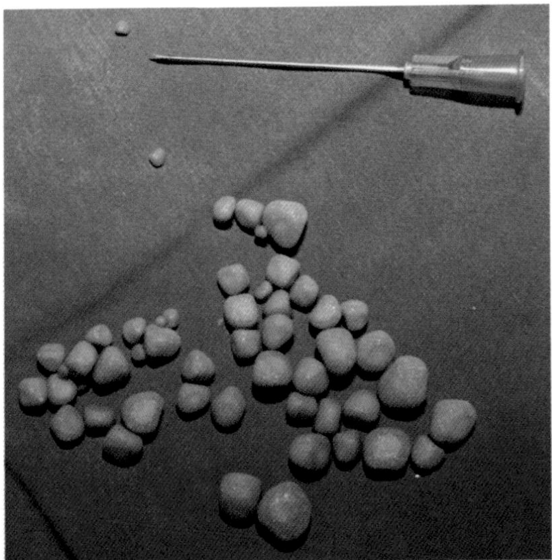

Figure 113.3 Cystine stone.

- *Cystine stones*: Found in patients with the congenital metabolic abnormality of cystinuria, these stones are rare (Fig. 113.3).

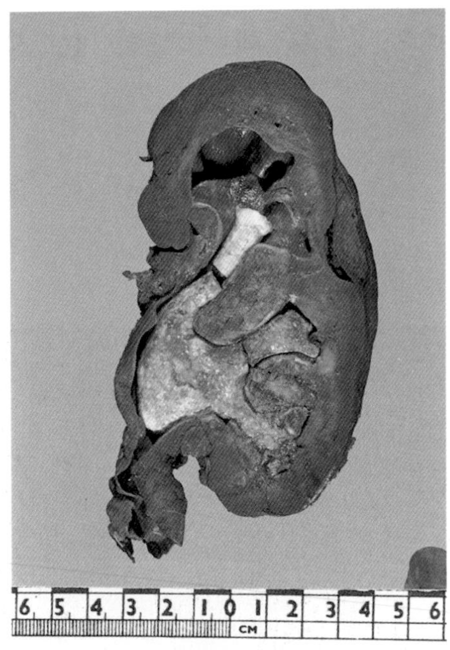

Figure 113.4 Staghorn calculus.

Under what circumstances do triple phosphate stones form?

This type of stone is found in infected and stagnant urine. It is, for example, the 'staghorn' calculus that forms in the pelvis and calyces of a pyonephrosis of the kidney (Fig. 113.4). This type of calculus may also form around foreign material left anywhere in the urinary tract – around non-absorbable sutures, a broken-off piece of catheter or any of the multitudinous strange objects such as hairpins or pieces of tubing that people may insert into their bladders.

What is the classical triad of symptoms that often occur in patients with bladder stone?

Urinary frequency, dysuria (pain on passing urine) and haematuria.

What special investigations are used to confirm the clinical diagnosis of bladder stone?

A plain X-ray of the abdomen often demonstrates the calculus because of its high calcium content. The X-ray in Fig. 113.5 shows a typical example – a large triple phosphate stone in the bladder of a north African woman who had previously had a vesico-vaginal fistula repaired. Cystoscopy enabled the stone to be directly visualized.

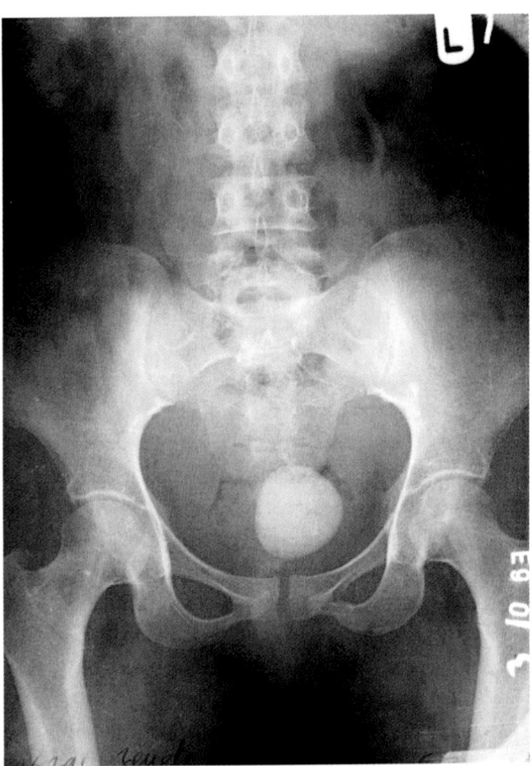

Figure 113.5 X-ray of a triple phosphate stone.

Case 114 An insidious cause of lumbago

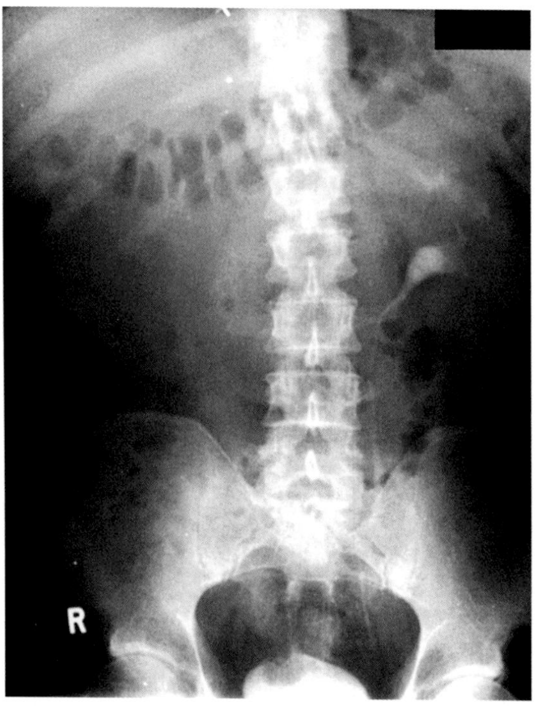

Figure 114.1

A house painter and decorator aged 62 years reported to his family doctor complaining of 'lumbago' for the past 4 or 5 weeks. When the doctor went carefully into the story, this was in fact a dull aching pain experienced in the right loin, which was getting worse, was present most of the time, disturbing his sleep, but was relieved somewhat with the proprietary analgesic tablets the patient was getting from his pharmacist. Apart from nocturia ×1, which he had been experiencing now for about a year, he denied any urinary symptoms; in particular, he had not noticed any change in the colour of his urine.

On examination, his GP found him to be a heavily built, overweight but otherwise healthy man. Nothing was found on abdominal examination but a dipstick test on his urine was positive for blood. He was therefore referred urgently to the local hospital, which had a special haematuria clinic.

At the clinic, the surgeon confirmed the above findings but there was deep tenderness, although no mass to feel, on deep bimanual palpation of the right flank. Rectal examination revealed a moderately enlarged, smooth-rubbery prostate. Microscopy of the urine, which was slightly turbid to the naked eye, showed numerous red blood corpuscles. An urgent intravenous urogram was ordered, and Fig. 114.1 shows the 15 min film of the series:

Describe the abnormal findings on this X-ray film (Fig. 114.1)

There is an irregular filling defect on the right side of the bladder, in the region of the right ureteric orifice. The right calyceal system and ureter are not visualized. The left kidney and ureter are normal.

What radiological diagnosis can be deduced from this investigation?

There is a tumour in the right side of the bladder that has obstructed the ureteric orifice. This has presumably resulted in hydronephrosis of the right kidney with gross functional impairment. The fact that the ureteric orifice is occluded is in favour of the tumour being malignant. Note that this is a good example of how a lesion in one part of the urinary tract may present with features in another part. Here, the bladder tumour presents with loin pain due to the resultant hydronephrosis.

What special investigation needs to be carried out in order to confirm the diagnosis?

Cystoscopy and transurethral biopsy. This was carried out under a general anaesthetic, which enabled a bimanual examination of the pelvis to be performed. A distinct mass was detected. Cystoscopy showed a sessile, superficially ulcerated mass overlying the right ureter. Biopsies were taken.

What would be the likely histological diagnosis of the tumour?

Transitional cell carcinoma is by far and away the commonest malignant tumour of the 'uroepithelium', which extends from the renal pelvis, along the ureter, the bladder and the urethra to just before the urethral orifice.

What factors predispose to the development of bladder cancer?

There is a raised incidence of bladder cancer in smokers. There is a high incidence of malignant change in the exposed mucosa of ectopia vesicae (see Case 112, p. 234) and in the bladder infected with schistosomiasis. Malignant change may also take place within a bladder diverticulum. Bladder tumours were once extremely common in aniline dye and rubber workers because of the excretion of carcinogens, such as β-naphthylamine, in the urine. Public health measures have eliminated this problem in the UK.

Examination of the tumour biopsy material revealed a poorly differentiated transitional cell carcinoma invading muscle. The patient was treated with platinum-based chemotherapy (cisplatin and gemcitabine) followed by radical cystectomy with formation of an ileal conduit, a loop of isolated ileum acting as a new bladder to which the ureters were anastomosed.

Case 115 A man with difficulty passing urine and with an interesting X-ray

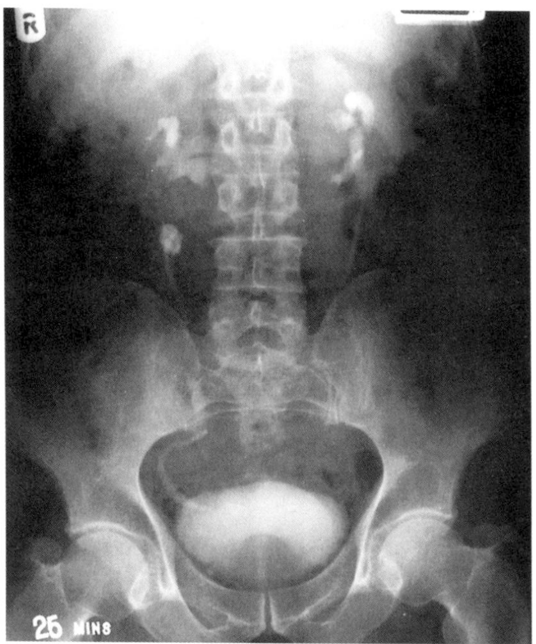

Figure 115.1

A retired postal worker aged 70 years was referred to the urological clinic with a history of increasing difficulty passing his urine. He first noticed increasing frequency of micturition about 5 years previously. This became progressively more marked, so that he was now passing urine every 2 or 3 h during the day and three or four times at night. There was a good deal of urgency, so that he now planned any journey away from home to ensure that there was a lavatory available in the vicinity. The stream was poor, there was dribbling and he was occasionally incontinent of urine. The urine itself was clear and he had never seen blood in it. Apart from this, his general health was good. He was a smoker and had a morning productive cough.

On examination, he was thin and appeared well. On abdominal examination there was a smooth swelling to feel three fingers above the pubis, which was dull to percussion. Pressure on this gave him the desire to pass urine. On rectal examination there was a considerable smooth, rubbery enlargement of the prostate.

His routine full blood count and biochemistry were normal, including his serum urea and creatinine. The chest X-ray was clear. His serum prostate-specific antigen (PSA) was 8 ng/ml. (Note that although the normal upper limit for this is less than 4 ng/ml, this may be increased in benign prostatic hypertrophy in the range of 4–12 ng/ml.)

An intravenous urogram was ordered and Fig. 115.1 shows the 25 min film.

What evidence can you see in Fig. 115.1 of prostatic enlargement?

Intravesical enlargement of the prostate is shown by the globular filling defect at the base of the bladder. The bladder outline itself is slightly irregular instead of being completely smooth. This suggests that it is thickened and trabeculated due to chronic obstruction.

What do you notice about the appearance of the lower ends of the ureters?

The terminations of the ureters are hooked upwards. This is caused by the enlarged prostate pushing up the trigone of the bladder.

Apart from the urinary tract, what else should you look for carefully on films in a patient with prostatic symptoms?

The lumbar spine and pelvis should be carefully studied on these X-rays for evidence of secondary deposits, frequently sclerotic, which are often present in patients with prostatic cancer (see Case 116, p. 241).

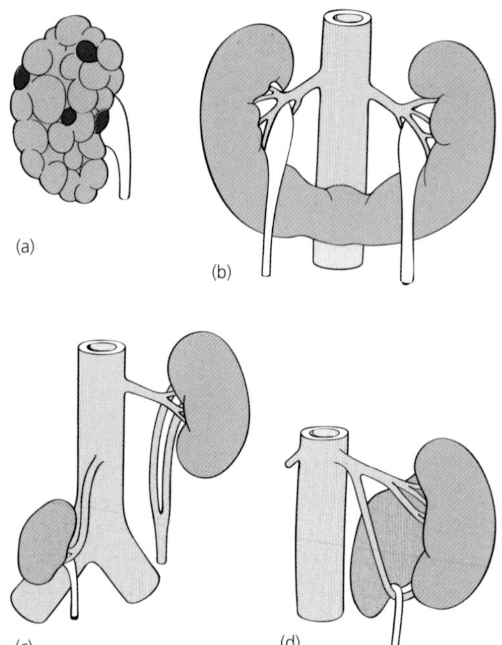

Figure 115.2 Renal abnormalities: (a) polycystic kidney, (b) horseshoe kidney, (c) pelvic kidney and double ureter, and (d) aberrant renal artery and associated hydronephrosis.

The renal pelvises on this film demonstrate a congenital renal abnormality. What is this?

Note that the renal pelvises are deviated laterally. This is the typical appearance of a horseshoe kidney, a diagram of which is shown in Fig. 115.2.

There is another abnormality to see on the X-ray, adjacent to the right ureter, which is not related to the urinary tract. What is it?

This area of speckled calcification is typical of a calcified tuberculous mesenteric lymph node, probably due to ingestion of contaminated milk as a child. It is sometimes mistaken for a radio-opaque ureteric stone.

Case 116 Sciatica with a sinister cause

A retired railway worker aged 82 years was referred to the orthopaedic outpatient clinic with a note that read 'Severe lumbago and right-sided sciatica, ? prolapsed intervertebral disc.'

Why did the surgeon discard the diagnosis of 'prolapsed intervertebral disc' on reading the referral letter and even before seeing the old gentleman?

A prolapsed intervertebral disc is prolapse of the nucleus pulposus, the jelly-like centre of the disc (Fig. 116.1). This becomes less differentiated from the surrounding annulus fibrosus as age progresses. By the age of 55, it has more or less disappeared as a distinct structure. A 'prolapsed disc' in the late fifties is rare – in the eighties it is an impossibility!

When a detailed history was taken in the orthopaedic clinic, the patient described the pain as being in the region of the lumbar spine, the pelvis and spreading down the back of the thigh to the level of the ankle. It had commenced 3 or 4 months previously, and was getting much worse. It was a severe, dull pain, which kept him awake at night, was aggravated by coughing and straining, and was no longer relieved by analgesic tablets. In addition, the patient was having problems passing his urine, with hesitancy, poor stream, dribbling and a frequency of every 3 or 4 h during the day and three or four times at night.

On examination he was in obvious pain. The lumbar spine was held rigid, with marked erector spinae spasm. Straight leg raising on the left was 70°, and on the right side 30°, and painful. There were no gross neurological anomalies. On rectal examination, the prostate was enlarged, irregular and woody hard.

What is now your clinical diagnosis?

The patient has marked prostatic symptoms and the clinical findings on rectal examination strongly suggest that he has a carcinoma of the prostate. The recent history of lumbar and pelvic pain, with sciatic radiation makes it likely that he has lumbar and pelvic secondary bone deposits.

The consultant urologist ordered X-rays of the chest, lumbar spine and pelvis. The chest X-ray was clear. Figure 116.2 is the film of the patient's lower lumbar spine, pelvis and hips. What does it demonstrate?

There are extensive osteosclerotic deposits in the lumbar vertebrae, upper sacrum and the pelvic bones. Prostatic secondary deposits typically produce osteosclerotic lesions, whereas other secondary deposits are usually osteolytic (compare Case 100, p. 207).

Give an anatomical explanation for the patient's lumbar pain and its radiation

Prostatic cancer spreads readily by Bateson's* valveless vertebral venous plexus from the prostatic venous plexus to the vertebrae and pelvic bones. Wedging and pathological fractures account for the lumbar pain. Involvement of the sacral nerve roots explains the pain radiating down the back of the thigh (S2, S3, S4). Coughing and straining increase the spinal cerebrospinal fluid pressure and aggravate the pain.

How may the diagnosis be confirmed in this patient?

His prostate specific antigen was estimated and was 30 ng/ml, which is well in the range of disseminated prostatic cancer. Tissue diagnosis can be obtained by performing a transrectal biopsy of the prostate under ultrasound guidance. However, this is an invasive procedure, nearly always accompanied by marked haematuria

*Oscar Bateson (1894–1979), Professor of anatomy, University of Pennsylvania, Philadelphia.

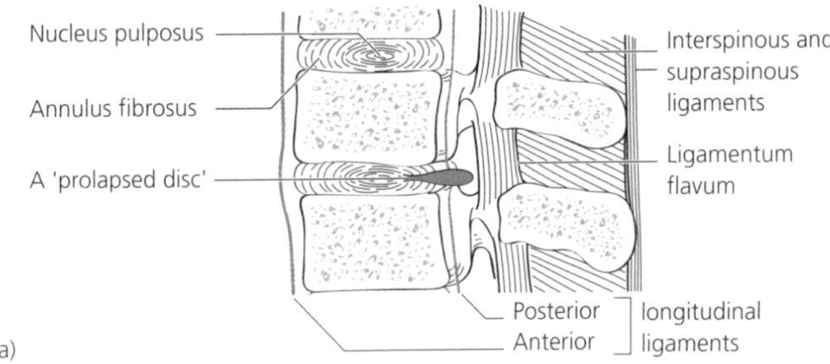

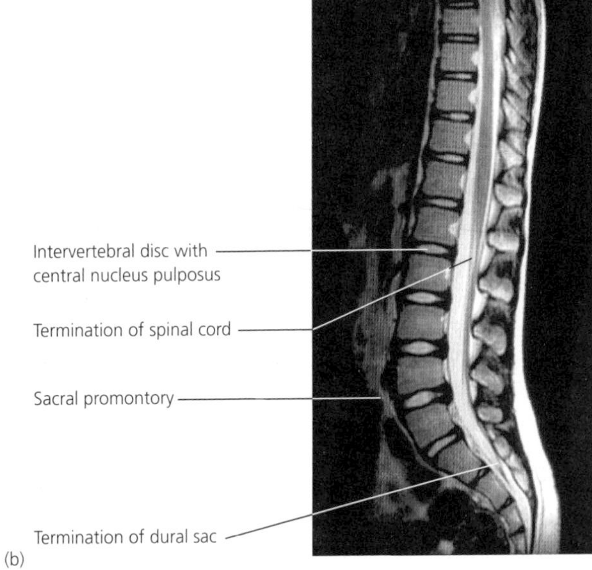

Figure 116.1 (a) Longitudinal section through the lumbar vertebrae showing a prolapsed intervertebral disc. (b) MR image through a normal lumbar spine and sacrum. Note the excellent anatomical details.

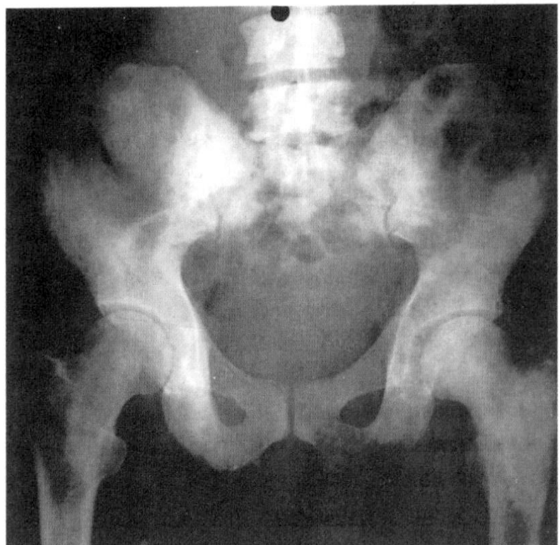

Figure 116.2 X-ray of the lower lumbar spine, pelvis and hips.

and with the risk of septicaemia, so that it needs to be covered by broad spectrum antibiotics. In this case, it was considered that the diagnosis was sufficiently established to merit avoidance of a biopsy.

What treatments are available for patients such as this with disseminated prostatic cancer?

- The mainstay of treatment is androgen suppression or the use of specific androgen antagonists, which will produce symptomatic relief in about 75% of cases.
- Radiotherapy may relieve the pain of bony deposits and can also be used for local control of the prostate to supplement hormonal therapy.
- Urinary obstruction due to the prostatic tumour may resolve on hormonal therapy; if not, a transurethral endoscopic prostatectomy may be required.

Case 117 A patient with a very distended bladder

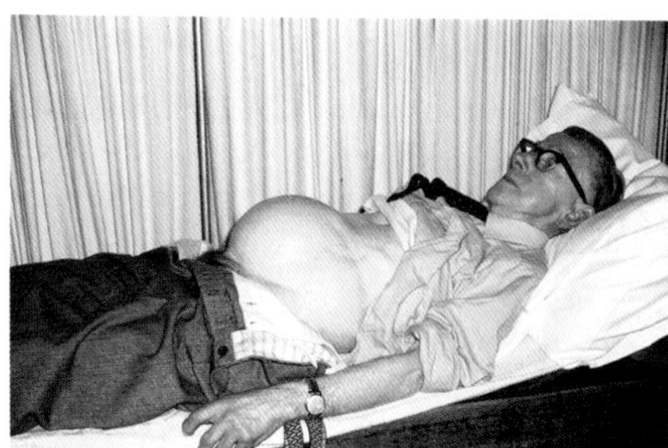

Figure 117.1

Figure 117.1 shows a 72-year-old grocer who is still running his own street corner shop. He walked into the surgical outpatient clinic complaining of some frequency passing his urine. This was the surprising appearance of his abdomen when he lay on the examination couch.

On taking a detailed history from the patient, he had experienced increasing frequency of micturition, dribbling and a poor stream for the past 5 or 6 years, but put this down to 'getting old' and did nothing about it. In the past 3 months this was becoming a real nuisance. He was now dribbling urine 30 to 60 min during the day and several times at night and sometimes wet himself, especially in bed and while asleep. Apart from this, he felt quite well and had come to the clinic straight from working in his shop.

On examination, as can be seen in Fig. 117.1, he looked well with a good colour and a moist tongue. Abdominal examination revealed this large smooth, painless swelling, which reached to just above the umbilicus and which was dull to percussion. On rectal examination, the prostate was considerably and smoothly enlarged and was rubbery in consistency.

What is your clinical diagnosis?

The patient has *chronic* retention of urine, due to a clinically benign prostatic hypertrophy. *Acute* retention is extremely painful, but, in the chronic case, the bladder becomes progressively and gradually distended.

The intense frequency in these patients is actually dribbling of urine from the full bladder, the so-called 'retention with overflow' or 'overflow incontinence'.

Apart from benign prostatic hypertrophy, what other local causes are there for retention of urine?

As with any obstructed tube in the body, think of 'causes in the lumen, in the wall and outside the wall':

- Within the lumen of the urethra: Stone or blood clot ('clot retention').
- In the urethral wall: Urethral stricture (see Case 113, p. 235).
- Outside the wall: Carcinoma of the prostate (see Case 116, p. 241) or occasionally pressure from faecal impaction or from a pelvic tumour.

What may be the causes of retention of urine in the absence of an actual urethral obstruction?

The 'general' causes of retention of urine may be classified into:

- Postoperative.
- CNS disease, e.g. paraplegia from trauma, tumour, etc., multiple sclerosis, diabetes mellitus.
- Drugs, e.g. anticholinergics, tricyclic depressants.

What clinical features might suggest renal damage (uraemia) in a patient such as this with chronic retention?

The patient with uraemia may complain of headache, anorexia and vomiting. He may have a dry coated tongue and be drowsy.

How would you further investigate and manage this patient?

He needs urgent admission to the urological unit and

prompt further investigations. The essentials are a chest X-ray and full blood count. Serum electrolytes, urea and creatinine should be ordered to investigate his urinary function, which may have been impaired by chronic back pressure on the kidneys. A prostate-specific antigen (PSA) estimation could well be elevated even in advanced benign disease and in the elderly subject, so it is by no means a diagnostic test for prostatic carcinoma. An intravenous urogram is valuable in demonstrating the anatomical details of his urinary tract (see Case 115, p. 239).

In this patient, the investigations were within normal limits, apart from a raised creatinine (154 μmol/L) and the ultrasound scan, which confirmed a large prostate, distended bladder and mild bilateral hydronephrosis.

A transurethral resection of the prostate was performed. He had a reasonably smooth postoperative course and his prostatic tissue was benign on histological examination.

Case 118 A foreskin problem in a child

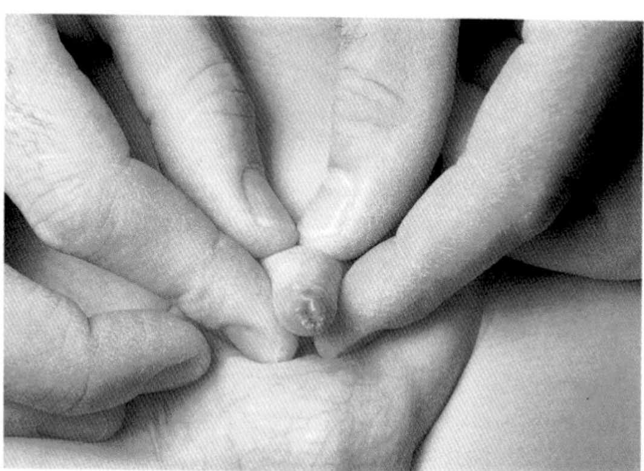

Figure 118.1

The parents brought this little boy, aged nearly 4 years, to the surgical clinic because they had never been able to retract his prepuce. Apart from this, the child was entirely well. His father had been circumcised as a baby.

What is your diagnosis?

Phimosis – the term implies gross narrowing of the preputial orifice.

What often leads to the development of this condition?

Although this may occur as a congenital condition, it often results from repeated trauma of forcible attempts to retract the baby's foreskin or may result from chronic balanitis.

What is the natural history of the prepuce in children?

The prepuce is normally non-retractile in the first few months of life, due to congenital adhesions between the glans and the prepuce. By the end of the first year, 50% can be retracted easily, and the great majority are retractile by the third or fourth year.

What is the function of the prepuce in the baby?

The prepuce protects the glans and the urethral orifice from the excoriation of ammoniacal dermatitis.

What are the indications for circumcision in children?

Circumcision may be requested by the parents on religious grounds. It is indicated when there is established organic phimosis, as in this case, or in those instances when the prepuce cannot be retracted after the age of 6.

Case 119 An ulcerated prepuce

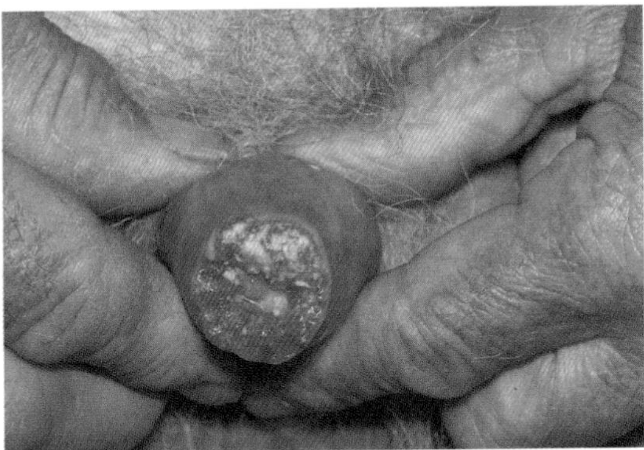

Figure 119.1

This 85-year-old retired labourer presented with a foul-smelling and ulcerated lesion of the penis, which had been getting progressively worse over the past year. He noticed blood-staining of his underpants. He had been treating the lesion with various proprietary ointments. On examination, the prepuce could only be retracted as far as can be seen in Fig. 119.1. The ulcer felt hard; it involved the glans itself, as well as the inner aspect of the prepuce.

What is the obvious clinical diagnosis, and what will be its likely histological appearance?

This is an ulcerating tumour of the penis. The vast majority of these are stratified squamous cell carcinomas.

How does this tumour spread?

- *Local*: The tumour may fungate through the prepuce and may spread along the shaft of the penis to destroy its substance. Surprisingly, it rarely occludes the urethra, so retention of urine does not occur.
- *Lymphatic*: To the inguinal lymph nodes on either side.
- *Blood-borne*: Spread to the lungs is late and is unusual.

In what group of men is this disease rarely seen?

It is virtually unknown in Jews, who are circumcised soon after birth. This eliminates the presence of retained smegma under the prepuce, which is the almost invariable pre-existing factor in this disease.

What is the cause of death in this disease?

Haemorrhage from the fungating involved inguinal lymph nodes.

How is this condition treated?

The diagnosis is first confirmed by biopsy. Early lesions are treated by radiotherapy, usually by implantation of iridium wires. If the urethra is invaded, as in this case, partial amputation of the penis is required, as the radiation therapy would result in a urethral stricture. Survival from early disease is good.

When the regional lymph nodes are involved but are still operable, radical amputation of the penis and bilateral block dissection of the inguinal nodes is required. Since the external urethral sphincter is preserved, the patient remains continent of urine, although he needs to micturate in the sitting position.

Inoperable fixed inguinal nodes are treated with palliative radiotherapy.

Case 120 A missing testis

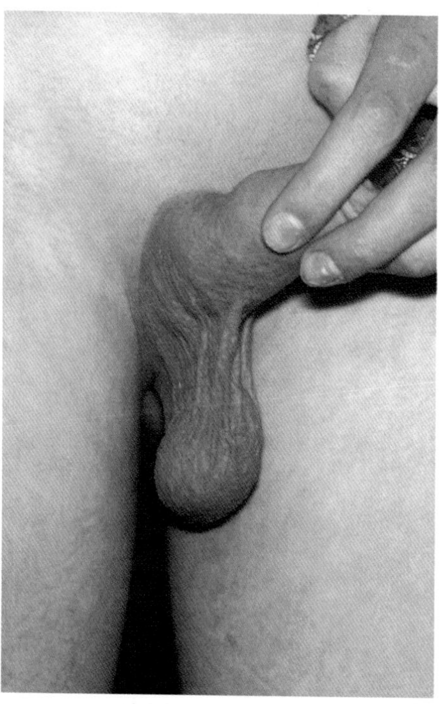

Figure 120.1

This 19-year-old college student, a keen footballer, was admitted to the orthopaedic unit for arthroscopic excision of a loose body from his left knee. When he was fully examined by the surgeon preoperatively, it was noted that the patient's right testis was absent, nor could a testis be felt along the line of the right inguinal canal, or at the base of the penis (Fig. 120.1). The left testis was normal in size and position. There was no history of previous surgery, nor was there any surgical scar. Surprisingly, the young man was completely unaware of the fact that he only possessed one testis.

What is this condition called?

The patient has a (previously undiagnosed) right undescended testis. The term cryptorchidism is often used to refer to the absence of a testis from the scrotum.

Apart from previous surgical removal, there are two other causes of an absent testis (or testes). What are these? And how are they differentiated from an undescended testis?

• *A retractile testis* (or testes): This is a normal testis where an excessively active cremasteric reflex draws the testis up to the apex of the scrotum or even to the external inguinal ring. It is a common phenomenon in babies and young children, but may be seen in adolescents. On careful examination, the testis can be coaxed into the scrotum. Moreover, the patient (or the parents, in young children) may notice that the testis is in its normal scrotal position when the subject is relaxed in a warm bath.

• *An ectopic testis*: The testis has emerged from the external inguinal ring but has strayed into an 'ectopic' position – the commonest is in the superficial inguinal pouch, which lies in front of the external oblique aponeurosis. Other rare situations are the groin, the perineum, the root of the penis or the femoral triangle.

Figure 120.2 is an example of the commonest variety of ectopic testis. This 7-year-old boy has a normally placed left testis, of normal size for his age. The right scrotum is empty, but there is an obvious bulge in his right groin, which can be seen (arrowed) immediately above the examiner's index finger. This testis cannot be coaxed into the scrotum. It has thus emerged from the external inguinal ring and has then passed, ectopically, to its position in front of the external oblique aponeurosis. At operation, it was mobilized and easily deposited into the scrotum.

What are the complications of an undescended testis?

• Defective spermatogenesis: Sperm production depends on the testis being at room temperature. If the testis is malpositioned the testicular tubules commence to degenerate in early childhood. Bilateral undescended

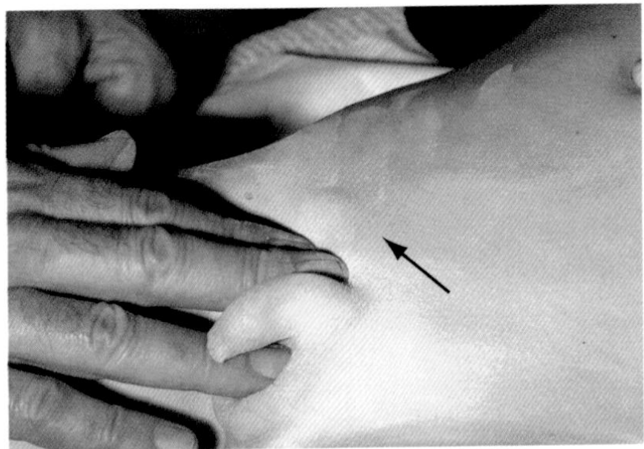

Figure 120.2 Ectopic testis.

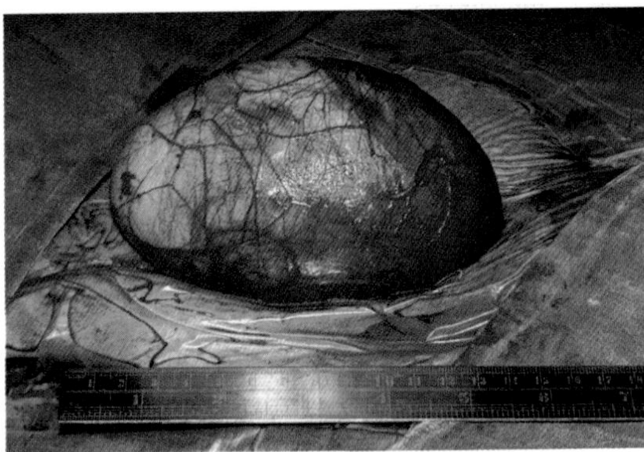

Figure 120.3 Seminoma of an ectopic testis exposed through an inguinal incision. Orchidectomy was performed.

testes, therefore, will result in sterility. In contrast, the interstitial cells of the testis, which secrete the male sex hormones, remain unaffected so secondary sexual characteristics develop normally at puberty in children with bilateral, untreated, undescended testes.

- Increased risk of testicular torsion.
- Increased risk of trauma: The tethered testis cannot slip away from a direct injury.
- Increased risk of malignant change, which remains true even if surgical correction is carried out. Figure 120.3 was taken at operation and shows a seminoma of an ectopic testis exposed in the groin of a man aged 32.
- Psychological: Even young boys can be embarrassed by their anomaly.

What is the treatment of this condition?

The ectopic or undescended testis must be placed in the scrotum and this must be done before damage is done to the spermatogenic tubules. The operation is carried out around the age of 2. This procedure, termed orchidopexy, comprises mobilization of the testis and its cord, removal of the coexisting congenital inguinal hernia sac and fixation of the testis in the scrotum without tension.

Case 121 A swelling in the scrotum

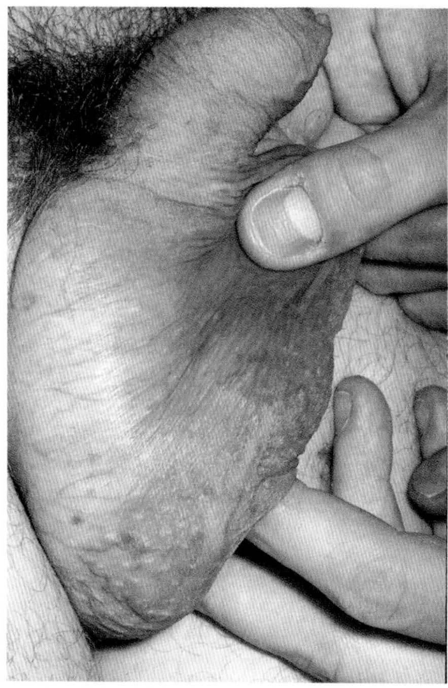

Figure 121.1

Figure 121.1 is of the scrotum of a man of 45 years who had noticed a lump in the right side of the scrotum about a year previously. This was entirely painless and did not really bother him. However, as it was slowly getting bigger, he decided to report to his doctor, who referred him to the surgical outpatient clinic.

Describe the steps you would take in the examination of a scrotal swelling such as this one

When examining any scrotal swelling, the following three points should be considered in turn:

1 Can your fingers meet above the swelling? If this is not possible, the swelling arises from within the abdomen, and the mass is an inguino-scrotal hernia.

2 If you can palpate clearly above the swelling, is the swelling cystic? If the mass is cystic on transillumination and the testis can be felt distinctly separately from the mass, the swelling is a cyst of the epididymis. However, if the testis cannot be felt separately because it is situated within the cyst, it is a hydrocele.

3 However, if the swelling is solid, the following must be considered:

- The swelling is a solid mass in the testis – it is a testicular tumour (today, a gumma of the testis is a rarity).
- The epididymis is involved – almost always an inflammatory condition, acute or chronic epididymitis. The latter is either tuberculous, which is uncommon in the UK, or the residual chronic thickening that may persist for many months after an acute pyogenic epididymitis which has been treated with an antibiotic.

This scheme of examination is shown in Fig. 121.2.

In this patient, the fingers could meet easily above the swelling, which was smooth, non-tender, cystic and which could be felt to be separate from the right testis, which lay inferiorly to it. The room was darkened and the scrotum transilluminated with a torch, as shown in Fig. 121.3.

What does this demonstrate, and what now is your diagnosis?

The mass transilluminates brilliantly – it is a cyst that is separate from the adjacent testis below it, and is therefore an epididymal cyst.

What may be the appearance of the contents of this cyst, and how does this contrast with the fluid in a hydrocele?

The fluid in an epididymal cyst may be water-clear or may be milky in appearance. It may occasionally contain

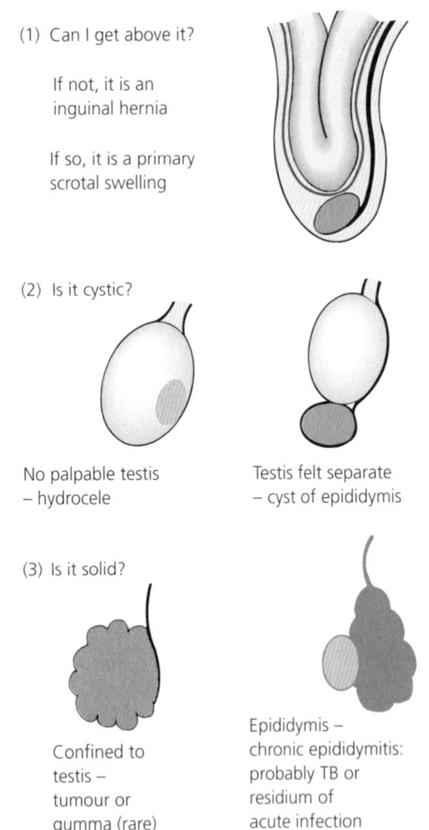

Figure 121.2 Scheme for the examination of a scrotal swelling.

sperm, hence the now discarded name of 'spermatocele'. In contrast, hydrocele fluid is yellow.

Can cysts of the epididymis be multiple, and can they be bilateral?

The answer to both questions is yes – and not infrequently so.

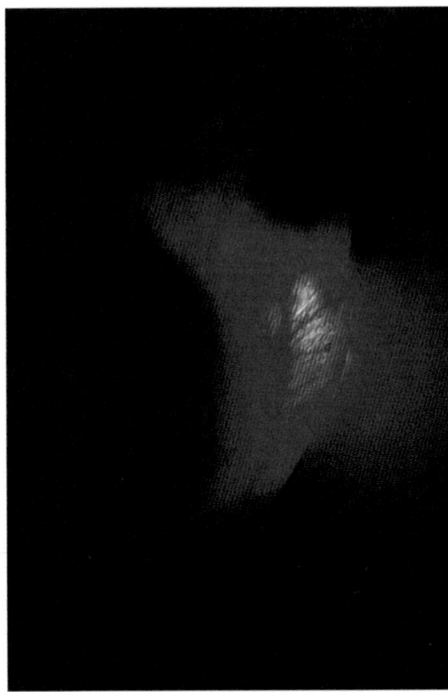

Figure 121.3 Transillumination of the scrotum.

What treatment would you advise in a patient with this condition?

A small cyst, which does not bother the patient, can be left alone. The patient is reassured that he has a simple benign cyst. If he is worried about the lump, it can be removed surgically, leaving the testis and epididymis intact. Simple aspiration of the cyst gives only temporary relief, as it invariably slowly refills.

Case 122 Two examples of testicular tumours

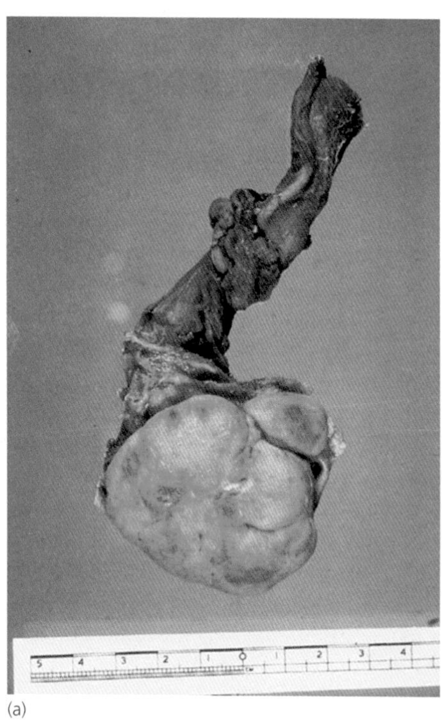
(a)

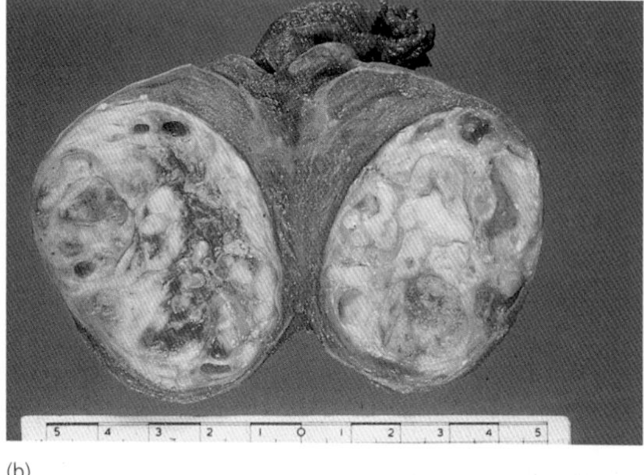
(b)

Figure 122.1

Figure 122.1 shows the cut surface of two testes, together with their spermatic cords, that were removed surgically. Figure 122.1a is from a man aged 37 years and Fig. 122.1b is from a student aged 17.

What is your diagnosis of the first tumour and what is its histological appearance?

Figure 122.1a has the typical appearance of a seminoma – rather like a cut potato. Histologically, it comprises sheets of cells, which may vary from well differentiated spermatocytes to undifferentiated round cells with clear cytoplasm. Some 10% arise in undescended tests (see Case 120, p. 247 and Fig. 120.3).

What is your diagnosis of the second specimen, and what is its microscopic appearance?

Figure 122.1b is a teratoma of the testis. It occurs usually in a younger age group, peaking at 20–30 years, in contrast to the age range of seminoma of 30–40 years. Macroscopically it usually has a cystic appearance, and areas of haemorrhage and infarction are common. Histologically, the appearance is very variable and the tumour may contain cartilage, bone, muscle, fat and other tissues. The rare variety of chorionepithelioma may contain syncytial tissue.

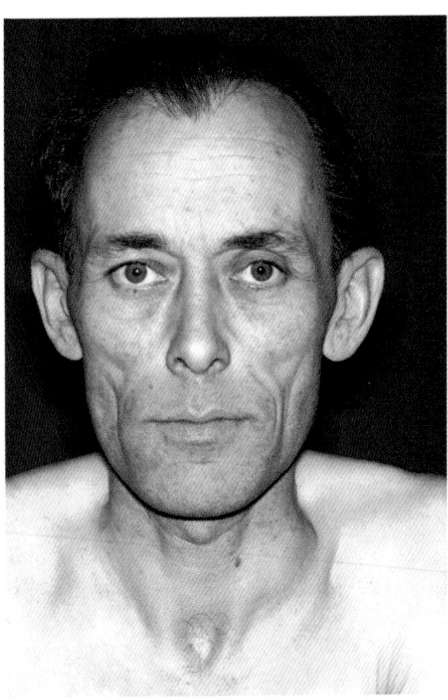

Figure 122.2 Lymph nodes in the left supraclavicular fossa.

What may be the local presenting features of a testicular tumour?

The tumour commonly presents as an enlarging painless mass in the testis. There is often an effusion of fluid into the tunica vaginalis, producing a secondary hydrocele, which may lead to misdiagnosis. The fluid in such a case is often blood-stained, unlike the clear yellow fluid of a primary hydrocele. Occasionally the tumour may manifest as a painful, rapidly enlarging swelling that is mistaken for an orchitis. Rarely a late case presents with the tumour ulcerating through the overlying scrotal skin.

Describe the pathways of dissemination of testicular tumours

Lymphatic spread is to the para-aortic lymph nodes via the lymphatics that accompany the testicular vein. Spread may then occur along the thoracic duct to the supraclavicular nodes, especially on the left side. Figure 122.2 is a photograph of a patient who presented with a hard, painless mass in the left testis who, on examination, had this obvious mass of hard, discrete lymph nodes in the left supraclavicular fossa.

Blood-borne spread from testicular teratoma occurs relatively early to the lungs and liver. In seminoma, this spread tends to be later in the natural history of the disease.

Discuss tumour markers in testicular tumours

Teratomas of the testis usually produce α-fetoprotein and may also produce β-human gonadotrophin (β-hCG). Some seminomas also secrete β-hCG. These are of use in making a diagnosis, but are also valuable in subsequent follow-up and in diagnosis of occult recurrence of the tumour.

Outline the initial diagnostic approach and operative management. Why is orchidectomy not performed through the scrotum?

Suspected tumours are investigated by ultrasonography. If they are suspicious of tumour, or if doubt exists, they are explored through a groin incision, through which the testis is delivered. An atraumatic clamp is placed across the cord. If the diagnosis is clear then an immediate orchidectomy is performed; if doubt exists a frozen section is performed and, if tumour is confirmed, an orchidectomy performed. Orchidectomy is performed through an inguinal rather than a scrotal approach to avoid tumour exposure to scrotal skin and lymphatics (which drain to the inguinal nodes, unlike the cord which drains to the internal iliac nodes). If this were done, radiation to the scrotum may be required to avoid local recurrence, with inevitable consequences to the contralateral testis.

Outline the different adjuvant therapies for the different tumour types. What is the prognosis for a young man with a testicular tumour confined to the scrotum?

- Seminomas are highly radio-sensitive, such that following orchidectomy radiotherapy is given to the ipsilateral iliac and para-aortic nodes. Chemotherapy is indicated for more extensive disease.
- Teratomas are not as radio-sensitive, and are best treated by combination chemotherapy usually involving one of the platinum compounds (e.g. cisplatin or carboplatin).
- In the absence of nodal spread a 5-year survival of near 100% is common; even with nodal spread a 95% 5-year survival is achieved.

Case 123 A renal transplant recipient with a gastrointestinal haemorrhage

A 23-year-old nulliparous female teaching assistant underwent a kidney transplant for glomerulonephritis. She had been waiting on haemodialysis for 3 years before she was called in for a transplant. She was told that the long wait was because she had previous blood transfusions, but couldn't understand why this was.

The kidney had come from a heart-beating donor, a 46-year-old lady who had suffered a subarachnoid haemorrhage and who died on a neurosurgical unit in another part of the country. Death was certified using brainstem criteria.

The recipient's principal immunosuppression was tacrolimus, azathioprine and prednisolone, and at the time of transplant she had received a course of a monoclonal antibody to the CD25 antigen. She made an uneventful recovery, being discharged 7 days later with a serum creatinine of 98 μmol/L.

Why can having a previous blood transfusion make it more difficult to get a suitable kidney?

Previous blood transfusions, transplants and pregnancies are associated with the production of antibodies against the foreign major histocompatibility antigens (human leucocyte antigens, HLAs) that are expressed on the donor cells. If a patient receives a transplant with any HLA antigens against which the recipient has preformed HLA antibodies, the kidney will be subject to hyperacute rejection and destroyed within minutes or hours. In order to avoid this, a cross-match test is performed whereby serum from the recipient, (which will contain any preformed antibodies), is mixed with donor lymphocytes, (obtained from donor blood, spleen or lymph nodes removed at the time of donation). If binding is observed, the cross-match test is deemed positive and the transplant cannot go ahead. Hence it can be seen that the presence of such antibodies makes it more difficult to find the patient a suitable matched kidney, avoiding any HLA antigens against which she has antibodies.

What are the brainstem criteria used to diagnose death in the organ donor?

Death may be certified either by the absence of a heart beat or by the absence of brainstem function. To be diagnosed as dead by brainstem criteria the patient must be in a coma and maintained on a ventilator with a clearly identified cause of death. Hypothermia, intoxication, sedative drugs, neuromuscular blocking drugs and severe electrolyte and acid–base abnormalities must be excluded. If the above criteria are met, the following tests are performed:

- Pupil reflexes: Dilated and do not respond to direct or consensual light.
- Corneal reflex: Absent.
- Vestibulo-ocular reflex: Absent. When the head is turned passively the eyes remain fixed relative to the head.
- Vestibulo-caloric reflex: Absent. Slow injection of 20 ml of ice cold water into each external auditory meatus does not cause eye movement.
- Cranial nerve motor responses: Absent in the presence of adequate stimulation of a somatic area.
- Gag reflex: Absent, even to bronchial stimulation with a suction catheter.
- Respiratory movements: Absent, even when disconnected from a ventilator long enough for the PCO_2 to rise above 6.65 kPa.

If the above criteria are satisfied the patient is declared dead. At that stage any prior wish to be an organ donor is ascertained, as in this case, and donation proceeds.

What is a monoclonal antibody? Where else are they of surgical importance?

A monoclonal antibody is an antibody that targets a specific epitope on a cell surface, in contrast to polyclonal antibodies which target many epitopes. In transplantation the common targets for monoclonal antibodies are on T-lymphocytes, including the CD3 antigen (e.g. mur-

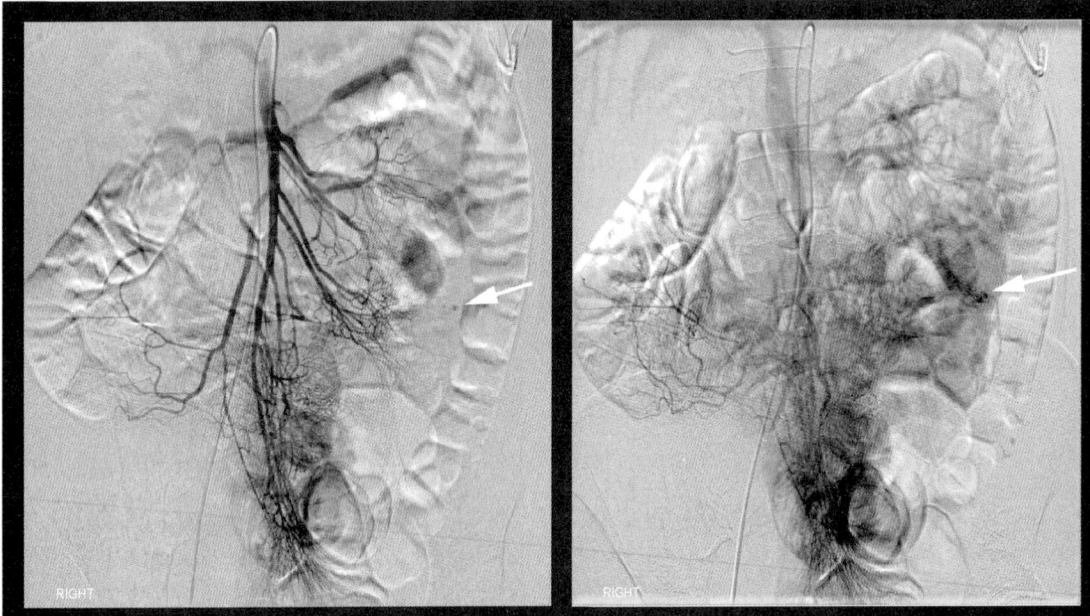

Figure 123.1 Selective superior mesenteric artery angiogram showing a bleeding point in the jejunum (arrowed).

omonab CD3), and the activated interleukin 2 receptor (the CD25 antigen, e.g. basiliximab and daclizumab).

In other fields of surgery they are important in the adjuvant treatment of malignancy (e.g. trastuzumab for breast cancer) and as anti-inflammatory treatment (e.g. infliximab, a tumour necrosis factor monoclonal antibody used for Crohn's disease). They have also revolutionized histopathological diagnosis (immunohistochemistry), identifying markers characteristic of certain diseases, such as CD117 in gastrointestinal stromal tumours.

What are the common complications of immunosuppression?

Patients on immunosuppression are at risk of complications of the drugs themselves, and the complications of being immunosuppressed:

1 *Complications of immunosuppressive drugs*:
  - Tacrolimus and ciclosporin: Nephrotoxicity, neurotoxicty, diabetes mellitus.
  - Mycophenolate: Diarrhoea, marrow suppression.
  - Azathioprine: Marrow suppression, liver disease.

2 *Complications of being immunosuppressed*:
  - Infections, particularly infections by the herpes family viruses such as herpes simplex, varicella zoster and cytomegalovirus. In addition, opportunist infections with organisms such as *Pneumocystis jiroveci* (formerly called *Pneumocystis carinii*) and *Candida albicans*.
  - Cancer, particularly skin cancers (related to the papilloma virus) and lymphomas (related to the Epstein–Barr virus). In addition, most other cancers are more common.

Six months after her transplant the patient presented with generalized lymphadenopathy. Biopsy of a groin node confirmed a lymphoma secondary to Epstein–Barr virus. She was treated with immunosuppressive reduction and a course of chemotherapy including the B-cell lytic monoclonal antibody rituximab. Two days later she experienced a brisk gastrointestinal (GI) bleed. Upper GI endoscopy and colonoscopy failed to identify the source of bleeding. She continued to bleed.

How would you investigate her next?

Most causes of GI bleeding will be picked up on endoscopy. If that is negative the bleeding point is somewhere between the second part of the duodenum and the ileocaecal valve. In the presence of active bleeding a mesenteric angiogram is the next investigation. In this woman, selective cannulation of the superior mesenteric artery suggested a bleeding point in the jejunum (arrowed on Fig. 123.1).

The patient was taken to theatre where multiple necrotic areas of small bowel were found (Fig. 123.2) and resected. The specific point of bleeding was not identified but was presumed to be in association with one of these areas. The necrotic areas represented lymphomatous deposits in the small bowel that had been destroyed by the chemotherapy, in particular the monoclonal antibody therapy. Necrotic mesenteric lymph node masses were also noted. Following surgery she completed her chemotherapy and made a complete recovery.

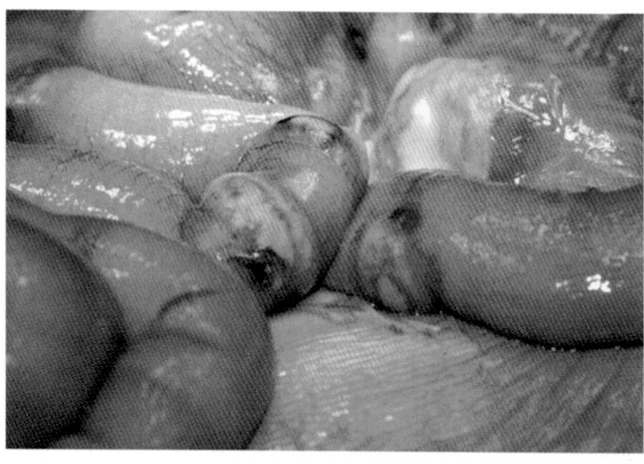

Figure 123.2 Necrotic areas of small bowel.

MCQs

For each situation, choose the single option you feel is most correct.

1 Malignant melanoma *Malignant melanomas are common tumours arising in junctional naevi.*

Which of the following correlates best with prognosis?

a. The thickness of the tumour
b. The diameter of the tumour
c. Variation in pigmentation
d. Bleeding from the tumour
e. Presence of the tumour on the hand

2 Shock *A 61-year-old man presents with abdominal pain and is found to be tachycardic and hypotensive. Management includes floating of a Swann–Ganz catheter, which reveals that the systemic vascular resistance is low.*

Which of the following conditions is likely to account for such a finding?

a. Myocardial infarction
b. Haemorrhage from a duodenal ulcer
c. Non-strangulating small bowel obstruction
d. A perforated diverticulum of the colon
e. Ruptured abdominal aortic aneurysm

3 Breathlessness *A 62-year-old female medical secretary underwent an anterior resection for carcinoma of the upper rectum under general anaesthetic. The anaesthetist placed an epidural for postoperative analgesia but unfortunately this fell out on transfer from theatre to the ward. Her pain was eventually controlled with a patient-controlled morphine pump. On the ninth day after surgery she became acutely dyspnoeic while opening her bowels. On examination she was tachycardic but her chest sounded clear. An electrocardiograph showed right axis deviation with evidence of right heart strain.*

What is the most likely diagnosis?

a. Myocardial infarction
b. Pulmonary collapse
c. Pulmonary embolism
d. Basal atelectasis
e. Anastomotic disruption

4 Lung cancer *A malignant tumour can manifest through the effects of the primary tumour, the effects of its secondary deposits, the general effects of malignant disease or by a paraneoplastic syndrome caused by a tumour cell product.*

When considering squamous carcinoma of the bronchus, which of the following is not a recognized manifestation?

a. Pneumonia
b. Fracture of the femur resulting from minimal trauma
c. Finger clubbing
d. Cushing's syndrome
e. Hypercalcaemia

5 Coarctation of the aorta *A medical student, while practising clinical examination on his 22-year-old girlfriend, observed that she had a blood pressure of 180/100 mmHg in the right arm and also noted a difference in the appearance of the radial and femoral pulses, the femoral pulse seeming a little weaker than the radial pulse. He diagnosed a coarctation of the aorta.*

Which of the following observations support the diagnosis?

a. Angiography showing a patent ductus arteriosus
b. Echocardiography showing a normal left ventricle
c. Notching of the ribs on chest X-ray
d. Normal plasma renin levels
e. A blood pressure of 100/60 in the left arm

6 Aortic dissection *A left-handed 52-year-old man with a long history of hypertension refused to take any antihypertensive drugs, preferring instead to rely on herbal remedies. He developed a severe retrosternal chest pain while watching his favourite football team lose. The pain moved to between the scapulae over the following minutes, and he lost consciousness for a couple of minutes and on coming round could not move his right arm. On examination he was shocked and he had a diastolic murmur at the right sternal edge. You could not palpate any pulses in the left arm. Over the next 4 h he passed no urine. You diagnose an aortic dissection.*

Which of the following statements is true and why?

a. The patient has experienced a type B dissection
b. The dissection always runs distally along the aorta
c. Surgery is only indicated in type B dissections
d. Transoesophageal echocardiography (TOE) is more sensitive than angiography in detecting dissections
e. Loss of function of the left arm is due to stretching of the brachial plexus over the dissecting aorta

7 Abdominal aortic aneurysm *A recently retired surgeon notices an abnormal pulsation in his abdomen while lying on the beach in the south of France. On his return home an ultrasound scan confirms the presence of an abdominal aortic aneurysm measuring 5.1 cm in anteroposterior diameter, and arising immediately caudal to the origin of the renal arteries.*

Which of the following statements is true and why?

a. Annual screening of his aneurysm is not necessary until he is 67 years old
b. There is a significant risk of gastrointestinal haemorrhage from an aorto-enteric fistula
c. Endovascular aneurysm stenting is only effective in patients with smaller aneurysms
d. Angiography is superior to ultrasound in assessing aortic diameter
e. The risk of rupture of his aneurysm is less than 5% per annum at that diameter

8 Carotid artery stenosis *A right-handed writer describes a curtain coming down across his right eye while out celebrating his 50th birthday. The blindness lasted no more than 10 min before resolving. A duplex scan of carotid arteries reveals a 75% stenosis of the ipsilateral carotid artery.*

Which of the following is true?

a. He is also at risk of an ipsilateral hemiparesis from an embolism into the cerebral circulation
b. Carotid endarterectomy is indicated and should be performed without delay
c. Hypoglossal neurapraxia is common in patients with stenosis of the carotid artery
d. Intravascular angiography is the investigation of choice
e. Aspirin is contraindicated due to the risk of retinal haemorrhage

9 Varicose veins *A woman aged 45 presents with a 5-year history of varicose veins in the left leg, which she claims are causing aching in her leg. Her past history includes a fractured left tibia and fibula in a skiing accident 7 years previously. On examination she has an incompetent left sapheno-femoral junction and varicosities along the course of the great (long) saphenous vein. There is evidence of deep venous insufficiency in the lower leg.*

Which of the following is correct?

a. Sapheno-femoral ligation and stripping of the greater saphenous vein is the treatment of choice in cases such as this
b. The evidence of deep venous insufficiency would typically include haemosiderosis and eczema affecting the lateral aspect of the lower leg
c. Long-term anticoagulation is indicated
d. Previous deep vein thrombosis is the likely cause of the varicose veins
e. Investigations should include venography to exclude an arteriovenous fistula

10 Pituitary tumour *A 48-year-old lawyer noted increased frequency of headaches in the 2 years prior to admission. On the day of admission he developed a rapid onset, severe retro-orbital headache. Over the previous 2 years he had also noted loss of body and axillary hair, and his 6 o'clock shadow had disappeared. He had also become more tired and was sensitive to the cold. There was no history of galactorrhoea (milky discharge from the nipples). Examination revealed a blood pressure of 105/85 mmHg and a pulse of 58/min. Magnetic resonance imaging confirmed haemorrhage (apoplexy) into a 4 cm diameter pituitary tumour.*

Which of the following is true?

a. The tumour is likely to be a thyroid-stimulating hormone (TSH) producing tumour of the anterior pituitary

b. The absence of galactorrhoea excludes a prolactinoma as the cause

c. Loss of body hair is due to low testosterone levels

d. Examination of the visual fields would reveal a homonymous hemianopia

e. Surgical excision is indicated for all pituitary adenomas

11 Head injury *You are called to the accident service to attend a 16-year-old who had stolen a motorcycle and crashed it into a parked car. He was not wearing a helmet. On examination he had a clear airway, was self-ventilating with a pulse rate of 120/min and a blood pressure of 80/30 mmHg. He was confused, mumbling incoherently, opening his eyes only when commanded and withdrawing his hand to pain. Primary skeletal survey was unremarkable as was chest examination. His abdomen was tense and there were no bowel sounds. Skull X-ray revealed a fractured left parietal bone, and chest X-ray suggested fractures to the left 8th, 9th and 10th ribs.*

Which of the following statements is true?

a. His Glasgow Coma Score is 12

b. Hypotension is unlikely to be explained by his head injury

c. A tachycardia occurs following head injury due to the Cushing reflex

d. The chest fractures should be managed by positive pressure ventilation

e. Since the patient is conscious a cervical spine X-ray is not required

12 Peripheral nerve injury *A 64-year-old woman on thyroxine for myxoedema complains of pain in her hand that is worse during the night, wakes her and is relieved by shaking her hand. On examination the thenar eminence is wasted. A diagnosis of carpal tunnel syndrome has been made.*

Which of the following is true?

a. Wasting of the muscles in the thenar eminence implies the median nerve compression is at a level proximal to the flexor retinaculum

b. Carpal tunnel syndrome occurs equally commonly in men and women

c. The sensory loss is likely to affect the thumb and lateral (radial) two fingers only

d. Carpal tunnel syndrome is more common in patients with myxoedema

e. Thumb abduction is preserved in carpal tunnel syndrome

13 Salivary glands *A 56-year-old lorry driver presents with a painless swelling anterior to his right ear. Examination confirmed a 2 cm firm swelling fixed deep but not to skin and you believe the lump to be parotid in origin. You also note that there is a lower motor neuron weakness of the facial muscles of the right side of the face, and a prominent hard jugulo-digastric lymph node.*

Which of the following is true?

a. Lower motor neuron lesions of the face are common in pleomorphic adenomas of the parotid

b. Mumps commonly affects the submandibular and parotid glands

c. Ten per cent of parotid tumours are adenolymphomas and these are associated with ipsilateral cervical lymphadenopathy

d. Pain in the ipsilateral ear commonly occurs with tumours of the parotid due the same branchial arch origin

e. Total parotidectomy with sacrifice of the facial nerve is the most appropriate treatment

14 Pharyngeal pouch *A 54-year-old man complained that after breakfast he would bring up the tablets that he had taken earlier in the morning. He also mentioned that his wife had complained that he had developed bad breath over the last 6 months. On examination you palpate a swelling posterior to the cricoid cartilage and suspect a pharyngeal pouch.*

Which of the following statements is correct?

a. Pharyngeal pouches are mucosal protrusions below the cricopharyngeus muscle, itself part of the inferior constrictor muscles of the pharynx
b. Pharyngeal pouches may present with recurrent episodes of aspiration pneumonia
c. Oesophagoscopy is the investigation of choice
d. The presentation is typical of the Plummer–Vinson syndrome
e. The diverticulum is best removed via a cervical incision because endoscopic diverticulotomy is associated with a high incidence of fistula formation

15 Oesophageal carcinoma *A 49-year-old builder presented with a 3-month history of progressive dysphagia and a weight loss of 5 kg. Prior to this he had suffered with reflux oesophagitis for over 15 years, which he treated with Gaviscon. On examination there was a palpable 3 cm lymph node in the left supraclavicular fossa.*

Which of the following statements is true?

a. Left supraclavicular lymphadenopathy is due to spread of tumour up the thoracic duct; it is called Troisier's sign
b. Longstanding reflux oesophagitis results in the oesophageal mucosa undergoing metaplasia from columnar epithelium to squamous epithelium, so-called Barrett's oesophagus
c. The pattern of oesophageal cancer is changing, and squamous carcinomas of the upper third are becoming most common
d. Barium swallow is the investigation of choice in this patient
e. Barrett's oesophagus, unlike Plummer–Vinson syndrome, is not premalignant

16 Congenital pyloric stenosis *A 5-week-old boy is admitted with a 2-day history of vomiting. The vomitus was not bile stained, nor did it resemble coffee grounds. On examination the child was dehydrated, floppy and irritable. A trial feed confirmed the presence of a palpable tumour in the right upper quadrant.*

Which of the following statements is likely to be correct?

a. Blood gases should confirm a metabolic alkalosis
b. Serum potassium is normal
c. Serum chloride is raised
d. Immediate surgery is indicated and a pyloromyotomy is the treatment of choice
e. Sixty per cent occur in males, usually first born

17 *Helicobacter pylori* *A 49-year-old publican complained of epigastric pain that was exacerbated by eating or drinking alcohol. He underwent an upper gastrointestinal endoscopy that confirmed the presence of a gastric ulcer.*

Which of the following statements is true?

a. Biopsies for *Helicobacter pylori* are placed in urea solution, which becomes alkali if positive
b. Biopsy of the ulcer is unnecessary if *Helicobacter* eradication therapy is commenced
c. Carcinoma of the stomach is best managed by a Bilroth I gastrectomy
d. *Helicobacter pylori* is eradicated by proton pump inhibitors such as omeprazole
e. A Bilroth II or Pólya gastrectomy is the procedure of choice for gastric ulcers

18 Obstruction *A 21-year-old student presents as an emergency with an 18 h history of vomiting and colicky abdominal pain. She says she feels bloated, and the pain has now become constant. Two years previously she underwent a laparoscopic appendicectomy. On examination she is pyrexial (38°C), tachycardic at 120/min, and has a leucocytosis of 19.3×10^9/L. Her abdomen is quiet on auscultation.*

Which of the following statements is likely to be correct?

a. She has simple intestinal obstruction secondary to adhesions; she is best managed by nasogastric aspiration and intravenous fluids in the first instance

b. Pelvic ultrasound is the most appropriate next investigation
c. She has strangulating obstruction, and should be operated on as soon as she is resuscitated
d. Small bowel obstruction is unlikely if she is continuing to pass flatus
e. Intussusception is common in patients who have previously undergone an appendicectomy

19 Appendicitis *John Murphy (1857–1916) and Charles McBurney (1845–1913) were American surgeons who made important contributions regarding appendicitis. Murphy described the classic triad of symptoms, namely central abdominal colicky pain, then nausea or vomiting, followed by movement of the pain to the right iliac fossa. McBurney's studies determined the position of the appendix in relation to the umbilicus and anterior superior iliac spine.*

Which of the following statements is correct?
a. McBurney's point is two-thirds of the way from the right anterior superior iliac spine to the umbilicus
b. Inflammation of a Meckel's diverticulum may be confused with the features described by Murphy
c. The normal time course of the progression of symptoms described by Murphy is 4–7 days
d. Pain in the right iliac fossa is due to irritation of the visceral peritoneum
e. In pregnancy the appendix moves lateral to McBurney's point as the uterus grows

20 Colonic stricture *An obese 68-year-old woman presents with a longstanding irregular bowel habit. She admitted to opening her bowels twice a week. On this occasion she has just experienced a single episode of profuse rectal bleeding, described as plum coloured with clots. It appeared to 'fill' the toilet pan. There was no associated pain. A haemoglobin estimation was 10.9 g/dL, with a mean cell volume of 92.*

Which of the following is the most likely diagnosis?
a. A bleeding gastric ulcer
b. Rectal carcinoma
c. Caecal carcinoma
d. Crohn's disease
e. Diverticular disease

21 Hernia *A 41-year-old man presents with a lump in the right groin. On examination it appears to originate above the inguinal ligament, and cannot be reduced.*

Which of the following statements is correct?
a. Inguinal herniae are more common in men, and the right side is more common than the left
b. A hernia such as this that cannot be reduced is termed an obstructed hernia
c. Inguinal herniae are less common in women than femoral herniae
d. The internal ring, through which a direct hernia passes, is palpated 1–2 cm above the mid inguinal point (midway between the symphysis pubis and anterior superior iliac spine)
e. The external spermatic fascia covers the cord structures within the inguinal canal

22 Jaundice *A 55-year-old teacher presented with a 2-month history of itching and 2 weeks previously had noted that her sclera were yellow. On direct questioning she admitted that she had been fatigued and lost a stone over the previous 6 months, but she had put this down to being diagnosed with diabetes at around the same time. She admitted to passing pale stools and having dark urine.*

Which of the following statements is likely to be correct?
a. The patient has carcinoma of the pancreas that is likely to be amenable to surgery
b. The pale stools are due to an absence of bilirubin glucuronide in the gut
c. The gallbladder will not be distended
d. The urine is dark due to the presence of urobilinogen
e. Her prothrombin time will be normal

23 Pancreatitis *A 32-year-old waitress on the oral contraceptive pill presents with severe epigastric pain that radiates to her back, and is associated with vomiting and retching. She denies a history of alcohol drinking, and gallstones are found on ultrasound.*

Which of the following findings is *not* a poor prognostic factor?
a. A haemoglobin of 10.1 g/dl

b. An arterial oxygen saturation of 7 kPa breathing air (FiO_2 21%)
c. A leucocyte count of 18.2×10^9/L
d. A C-reactive protein concentration of 200 mg/L
e. A blood glucose of 11 mmol/L

24 Splenectomy *A 35-year-old stable lad falls from his horse onto his left side and ruptures his spleen. He undergoes a splenectomy later the same day.*

Which of the following is correct?

a. In the future he will be at increased risk of infection from capsulated organisms such as *Haemophilus influenzae*
b. Thrombocytosis (an increased platelet count) following splenectomy suggests an underlying haematological disorder
c. Post-splenectomy syndrome is as likely after splenectomy for trauma as it is for non-trauma indications
d. Penicillin prophylaxis is necessary for children, but not adults, following splenectomy
e. Annual immunization against the influenza virus is unnecessary

25 A solitary breast lump *A 25-year-old office cleaner noticed a lump in the upper outer quadrant of her left breast while examining herself in the shower. She has no family history of breast disease, and is nulliparous. The lump is 2 cm across and highly mobile, and her specialist can find no evidence of other lumps nor of any lymphadenopathy.*

Which of the following statements is correct?

a. The lump is highly likely to be a fibroadenoma and so no further investigation or treatment is indicated
b. Mammography is indicated to exclude a carcinoma
c. The patient should be re-examined immediately after her next menstrual period
d. Ultrasound and core needle biopsy are indicated
e. Fibroadenomas are premalignant

26 Breast cancer *A 45-year-old medical secretary noted a fullness in her left breast associated with a dull dragging pain. Twenty-five years previously she had received radiotherapy for treatment of Hodgkin's disease, which had presented with left cervical lymphadenopathy. There was no family history of breast disease. Clinical examination confirmed the presence of a 6 cm lump with several 2 cm firm lymph nodes palpable in the axilla. Peau d'orange was visible, and skin tethering could be demonstrated when the patient raised her arms above her head.*

Which of he following statements is correct?

a. Mantle radiotherapy for Hodgkin's disease is associated with an increased risk of breast cancer
b. Invasive lobular carcinoma of the breast is the most common type
c. Skin tethering implies tumour invasion into the underlying pectoralis major
d. Early menarche and early menopause are both risk factors for carcinoma of the breast
e. Clinically this tumour can be staged as a T2N0 tumour

27 Thyroid swelling *A 38-year-old plumber presented to his doctor with a 3-week history of a lump in the left side of his neck. He had no dysphagia, but commented that swallowing was uncomfortable. He continued to sing in his local choir and had not noticed any hoarseness. On examination there was a swelling on the left side of the neck that moved with swallowing. There were no palpable lymph nodes in his neck. Indirect laryngoscopy revealed full vocal cord movement. Thyroid function tests were normal, and an ultrasound of the thyroid confirmed this to be a solid lump.*

Which of the following statements is correct?

a. The diagnosis is likely to be a multinodular goitre
b. A diagnosis of thyroid cancer is likely which, at his young age, is likely to be an anaplastic carcinoma
c. Surgical excision, by either hemi- or total thyroidectomy, is the treatment of choice
d. Radioiodine treatment is effective in the ablation of the thyroid bed and also in the treatment of occult metastases, but causes hypoparathyroidism
e. Exogenous levothyroxine should not be given post-operatively to patients following thyroid lobectomy for differentiated tumours

28 Ureteric colic *A 32-year-old surgical trainee presents with severe right loin pain that radiates to the groin and right hemiscrotum. It is colicky in nature and is relieved in part by pacing up and down the corridor outside the emergency room. He believes himself to have ureteric colic and is relieved to see the plain X-ray of his abdomen, which confirms a stone in the lower ureter.*

Which of the following is *not* associated with the formation of renal calculi?

a. Gout
b. Crohn's ileitis
c. Raspberries
d. Hyperparathyroidism
e. Chemotherapy for cancer

29 Urinary retention *A 66-year-old retired schoolteacher presents with a 6-month history of poor stream, hesitancy, terminal dribbling, frequency and nocturia, getting up every hour. Examination confirms a smoothly enlarged prostate. The prostate-specific antigen (PSA) concentration is 3.8 ng/ml (normal).*

Which of the following statements is true?

a. Finasteride is an α_1-adrenergic antagonist. As such it causes relaxation of the smooth muscle in the bladder neck and is an effective treatment for such symptoms
b. Like α_1-adrenergic antagonists, inhibitors of 5α-reductase have an immediate beneficial effect
c. Urinary flow rate assessment is useful in assessing outflow obstruction, but only if the volume voided is over 200 ml
d. Intravenous urography is the best modality to assess upper tract dilatation secondary to outflow obstruction
e. Absence of a mass on digital rectal examination rules out the presence of prostatic malignancy

30 Testis *An 18-year-old boy complains of dissimilar sized testes. Careful clinical examination revealed that the left testis was smooth and soft, but smaller than the right, and the left hemiscrotum felt like a bag of worms. The right testis was larger than the left, and felt hard and irregular.*

Which of the following is likely to be true?

a. There is a varicocele of the left testis, a condition that is thought to be due to the way the testicular vein drains obliquely into the vena cava on the left
b. Testicular tumours are usually found in ectopic and undescended testes
c. At this age seminoma is the most common cell type of testicular tumour
d. Lymphatic spread is to the para-aortic lymph nodes via the ipsilateral inguinal nodes
e. Unlike lymphatic spread from most cancers, even lymphatic spread from a testicular tumour can be associated with a good prognosis at 5 years in 95% of patients

EMQs

1 Postoperative pyrexia

a. Wound infection
b. Thrombophlebitis
c. Pulmonary collapse
d. Pulmonary embolism
e. Pelvic abscess
f. Urinary infection
g. Pneumonia
h. Drug reaction
i. Infective endocarditis
j. *Clostridium difficile*

For each of the following patients with a pyrexia select the correct diagnosis from the list above.

1. A 27-year-old diabetic woman presents with a fluctuating pyrexia and raised blood sugars 6 days after laparoscopic removal of a perforated appendix. The wounds were all healing well, but on rectal examination she was very tender anteriorly.
2. A 67-year-old man underwent an anterior resection of a carcinoma of the rectum. Eight days after surgery he developed a low grade fever and tachypnoea. He had been slow to mobilize because of abdominal pain but his abdominal CT scan had been unremarkable. He had no dysuria, urine cultures were clear and auscultation of his heart and lungs was also unremarkable. A plain chest X-ray showed clear lung fields.
3. A 54-year-old man had been on total parenteral nutrition for 2 weeks following a Whipple's procedure for an ampullary carcinoma. He developed a persistent pyrexia. Examination revealed an ejection systolic murmur at the left sternal edge, a normal chest and a soft abdomen. Urine testing revealed red cells but no growth.
4. A 73-year-old woman presented 6 days after been treated with cephradine (a cephalosporin antibiotic) by her general practitioner for acute cholecystitis. She had a pyrexia and distended abdomen, and was incontinent of faeces.
5. An obese 53-year-old woman with type 2 diabetes presented a week after a paraumbilical hernia repair with a pyrexia and increasing wound pain.

2 Diagnosis of jaundice

a. Gallstones
b. Primary sclerosing cholangitis
c. Carcinoma of the pancreas
d. Cholangiocarcinoma
e. Primary biliary cirrhosis
f. Ascending cholangitis
g. Haemolytic anaemia
h. Biliary colic
i. Periampullary carcinoma
j. Acute cholecystitis

For each of the following patients with jaundice select the likely diagnosis.

1. A 62-year-old man presents with a 2-month history of lethargy and 2-week history of painless jaundice. He was diagnosed with diabetes 2 months previously.
2. A 49-year-old diabetic presents acutely with a history of rigors, right upper quadrant pain and jaundice.
3. A 58-year-old woman presents with a short history of relapsing jaundice. She has intermittently dark urine and pale stools that appear slightly silver.
4. A 28-year-old multiparous woman presents with right upper quadrant pain that radiates through to the inferior angle of her right scapula. The pain came on 2 h after her evening meal, and lasted 3 h before waning. She had one previous episode during her last pregnancy. On examination she is afebrile.
5. A 31-year-old man with ulcerative colitis presented with a history of pruritus, non-specific upper abdom-

inal pain, fevers and jaundice. Magnetic resonance cholangio-pancreatography (MRCP) demonstrated multiple intrahepatic strictures, giving the appearance of a string of beads.

3 The acute abdomen

a. Salpingitis
b. Acute diverticulitis
c. Appendicitis
d. Ruptured ectopic pregnancy
e. Small bowel obstruction
f. Pancreatitis
g. Perforated duodenal ulcer
h. Acute pyelonephritis
i. Ruptured abdominal aortic aneurysm
j. Crohn's disease

For each of the following patients presenting with an acute abdomen select the most likely diagnosis.

1. A 28-year-old female with an intrauterine contraceptive device presents with a history of rapid onset, right-sided abdominal pain, which became generalized over the following 6 h. There was no history of nausea or vomiting, and her last period was on time but lighter than normal. There was no history of vaginal discharge. Following pelvic examination she became profoundly hypotensive.
2. A 31-year-old woman on the oral contraceptive pill developed lower abdominal pain and nausea and urinary frequency. The pain moved to the right side radiating round to her right loin and she suffered an episode of rigors. Hip extension did not affect the severity of the pain.
3. A 32-year-old theatre sister presented with a history of colicky central abdominal pain that had moved to the right iliac fossa and was now constant; she had also suffered nausea and vomiting, and abdominal distension. She has had recurrent episodes of pain over the last 6 months, and had lost 6 kg over the same period.
4. A 78-year-old woman with osteoarthritis presented in shock having had a sudden pain in her epigastrium. An erect chest X-ray revealed a trace of free air under he diaphragm. Her amylase was 790 units/L (a normal level is less than 350 units/L).
5. An obese 52-year-old woman presented with a history of central lower abdominal pain that localized to the left iliac fossa. She had vomited and on examination was flushed, pyrexial and had tenderness and rebound in the iliac fossa.

4 A breathless patient

a. Myocardial infarction
b. Thromboembolism
c. Pulmonary collapse
d. Paradoxical embolism
e. Aortic dissection
f. Haemopneumothorax
g. Flail chest
h. Fat embolism
i. Cardiac tamponade
j. Tension pneumothorax

For each of the following breathless patients select the most likely diagnosis from the list above.

1. A 46-year-old lorry driver was involved in a road traffic accident and sustained a fractured left femur. This was treated by immobilization on traction. No other injuries were sustained. The following day he became dyspnoeic, and on examination was tachycardic with an oxygen saturations of 85%. Arterial blood gases showed hypoxia and hypercapnia. A chest X-ray showed diffuse bilateral shadowing.
2. An 18-year-old rugby player felt his ribs crack and he developed severe pain in the left side of his chest after being caught at the bottom of a scrum. Over the next few minutes he became progressively breathless and lost consciousness. Observers noted progressive cyanosis. On examination he was tachycardic and hypotensive, and his trachea appeared to be shifted to the right.
3. A 61-year-old woman was admitted with a swollen right leg 9 days after a hysterectomy for endometrial carcinoma. She was breathless on arrival, and went on to develop a right hemiparesis later on the day of admission. A cranial CT scan suggests an infarct in the middle cerebral artery territory. The following day she developed a painful right leg, which on examination was pale and cool and no pulses were palpable.
4. A 24-year-old salesman was involved in a road accident when his car left the road and drove headlong into a wall. He suffered a blow to his chest from the steering wheel. In the emergency department he complained of chest pain, had difficulty breathing – taking rapid shallow breaths – and was shocked with

a tachycardia and blood pressure of 80/60 mmHg. His neck veins were engorged, and heart sounds quiet.

5. A 58-year-old librarian with ankylosing spondylitis underwent an emergency laparotomy for a perforated peptic ulcer, presumed secondary to the non-steroidal anti-inflammatory drugs he was taking. The following day he developed a pyrexia of 37.5°C and became dyspnoeic and tachycardic, with reduced oxygen saturations on pulse oximetry.

5 Neck swellings

a. Multinodular goitre
b. Pharyngeal pouch
c. Branchial cyst
d. Virchow's lymph node
e. Parathyroid adenoma
f. Sternomastoid tumour
g. Papillary carcinoma of thyroid
h. Cervical rib
i. Chemodectoma
j. Thyroglossal cyst

For each of the following patients with swelling select the most likely diagnosis from the list above.

1. A 34-year-old teacher presented with a swelling in the anterior triangle of her right neck. The autumn school term had begun 3 weeks earlier and she blamed the children for a cold she had caught at that time. On examination there was a smooth 5 cm diameter swelling emerging in front of the anterior border of sternomastoid.
2. A 30-year-old woman presented complaining of an intermittent cold and numb left arm, and a lump in the left side of her neck. On further questioning it was clear that the numbness was in the T1 distribution. Examination confirmed a hard 2 cm mass in the left supraclavicular fossa and wasting of the small muscles of the hand.
3. A 19-year-old medical student was found to have a lump in his neck by his colleague while they were practising neck examination. This was a small (1.5 cm) midline lump, which moved on swallowing and on protrusion of the tongue.
4. A 28-year-old mother of three presented to her GP having noticed a lump in her neck, which was more prominent when she swallowed. On examination she was clinically euthyroid, and had a 4 cm swelling on the right anterior triangle of her neck that moved on swallowing. In addition there was a 1.5 cm firm lump in the area of the jugulo-digastric lymph node, which was mobile.
5. A 62-year-old postman presented with a history of dysphagia, with a sensation of food sticking in his chest. He had lost a stone in weight over the last 3 months.

6 Intestinal obstruction

a. Femoral hernia
b. Meconium ileus
c. Adhesions
d. Intussusception
e. Sigmoid volvulus
f. Gallstone ileus
g. Obturator hernia
h. Colonic diverticular disease
i. Crohn's disease
j. Caecal carcinoma

For each of the following patients with intestinal obstruction select the most likely diagnosis from the list above.

1. A 64-year-old shopkeeper presented with a 3-month history of increasing abdominal distension, and a 1-week history of vomiting and crampy abdominal pain. Examination revealed a 5 cm mass in the right iliac fossa.
2. A 75-year-old woman presented with a day's history of colicky central abdominal pain, vomiting and distension. She continued to pass flatus. Abdominal examination confirmed distension and tinkling bowel sounds were audible. A 3 cm mass was palpable just below the medial end of the left inguinal ligament.
3. A 25-year-old junior doctor presents with a 24 h history of colicky central abdominal pain and nausea and vomiting. She gave a 6-month prior history of intermittent abdominal pain and diarrhoea leading up to this episode. On examination she was a thin woman, pyrexial at 38.2°C, and there was a tender 4 cm mass in the right iliac fossa.
4. A 35-year-old diabetic patient underwent a combined kidney and pancreas transplant 12 months previously, during which the kidney was placed extraperitoneally and the pancreas intraperitoneally, with exocrine drainage via a Roux-en-Y duodeno-jejunsotomy. He now presents with colicky central abdominal pain and

vomiting. Examination confirmed abdominal distension with tinkling bowel sounds, and investigation revealed normal blood glucose, amylase and creatinine.

5. An 8-month-old previously healthy infant boy presented with a history of vomiting and colic. Between bouts of pain he seemed normal, but the pains increased in frequency. Twelve hours later he started to pass blood and mucus rectally. On examination his abdomen was distended, and there was a suggestion of a sausage-shaped mass in the right upper quadrant.

7 Skin lumps

a. Basal cell carcinoma
b. Squamous carcinoma
c. Calcifying epithelioma of Malherbe
d. Sequestration dermoid
e. Sebaceous cyst
f. Solar keratosis
g. Kaposi's sarcoma
h. Hutchinson's freckle
i. Malignant melanoma
j. Implantation dermoid

For each of the following patients with skin lumps select the most likely diagnosis from the list above.

1. A 40-year-old waitress reports that her hairdresser is having difficulty cutting her hair because of two lumps she has in her scalp. On examination there are two similar 2 cm lumps that are fixed to the skin and move freely over the underlying skull. Each has an umbilicated surface suggestive of a punctum. There is no associated lymphadenopathy.
2. A 34-year-old professional cricketer presents with a 5 mm lump on the dorsum of his hand, which he first noticed when it was smaller at the start of the season, 2 months ago. It is pigmented, slightly raised, fixed to the skin but not deeply, and has recently bled. Two centimetres proximally is a second pigmented lesion 2 mm across and also raised.
3. A 48-year-old gardener and prize-winning rose grower presents with a 5 mm lump on the pulp of the distal phalanx of his right index finger. He says it has been there for a year, and has increased in size over that time. It appears to be deep to the skin, but is not fixed deeply. There is no associated lymphadenopathy.
4. A 29-year-old Egyptian man had undergone a successful renal transplant 18 months previously. He now presents with a 3-week history of a painless, raised, purple, plaque-like lesion, 1 cm across, on his chest wall. Infectious screening confirmed that he was negative for HIV (human immunodeficiency virus), but had antibodies to HHV8 (human herpes virus 8).
5. A 12-year-old is brought to see you with a lump at the outer angle of the left eye, which the parents believe may have been there since she was very young. On examination there is a 1.5 cm cystic swelling that is deep to skin, fixed deep and smooth and soft in consistency. There is the sensation that the underlying outer aspect of the orbit is scalloped out. There is no associated lymphadenopathy.

8 Breast disease

a. Phylloides tumour
b. Carcinoma of the breast
c. Intraduct papilloma
d. Duct carcinoma in situ
e. Tietze's syndrome
f. Galactocoele
g. Inflammatory breast cancer
h. Duct ectasia
i. Breast abscess
j. Fibroadenoma

For each of the following patients select the most likely diagnosis from the list above.

1. A 28-year-old woman presents with a 6-week history of a lump in the right breast. She has no family history of breast disease and on examination you find a mobile 2 cm lump which is neither attached to skin or to the underlying fascia.
2. A 35-year-old woman gave birth to a baby girl 4 months previously and stopped breastfeeding 2 weeks later. She noticed a swollen left breast and on examination there is indeed a smooth swelling in the upper outer quadrant of the left breast.
3. A 35-year-old woman presents with a 2-week history of a lump in the upper outer quadrant of the right breast. It is 5 cm in diameter, intimately associated with the skin, which appears tethered when she puts her hands on her head. It is not fixed to the underlying fascia. At the age of 18 she had developed Hodgkin's

disease and was successfully treated. There is no family history of breast disease.

4. A 38-year-old diabetic woman presents with a swollen, painful left breast that had come on about 48 h previously, but had got progressively worse since. On examination she was pyrexial (38.4°C) and the whole of the breast was inflamed, although there was no obvious area of fluctuation. There was tender lymphadenopathy in the axilla.
5. A 55-year-old woman develops a discharge from the left nipple. It is dirty brown in colour, and appears to arise from three separate points on the nipple. There is a palpable discrete lump.

9 Haematuria

a. Acute pyelonephritis
b. Glomerulonephritis
c. Acute papillary necrosis
d. Renal cell carcinoma (adenocarcinoma)
e. Transitional cell carcinoma of the bladder
f. Ureteric calculus
g. Haemophilia A
h. Polycystic kidney disease
i. Neuroblastoma
j. Nephroblastoma

For each of the following patients select the most likely diagnosis from the list above.

1. A 46-year-old woman presents with a pulmonary embolism. Investigation reveals her to have haematuria, which had been asymptomatic, and polycythaemia.
2. A 50-year-old man presented to the neurosurgeons following a subarachnoid haemorrhage. He had a past history of hypertension and had one previous episode of frank haematuria associated with right loin pain, but had not sought attention for this since his father suffered the same symptoms before he died suddenly aged 46.
3. A 50-year-old asymptomatic smoker presented having had haematuria detected by his family doctor at a recent health check. Investigation revealed left hydronephrosis.
4. A 4-year-old girl presented with a rapidly enlarging mass palpable in the left loin. Microscopic haematuria was detected on screening.
5. A 28-year-old man presented with colicky right loin pain radiating to the right testicle.

10 Investigation of abdominal pain

a. Abdominal ultrasound
b. Oesophago-gastro-duodenoscopy (OGD)
c. Endoscopic retrograde cholangio-pancreatography (ERCP)
d. Plain abdominal X-ray
e. Abdominal CT scan
f. Serum amylase
g. Laparoscopy
h. Erect chest X-ray
i. Intravenous urogram (IVU)
j. Mesenteric angiography

For each of the following patients select the single most appropriate investigation.

1. A 56-year-old female presents with a history of recurrent bouts of right upper quadrant pain, radiating to the inferior angle of the right scapula. They usually occur at night, 2–3 h after her evening meal and last from 2 to 6 h. She denies any features of jaundice.
2. A 71-year-old man presents with a history of sudden onset left loin pain radiating into his groin. He felt faint when the pain occurred, and had to lie down.
3. A 23-year-old woman presents with a day's history of sudden onset right iliac fossa pain. She has no history of vomiting or disturbance of her bowel habit, and her last period finished 8 days previously and was normal. She was apyrexial but extremely tender in the right iliac fossa.
4. A 45-year-old man with known gallstones and awaiting cholecystectomy presented with a 12 h history of epigastric pain and vomiting. The pain radiated through to his back. On examination he was retching, sitting forwards, cold and clammy.
5. A 41-year-old alcoholic man complains of generalized abdominal pain. He says he was queuing at the off license to buy some more cigarettes when the pain came on suddenly. He is cold and clammy, and his abdomen is rigid.

SAQs

1 A 69-year-old man attends his GP asking for a test to see if he has an abdominal aortic aneurysm. His brother died aged 64 from a ruptured aneurysm. He is otherwise well, smokes 20 a day with a 40 pack year exposure, and is on lisinopril for hypertension.

a. What are the requirements of an effective screening programme?
b. When should an abdominal aortic aneurysm be repaired?
c. What treatment modalities exist for patients with abdominal aortic aneurysms and what are the relative merits of each approach?
d. What are the complications of an abdominal aortic aneurysm?

2 A 53-year-old man is referred with a 3-week history of jaundice. He has been otherwise of good health and rarely consults his doctor.

a. Classify the causes of jaundice.
b. What facts do you need to elicit from the history?
c. What features on examination would you look for in someone with jaundice?
d. Outline three basic tests that would help you to determine the likely cause of the jaundice.

3 A 21-year-old student presents with a 6 h history of severe epigastric pain radiating to his back following an alcoholic binge the previous night. He is vomiting and retching, but has not vomited blood. On examination he is shocked, with generalized abdominal tenderness and guarding in the upper abdomen and right iliac fossa.

a. What is the likely diagnosis and how would you prove it? What would be your differential diagnosis?
b. What are the two common causes of this condition, and what others do you know?
c. How can you estimate the severity of pancreatitis?
d. What else can cause a raised amylase?

4 A 52-year-old motor mechanic with type 1 diabetes complains of a painful lump in the left groin when he lifts things at work. The lump disappears overnight and reappears in the morning. He has previously had a right inguinal hernia repaired.

a. What factors would predispose this patient to getting a hernia?
b. Recurrent hernias are uncommon. What factors might predispose him to get a recurrence following repair?
c. In getting this patient's consent for hernia repair, what should he be told?
d. How would his diabetes be best managed during his admission for surgery?

5 A 12-year-old boy was trying to light a barbecue using petrol he found in his garage. He sustained burns to his right arm, face and upper body. On arrival in the emergency department he is in severe pain. The burned area is extensive, and some areas appear to be partial thickness while other areas are full thickness.

a. How do you distinguish full thickness from partial thickness burns?
b. He needs to be resuscitated with intravenous fluids. How do you work out his fluid requirement, and what sort of fluids would you give?
c. What features would suggest that he has airway involvement?
d. Outline the likely course of management following resuscitation over the next few days. Consider what other treatments and interventions he might require.
e. What factors are likely to influence his prognosis?

6 A 17-year-old girl is admitted with abdominal pain and vomiting and undergoes a laparoscopy at which a perforated appendix is found; a laparoscopic appendicectomy is performed. The peritoneum is washed out. Five days later she develops a pyrexia and is unwell.

a. What are the possible causes of the postoperative pyrexia?
b. How would you investigate the patient?
c. What measures could be taken to reduce the likelihood of postoperative infective complications?
d. What late complications might the girl suffer?

7 A 55-year-old schoolteacher is due to have a total hip replacement but she has heard about hospital-acquired infections and is now considering cancelling her operation.

a. What is understood by the term 'hospital-acquired infection'?
b. What predisposes to such infections?
c. What are the common such infections seen in a surgical ward?
d. How can such infections be prevented?

8 Discuss the role of balloons in surgery. Answer by classifying the ways in which balloons are used, with appropriate examples.

9 A 34-year-old male nurse presented with a 2-week history of a swollen left testicle. There were no urinary symptoms and palpation of the scrotum revealed a normal right testis with a smoothly swollen, firm testis with a small flaccid surrounding hydrocoele. As an infant he had the left testis replaced in the scrotum.

a. What is the likely diagnosis and differential diagnosis?
b. What are the different types of testicular tumour?
c. What are the different macroscopic appearances of the two common sorts of testicular tumour?
d. What investigations are appropriate for this patient?
e. What treatment is given for testicular cancer? Detail the surgical approach.
f. What is the prognosis for testicular tumours?

10 A 55-year-old cleaner attends her family practitioner with a change of bowel habit and passing blood per rectum. She previously had an aortic valve replacement for aortic stenosis. Investigations confirm an adenocarcinoma of the rectum at 6 cm from the anal verge. Abdominal CT suggests that the disease is confined to the rectum. A barium enema does not show any abnormality in the rest of the colon.

a. What are the possible causes of aortic stenosis?
b. At her age, what type of valve replacement is she likely to have had, and why?
c. Assuming she is on warfarin, how would you manage her anticoagulation perioperatively?
d. What are the surgical options for the treatment of her rectal carcinoma?
e. Describe the eponymous classification of rectal carcinoma. Who was the man who described this system of classification?

MCQs Answers

1. a. Prognosis relates to the thickness of the tumour, known as the Breslow depth, measured vertically from the top of the granular layer to the deepest point of tumour invasion. Prognosis is good when the depth is less than 1.5 mm (90% 5-year survival), and poor when the depth is over 4 mm (less than 50% 5-year survival). Prognosis does not relate to the diameter of the melanoma. Variation in pigmentation and bleeding are both signs that a melanoma might be malignant, but have no prognostic significance. Acral melanomas, as tumours occurring on the extremities are known, have a better prognosis than melanomas that occur on the trunk.
2. d. The patient presents in a state of shock and all the possible answers are associated with shock. Patients suffering myocardial infarction can experience abdominal pain and develop cardiogenic shock as the cardiac output falls. The physiological response is sympathetic stimulation – the patient is pale and cold (vasoconstrictor) and clammy (sudomotor); the vasomotor response raises peripheral vascular resistance. Similarly haemorrhage, whether from a ruptured aneurysm or duodenal ulcer, results in reflex vasoconstriction. Small bowel obstruction, in the absence of strangulation, is associated with volume depletion due to vomiting and loss into the dilated intestine and the patient behaves as above. A patient with perforated diverticulitis of the colon is septic as a consequence of contamination of the peritoneum with faecal organisms. The sepsis results in vasodilatation with a consequent fall in peripheral vascular resistance. This latter patient would benefit from norepinephrine (noradrenaline), whose predominant actions cause vasoconstriction, in addition to fluid resuscitation. Patients with fluid loss (b, c and e) need aggressive fluid replacement and the patient in cardiogenic shock (a) would benefit from an inotrope, such as dobutamine, whose $\beta 1$ actions cause increased myocardial contractility and rate.
3. c. Pulmonary embolism typically occurs around the 10th day postoperatively, but may occur sooner. It is more common in patients who have had pelvic surgery, and often occurs in association with straining at stool, as in this case. The manifestation may range from sudden death to mild dyspnoea, and is associated with a tachycardia, low grade temperature and low oxygen saturation. Right axis deviation and right heart strain (ST depression in leads V1 to V3, III and AVF) is typical and is due to the right ventricle pumping against an obstructed pulmonary arterial tree.

   Pulmonary collapse (due to mucus plugging of the main airways) and basal atelectasis (collapse of the basal segments) usually occurs in the first 48 h postoperatively. Myocardial infarction affects the left ventricle and has characteristic electrocardiograph changes and is associated with central chest pain. Anastomotic disruption (leak) is associated with abdominal pain and not dyspnoea.
4. d. Squamous carcinoma of the lung often gives rise to metastases in the suprarenal gland that result in adrenocortical failure, rather than excess suprarenal activity. Small cell (oat cell) carcinomas of the lung can produce adrenocorticotrophic hormone (ACTH) and might be associated with Cushing's syndrome.

   Like breast, prostate, kidney and thyroid cancers, carcinoma of the bronchus commonly spreads to bone and may present with a pathological fracture. Multiple myeloma is also associated with skeletal metastases. Finger clubbing and hypertrophic osteoarthopathy are features of squamous lung cancers, as is hypercalcaemia secondary to ectopic parathyroid hormone production by the tumour. Lastly the primary tumour might partially occlude the bronchus, resulting in repeated bouts of pneumonia.

5. c. In coarctation of the aorta blood reaches the distal aorta via collaterals between branches of the subclavian, scapular and intercostals arteries. The observed rib notching on the chest X-ray is due to the enlarged intercostal arteries. Coarctation often presents with the complications of hypertension, such as cardiac failure and cerebral haemorrhage. Echocardiography usually demonstrates left ventricular hypertrophy secondary to the hypertension. The coarct is demonstrated as a narrowing in the descending aorta just distal to the left subclavian artery on angiography, not a patent ductus. Because the narrowing is distal to the left subclavian artery, there is no gradient between the arms, with both arms showing the same high blood pressure. The pressure in the lower limbs is usually much reduced. It is the low blood pressure distal to the coarct that results in excess renin production by the kidney to maintain renal perfusion, hence the high upper body blood pressure.
6. d. The patient has experienced an aortic dissection during which blood enters the media of the aorta and strips through that layer producing a false lumen, often returning to the true lumen further down the aorta. Aortic branches arising from the true lumen are deprived of blood since it is now flowing down the false lumen. In this case the loss of consciousness and loss of function in the right arm is probably due to the origins of the left common carotid artery and left subclavian artery being excluded from the circulation by the dissection, causing ipsilateral cerebral ischaemia. Were he right-handed you might have expected disturbances in his speech as well since the left hemisphere would have been the dominant hemisphere; in this left-handed man it is the right hemisphere that is dominant. The weakness is due to the cerebral ischaemia – the brachial plexus is some distance from the aorta and is not affected by aortic dissection. The anuria is ominous and suggests that both renal arteries are also excluded from the circulation. A dissection that occurs in the ascending aorta or arch of aorta, such as this one, is a type A dissection; Type B dissections occur in the descending aorta and seldom need surgery. In contrast, type A dissections usually do require surgery because the dissection can progress retrograde and through the aortic valve ring producing aortic regurgitation (as suggested in this case by the diastolic murmur), or into the pericardium causing acute cardiac tamponade and death. This patient requires an aortic valve replacement and repair of the aortic root with a prosthetic aortic graft.

   Investigation of a patient with a possible dissection usually involves CT scanning, which shows a characteristic flap across the lumen. Angiography is less useful since it tends to outline the true lumen and may miss a false passage. Transoesophageal echocardiography is the investigation of choice, since not only can it demonstrate the dissection in the aorta, but it can also accurately assess the aortic valve.
7. e. The annual risk of rupture of an aneurysm less than 5.5 cm in diameter is less than 5%. Once an aneurysm is detected it needs to be either repaired if it is large (over 5.5 cm) or followed by regular screening if it is small (less than 5.5 cm). The average rate of growth of an aneurysm depends upon its size, but at 5.1 cm an annual growth rate between 2 and 4 mm is likely. Therefore it will quickly reach the threshold for repair so the patient should be scanned every 6 months or so.

   Aorto-enteric fistulae are uncommon (1%) in patients who have previously had an aneurysm repaired, but very uncommon in patients with an aneurysm per se. When they do occur, they present with massive gastrointestinal haemorrhage.

   Endovascular stenting can be performed in large aneurysms and is not confined to small aneurysms. Angiography demonstrates the lumen of the aneurysm, which is often smaller by virtue of thrombus lining the wall of the aneurysm (mural thrombus). Thus it underestimates the diameter of the aorta. Ultrasound is the investigation of choice for assessing an aneurysm, permitting accurate measurement of the diameter of the aorta and documenting its relation to the left renal vein.
8. b. Endarterectomy is indicated and should be performed as soon as possible lest further embolic

events occur. Until then the patient should be started on low dose (75 mg/day) aspirin to reduce the likelihood of emboli. Emboli may either result in a further episode of ipsilateral amaurosis fugax (fleeting blindness) or contralateral hemiparesis due to an embolism into the ipsilateral cerebral hemisphere causing a transient ischaemic attack or complete stroke. Hypoglossal neuropraxia is a complication of endarterectomy, and not of the stenosis. The hypoglossal nerve crosses the upper part of the incision and may be damaged during surgery, resulting in protrusion of the tongue ipsilaterally (i.e. it points towards the side of the injury).

Intravascular angiography gives an accurate delineation of the stenosis, but is associated with a small incidence of emboli. Duplex imaging is thus the investigation of choice, with MR angiography where duplex produces equivocal results.

9. d. The patient gives a history typical of deep venous insufficiency secondary to deep vein thrombosis, which is likely to have occurred following the fracture of the tibia and fibula. Surgery to the superficial veins would be appropriate only if the deep system was known to be patent, which is not known in this case. This would be best assessed by duplex scan, rather than venography, which is invasive and can cause venous thrombosis. Arteriovenous fistulae can occur following fractured limbs and may cause prominent superficial veins. It is very uncommon, and is assessed by arteriography, not venography. Long-term anticoagulation is not warranted in patients with deep venous insufficiency; it is indicated in patients with recurrent venous thromboembolism. Haemosiderosis, eczema and lipodermatosclerosis are features of deep venous insufficiency but occur in the medial gaiter area (above the medial malleolus), not the lateral area.

10. c. Pituitary tumours present with local effects of the tumour, effects of excess hormone production by a hormone-secreting tumour, and effects of low hormone production from the rest of the anterior pituitary. The local effects include headache due to encroachment on the paranasal sinuses, and bitemporal hemianopia due to compression of the optic chiasma. Bleeding into large tumours (apoplexy) may also exacerbate local symptoms, as in this case. Homonymous hemianopia is due to interruption of the visual pathway between the chiasma and the occipital cortex, and does not occur with chiasmal compression.

The patient has a pituitary adenoma, half of which are likely to be prolactinomas. In a female this may be associated with galactorrhoea, but this is rarely a symptom in a man. The normal pituitary is compressed, resulting in reduced production of luteinizing hormone (LH), follicle-stimulating hormone (FSH), growth hormone, thyroid-stimulating hormone (TSH) and adrenocorticotrophic hormone (ACTH), producing hypogonadism with low testosterone production, hypothyroidism with low thyroxine production, and hypoadrenalism with low cortisol production. This patient's hair loss is compatible with a reduction in testosterone, and his tiredness, sensitivity to cold and bradycardia are all compatible with hypothyroidism (low TSH, rather than high TSH).

In patients presenting with a pituitary tumour and visual disturbances the possibility of chiasmal compression needs to be excluded. Surgical decompression by trans-sphenoidal hypophysectomy should be considered if found. Otherwise surgery is indicated to remove all pituitary tumours except prolactinomas, which can usually be managed with dopamine agonist therapy such as bromocriptine or cabergoline.

11. b. The Glasgow Coma Score (GCS) is E3V2M5 = 10 (see p. 71). Head injuries with increased intracranial pressure are associated with a bradycardia and hypertension (Cushing's reflex). Hypotension is unlikely to be due to the head injury and in this patient, with fractures to the ribs on the left side, a ruptured spleen would be a distinct possibility and would mandate an urgent CT scan if stable, or laparotomy if unstable. Only a flail chest is managed by positive pressure ventilation. Isolated rib factures require analgesia or intercostal anaesthetic blocks to ensure that the underlying lung is well ventilated. This patient has an impaired conscious level

(GCS 10) and a history that would be compatible with a cervical spine injury. His neck should be stabilized in a stiff collar and a fracture/dislocation excluded either by plain X-rays or CT scan.

12. d. Carpal tunnel syndrome is four times more common in women than men, and is associated with pregnancy, rheumatoid arthritis, myxoedema, acromegaly and wrist fractures. The motor supply to the muscles of the thenar eminence arises distal to the flexor retinaculum and so is compromised in carpal tunnel syndrome; thumb abduction is thus also lost. The sensory loss affects the thumb and radial three and a half fingers – the ring finger is usually supplied by the median nerve on its radial border, and the ulnar nerve on its ulnar border.
13. e. Only carcinoma of the parotid causes a lower motor neuron palsy as it infiltrates the facial (VII) nerve. Benign tumours like a pleomorphic adenoma or adenolymphoma do not affect the facial nerve. The treatment of carcinoma of the parotid is radical excision with sacrifice of the facial nerve and block dissection of the ipsilateral cervical nodes if these are involved. Adenolymphoma is a benign tumour and so would not be associated with lymphadenopathy. Mumps commonly affects the parotid glands, but only occasionally are the submandibular glands involved. The parotid glands are not derived from any branchial arch, and parotid tumours do not cause ear pain.
14. b. Pharyngeal pouches arise between the two parts of the inferior constrictor muscle, with the thyropharyngeus superiorly and cricopharyngeus inferiorly. They are often associated with recurrent episodes of pneumonia as pouch contents are aspirated. The diagnosis is best proven by barium swallow, since oesophagoscopy may inadvertently perforate the pouch. Endoscopic diverticulotomy, where the wall between the pouch and oesophagus is divided using an endoscopic stapling device, is the treatment of choice and has replaced the open exposure using a cervical approach, since the latter was associated with cervical fistulae. Plummer–Vinson syndrome, also called Paterson–Brown Kelly syndrome, is common in elderly females and is characterized by dysphagia, iron deficiency anaemia and an oesophageal web.
15. a. Troisier's sign is the presence of enlarged left supraclavicular nodes (Virchow's nodes) secondary to lymphatic spread from tumours in the lung, mediastinum or gastrointestinal tract. The most common oesophageal tumours are adenocarcinomas of the lower third. Many occur in areas where the oesophageal squamous epithelium has undergone metaplasia into a gastric columnar-type epithelium, so-called Barrett's oesophagus. Like Plummer–Vinson syndrome, Barrett's oesophagus is premalignant. A history like this that is suggestive of oesophageal carcinoma is best investigated initially with endoscopy, at which a biopsy may be taken to confirm the diagnosis.
16. a. Infants presenting with pyloric stenosis, like this child, need resuscitating with intravenous saline with added potassium to compensate for the lost chloride and potassium. Only when they have been fully resuscitated should they be operated on – there is no indication for urgent surgery. The procedure of choice is longitudinal division of the pyloric muscle down to the mucosa (Ramstedt's operation) (see Fig. 51.2, p. 105). Loss of gastric acid in the vomit results in a metabolic alkalosis. The condition is much commoner in males than females (80%), with half being the first-born child.
17. a. *Helicobacter* possess a powerful urease enzyme that splits urea-liberating ammonia. The urease test for *Helicobacter* relies on the fact that the urea solution becomes alkali. A gastric ulcer may be benign or malignant; biopsy is always indicated to confirm the nature of the ulcer. *Helicobacter* eradication therapy comprises a combination of anti-*Helicobacter* agents, either antibiotics or bismuth preparations, in addition to a proton pump inhibitor or histamine-2 receptor blocker (e.g. cimetidine) for symptomatic relief. In the case of a gastric carcinoma some pain relief may be gained by acid suppression, thus misleading the clinician that the ulcer was benign.

    Nowadays a benign gastric ulcer is best managed medically, and a malignant ulcer will need a more radical gastrectomy than a Bilroth I – this latter was the treatment of choice for peptic ulcers before medical therapy became so efficient. Bilroth II and Pólya gastrectomies were for duodenal ulcers, and involved removing the acid-producing antrum and body of the stomach.

18. c. Simple obstruction is characterized by colicky central abdominal pain, distension, vomiting and absolute constipation. In small bowel obstruction absolute constipation is a late occurrence, and patients often continue to pass flatus. Signs that an obstruction has become strangulating, where the viability of the bowel is jeopardized, are that the pain becomes constant, the patient becomes tachycardic, pyrexial and on examination there are features of peritonism. Bowel sounds become absent, and a leucocytosis develops.

    Pelvic ultrasound does not have a place in the diagnosis or management of obstruction, whereas CT is useful both to identify the site of obstruction as well as to exclude unusual herniae such as an obturator hernia. Intussusception sometimes occurs with the appendix at the apex of the intussusception. Following surgery to remove the appendix the ensuing adhesions are likely to make intussusception less likely.

19. b. An inflamed Meckel's diverticulum can mimic appendicitis completely. McBurney studied patients with appendicitis and found that the usual site of maximal tenderness was 'between an inch and a half to two inches from the anterior spinous process of the ilium' towards the umbilicus; nowadays we refer to McBurney's point as being one-third of the way from the anterior superior iliac spine to the umbilicus. In the pregnant female the appendix is displaced cranially, not laterally. Appendicitis general develops within 12–24 h; after 5 days one might expect to find an appendix mass in the right iliac fossa. Migration of the pain is due to the central visceral pain being replaced by a more severe pain in the right iliac fossa due to irritation of the parietal peritoneum.

20. e. Haemorrhage from a colonic diverticulum is typically profuse with plum-coloured blood and clots that appear to fill the pan. A bleeding gastric ulcer would present with haematemesis, and the rectal blood loss would be melaena. Rectal carcinoma is usually bright red and mixed in with the stool, rather than separate from it. Caecal carcinoma usually presents with iron deficiency anaemia, not present in this case. Crohn's disease may cause a colitis or perianal disease such as fissure and fistula in ano; it rarely presents with bleeding.

21. a. A hernia that cannot be reduced is termed irreducible. An obstructed hernia is one causing intestinal obstruction, and is usually irreducible. Inguinal herniae are more common than femoral herniae in women, although femoral herniae are more common in women than men. Indirect herniae pass through the internal (deep) ring; direct herniae pass directly through the floor of the inguinal canal. The external spermatic fascia is an extension of the external oblique aponeurosis beyond the external ring – it does not exist in the inguinal ring.

22. b. The patient is likely to have carcinoma of the pancreas. However, the recent diagnosis of diabetes and history of weight loss suggest that this tumour arose in the body some time previously and has spread to the head of pancreas, where it is causing obstructive jaundice. As such it is unlikely to be resectable. In obstructive jaundice bilirubin glucuronide from the liver cannot get into the gut; it is the absence of this that results in pale stools. Instead the bilirubin passes in the urine to give it the typical brown colour. The gallbladder is typically distended in obstructive jaundice not due to stones. Loss of bile from the gut impairs absorption of fat and the fat-soluble vitamins A, D, E and K. The absence of vitamin K impairs hepatic production of clotting factors, resulting in a prolonged prothrombin time.

23. a. Haemoglobin concentration is not a risk factor for severity in acute pancreatitis. A low PO_2, raised leucocyte count and hyperglycaemia are all factors in the Glasgow criteria predicting severity; a C-reactive protein over 140 mg/L is an independent predictor of severity.

24. a. The spleen is particularly important in patients with infections with capsulated organisms like *Haemophilus influenzae*, *Meningococcus* and *Pneumococcus*. Following splenectomy, patients are more susceptible to infections from such organisms, such that immunization

is recommended in addition to a 2-year course of penicillin prophylaxis. Prophylactic penicillin is indicated for longer in childhood. Annual immunization against influenza is recommended to minimize risks from bacterial superinfection following flu. Post-splenectomy sepsis is less common when the spleen has been removed following trauma, possibly because of seeding of splenic tissue throughout the peritoneum. Thrombocytosis is very common after splenectomy for whatever indication and does not indicate an underlying haematological disorder.

25. d. A mobile lump in a female of this age is likely to be a fibroadenoma. These are now believed to be aberrations of normal development, rather than neoplasms. They are not premalignant. Nevertheless as a solitary breast lump it requires triple assessment of clinical examination, ultrasound and core biopsy in order to rule out malignancy. In patients under 35, ultrasound is preferred to mammography. A discrete painless lump is not a typical presentation of cyclical mastalgia, which is better characterized by tender nodularity of the breasts that regresses following menstruation.
26. a. Mantle radiotherapy, especially if given before the age of 20, increases the risk of later breast cancer. Invasive duct carcinoma is the most common type of breast cancer. Skin tethering implies the tumour involves the skin or subcutaneous tissues. Peau d'orange is caused by invasion of the dermal lymphatics with tumour. Deep fixation implies that the tumour may have invaded the underlying pectoralis major muscle. Early menarche (less than 11 years) and late menopause (older than 51 years), resulting in prolonged oestrogen exposure, are risk factors for breast cancer. This tumour is over 5 cm (T3) and the nodes are palpable (N1). Distant spread has not been assessed (MX).
27. c. A solitary solid lump is a thyroid tumour and needs to be evaluated by ultrasound-guided core biopsy. Anaplastic carcinomas occur in the elderly, and are often associated with dysphagia and vocal cord palsies. This tumour is likely to be a follicular carcinoma. Thyroid lobectomy is generally used for papillary tumours, where the tumour is often confined to the lobe; follicular tumours require total thyroidectomy. Total thyroidectomy may result in the sacrifice of all parathyroid tissue, causing hypoparathyroidism. Radioiodine does not damage parathyroid tissue, but is given for its effects on the remaining thyroid tissue and metastases. Levothyroxine is given to all patients with differentiated thyroid tumours to suppress thyroid-stimulating hormone (TSH) production, and so reduce the stimulus to differentiated thyroid tumour cells.
28. c. Strawberries, not raspberries, have a high oxalate content and are associated with the formation of oxalate stones. Crohn's disease, where the terminal ileum is involved, or ileal resection also result in increased oxalate excretion. Increased uric acid secretion, and thus urate stone formation, is seen in patients with gout, but may also complicate chemotherapy for leukaemia or lymphoma, such that patients are often prescribed allopurinol as part of their treatment regimen. Hyperparathyroidism causes hypercalcaemia and hypercalciuria, resulting in calcium phosphate stones. Surgeons have a higher incidence of stone formation presumably through the passage of concentrated urine, a consequence of long operations.
29. c. Finasteride is a 5α-reductase inhibitor, which works by blocking the conversion of testosterone to its active metabolite dihydrotestosterone in the prostate. It results in reduction in size of the prostate, a beneficial effect that may take 6 months to appear. Tamsulosin is an example of a selective α1-adrenergic antagonist. Ultrasound has replaced intravenous urography in the assessment of the renal tract in patients with outflow obstruction, being able to demonstrate hydronephrosis and hydroureter, as well as estimating the post-micturition residue. Small T1 prostate cancers are impalpable, by definition.
30. e. The left testicular vein drains directly into the left renal vein, unlike the right testicular vein, which drains obliquely into the inferior vena cava. Testicular tumours are more common in testes in abnormal positions, but most are found in testes that have undergone normal descent. Teratoma is commoner in young patients, with seminoma more common in the 30–40-year age group. Lymphatic

spread is via the iliac lymph nodes to the para-aortic nodes; the scrotal skin drains to the inguinal nodes but not the scrotal contents. This is important where surgical exploration is concerned, since the testis is exposed through a groin incision not a scrotal incision. Mistaken removal of a testicular tumour via the scrotum would necessitate scrotal irradiation, and consequent infertility. Even in the presence of para-aortic lymphadenopathy, survival from teratoma remains good.

EMQs Answers

1

1. e. Pelvic abscess. Perforated appendicitis results in soiling of the peritoneum and pus collecting in the pouch of Douglas (female) or recto-vesical space (male). A pelvic abscess forms, and is diagnosed by a boggy mass anteriorly on rectal examination. Treatment is with antibiotics, with which the abscess may resolve or may point and discharge into the rectum, something that may be hastened by judicious rectal examination.
2. d. Pulmonary embolism. Bowel preparation for an anterior resection can result in dehydration in a patient who then spends some time in an operating theatre having pelvic surgery. Such patients are at high risk of deep vein thrombosis, which may embolize, either presenting as a massive pulmonary embolism with circulatory collapse or death, or multiple smaller emboli may occur. In this latter setting patients may be tachypnoeic, or breathless on exertion. Often, however, they just have a grumbling fever, the cause of which may be revealed after some searching by performing a thoracic CT scan.
3. i. Infective endocarditis. The presence of an indwelling intravenous catheter of any sort puts a patient at risk of infective endocarditis. Transthoracic echocardiography will confirm the presence of vegetations in most cases. If suspicion is high, but transthoracic echocardiography is normal then transoesophageal echocardiography (TOE) should be performed, since this is more sensitive, particularly for tricuspid involvement. Microscopic haematuria is common in endocarditis, as would be the presence of subungual splinter haemorrhages in the fingers and toes.
4. j. *Clostridium difficile*. Broad spectrum antibiotics such as cephalosporins predispose patients to infection with *C. difficile*, which usually presents with diarrhoea, often causing incontinence in the elderly, but may occasionally present with a toxic dilatation of the colon. Confirmation is by examination of the faeces for the toxin, although the presence of pseudomembranes at sigmoidoscopy is strongly suggestive.
5. a. Wound infection. Obesity and diabetes are both risk factors for postoperative wound infection, something that the wound pain also suggests. One week after surgery the wound should be becoming less painful.

2

1. c. Carcinoma of the pancreas. Recent onset of diabetes is a recognized feature of patients presenting with pancreatic carcinoma as the tumour invades the pancreas and destroys the islets. The jaundice is typically painless and progressive.
2. f. Ascending cholangitis. Rigors are typically associated with biliary tract and renal tract sepsis. The triad of rigors, jaundice and pain was described by Charcot and is typical of acute cholangitis.
3. i. Periampullary carcinoma. Carcinoma of the ampulla of Vater typically presents early with jaundice. As necrotic tumour sloughs the obstruction is relieved, hence the jaundice gives the impression of relapsing. The dark urine and pale stools suggest an obstructive jaundice. The silvery appearance is attributable to altered blood on the surface of the stool and is said to be pathognomic of ampullary carcinoma.
4. h. Biliary colic typically presents a couple of hours after a fatty meal and is due to sustained contraction of the gallbladder (stimulated by cholecystokinin) against an obstruction. If, as in this case, the patient is jaundiced, that obstruction lies within the common bile duct or ampulla. Unlike acute cholecystitis, the patient is usually not pyrexial, and the pain resolves spontaneously after a few hours, but its disappearance is hastened by opiate analgesia.

5. b. Primary sclerosing cholangitis is associated with inflammatory bowel disease (Crohn's disease and ulcerative colitis) and is more common in men. It often presents with non-specific symptoms and is diagnosed at magnetic resonance cholangio-pancreatography (MRCP) or endoscopic retrograde cholangio-pancreatography (ERCP) by the beaded appearance of the bile ducts, with typical changes on liver biopsy. It is associated with other autoimmune phenomena.

3

1. d. Ruptured ectopic pregnancy. An intrauterine contraceptive device is associated with a higher incidence of pelvic infection and also of extrauterine pregnancy. A history of an abnormal last period, whether it is lighter than normal, or fails to happen is suspicious of a pregnancy. In this context a history of rapid onset right iliac fossa pain is highly suggestive of a ruptured ectopic pregnancy. That being the case, the diagnosis is best confirmed by the presence of a raised β-human gonadotrophin (βhCG); a full blood count may reveal anaemia but this is unlikely in an acute bleed. In this setting a pelvic examination should be deferred because of the risk of disrupting the pregnancy and causing further haemorrhage, as has happened in this case. It is best to perform this examination in the anaesthetic room, or preferably not at all until the diagnosis of ectopic pregnancy has been excluded.
2. h. Acute pyelonephritis. Urinary frequency suggests a urinary infection in a young woman who is sexually active – indeed it often follows the act of copulation. The movement of this pain to the right loin suggests pyelonephritis. Rigors typically occur with infection of the biliary or renal tracts. Had this been a retrocaecal appendicitis causing loin pain then hip extension, which tenses the psoas muscle (the psoas stretch test), would be expected to cause pain.
3. j. Crohn's disease. While central colicky abdominal pain that moves to the right iliac fossa would be a typical history of appendicitis, the past history of abdominal pains is not typical and might be more suggestive of Crohn's ileitis. A history of weight loss, distension and vomiting, suggesting obstruction, would further support a suspicion that this might be an acute presentation of Crohn's disease. CT imaging would be the quickest way to support a diagnosis of Crohn's disease or appendicitis, and laparoscopy could also confirm appendicitis.
4. g. Perforated duodenal ulcer. Sudden onset pain is typical of a perforated viscus. Elderly women with arthritis usually take non-steroid anti-inflammatory drugs to control the discomfort, and these drugs are associated with peptic ulcer formation. The presence of subdiaphragmatic air supports the suspicion of a perforated viscus. Following perforation of a duodenal ulcer the contents of the duodenum, including the pancreatic secretions, are lost into the peritoneum. The amylase-rich pancreatic fluid is reabsorbed, resulting in a raised serum amylase.
5. b. Acute diverticulitis. Left iliac fossa pain in an elderly patient is frequently, but not exclusively, due to diverticulitis. If the condition does not settle on antibiotics within 48 h, or if there is a suspicion that the presentation is not simple acute diverticulitis, a CT scan is appropriate to exclude a complication such as abscess formation or perforation, as well as to exclude any other pathology.

4

1. h. Fat embolism. Long bone fractures are commonly associated with fat emboli, which may occur 24–48 h after injury, unlike blood clots, which tend to embolize later following immobilization (10 days). Typically, patients become hypoxaemic and dyspnoeic. The occurrence of emboli may be associated with the occurrence of reddish-brown petechiae over the upper body and axillae. Diagnosis is usually made from the presence of otherwise unexplained hypoxia. The presence of fat in the urine is common in trauma and is an unreliable indicator of embolism, although anaemia, thrombocytopaenia and hypofibrinogenaemia are suggestive, though non-specific.
2. j. Tension pneumothorax. Cracked ribs are a common cause of pneumothorax. However, the progressive breathlessness and developing cyanosis is more in keeping with the development of a tension pneumothorax. This is supported by the tracheal deviation to the opposite side as the left pleural space fills with air, together with the tachycardia and hypotension as the venous return to the heart is inhibited by the increased intrathoracic pressure.
3. d. Paradoxical embolism. Pelvic surgery and malignancy are risk factors for the development of deep venous thrombosis, which is the explanation

for the swollen right leg. The presence of breathlessness suggests that some of the clot has embolized to her lungs. This results in increased pulmonary artery pressure, and may cause shunting of blood (and clot) through a longstanding persistent foramen ovale. Once through the foramen, the clot embolizes to the systemic circulation. In this patient it first manifested as a hemiparesis, and later the clot caused an acutely ischaemic lower leg – pale, pulseless and cold. The diagnosis is confirmed by the presence of a pulmonary embolism, which was confirmed on thoracic CT, and transoesophageal echocardiography, confirming the presence of a patent foramen ovale.

4. i. Cardiac tamponade. Cardiac tamponade occurs following the rupture of an aortic dissection into the pericardium, the rupture of necrotic myocardium following a myocardial infarct, pericarditis or trauma. Chest pain, typically radiating to the neck, shoulder or back, and difficulty breathing are the initial presenting features, and on examination the characteristic triad of features are hypotension, distended jugular veins and muffled heart sounds. Diagnosis is rapidly made by echocardiography, although an enlarged cardiac silhouette in the context of trauma is highly suggestive. The pericardial fluid, which in the case of trauma is blood, needs evacuating as a matter of urgency.
5. c. Pulmonary collapse. Upper abdominal surgery typically causes reduced ventilation because breathing is painful. In a patient with ankylosing spondylitis the vertebrae become fused, often causing a kyphosis, compromising the lung volumes. Most of the normal respiratory effort in such patients derives from diaphragmatic contractions, and upper abdominal surgery is likely to make this extremely painful. Coughing is also inhibited by pain. The stage is thus set for pulmonary collapse, which usually occurs early postoperatively and is the result of mucus plugging of small airways. The resultant collapsed lung continues to be perfused by blood and acts as a shunt, returning deoxygenated blood to the left atrium. The collapsed lung segment frequently becomes secondarily infected.

5

1. c. Branchial cyst. Typically presentation follows an upper respiratory tract infection, an occurrence that is thought to be related to the lymphoid tissue within the cyst. The swelling emerges from behind the lower third of the sternomastoid muscle. They are believed to be derived from the second branchial cleft.
2. h. Cervical rib. The presentation with an intermittent cold hand and neurological symptoms is suggestive of thoracic outlet syndrome due to compression of the brachial plexus and subclavian artery. One cause is a cervical rib, which is sometimes felt as a swelling in the neck arising from the seventh cervical vertebra. Confirmation of thoracic outlet syndrome can be made by asking the patient to raise (abduct and externally rotate) their arms following which the radial pulse disappears (Adson's sign).
3. j. Thyroglossal cyst. Thyroglossal cysts arise from the thyroglossal duct, which passes from the foramen caecum in the tongue around the hyoid bone to the isthmus of the thyroid gland. Typically they are midline, just caudal to the hyoid bone, and move up on protrusion of the tongue.
4. g. Papillary carcinoma of thyroid. A swelling that moves with swallowing is usually of thyroid origin. This swelling is associated with lymphadenopathy suggesting a malignancy. Papillary thyroid cancer occurs in adolescents and young adults, and it is often associated with cervical lymph node spread at diagnosis. Ultrasound would confirm that this was a solid lesion, and fine needle aspiration confirms its histology.
5. d. Virchow's lymph node. Thoracic and intraperitoneal malignancy may present with lymphadenopathy in the left supraclavicular fossa due to lymphatic tumour spread up the thoracic duct, which drains into the subclavian vein on that side. The lymph node was described by Virchow, and Troisier made the association with malignancy. In this patient's case the history of dysphagia and weight loss would be suspicious of an oesophageal carcinoma until proven otherwise.

6

1. j. Caecal carcinoma. While caecal carcinomas typically present with a history of progressive iron deficiency anaemia, when the tumour impinges on the ileocaecal valve presentation with small bowel obstruction may occur. At the age of 64, the commonest causes of obstruction in a patient

without a history of previous surgery are a hernia or a malignancy. The presence of a right iliac fossa mass points to a caecal neoplasm in this case.

2. a. Femoral hernia. Femoral herniae are common causes of obstruction in elderly females, and are often found undiagnosed on the medical wards. The finding of a mass below the medial end of the left inguinal ligament (the femoral canal) suggests the presence of a femoral hernia in this case. Such herniae are often of the Richter type, with only part of the bowel wall caught up and rendered ischaemic, while features of obstruction might be absent.
3. i. Crohn's disease typically manifests in young adults, and is suggested by a history of intermittent abdominal pains and diarrhoea leading up to the presentation. At laparotomy multiple inflammatory strictures in the terminal ileum are found.
4. c. Adhesions. Anyone presenting with features of intestinal obstruction who has had previous abdominal surgery, whether or not it is surgery you are familiar with, is at risk of intestinal obstruction. In this case extensive surgery had been performed within the peritoneal cavity to expose the right common iliac vessels by mobilizing the caecum, and a Roux loop had also been fashioned. Adhesions are therefore likely. Patients with previous transplants, be it heart, lung, liver or kidney and pancreas, as here, get common conditions and suffer from delayed diagnosis. This patient should be examined to exclude evidence of strangulation, and then managed in a standard manner, taking care to continue his immunosuppressive therapy by giving it intravenously.
5. d. Intussusception. The classical presentation with redcurrant jelly stools occurs in about 20% of cases. Most occur in infants aged between 6 and 12 months, boys being more often affected than girls. Predisposing factors include recent respiratory tract infections or diarrhoeal illness.

7

1. e. Sebaceous cyst. Lumps on the scalp are usually sebaceous cysts, and the embarrassment of a hairdresser's comments often prompts referral. The presence of a punctum usually confirms the diagnosis.
2. i. Malignant melanoma. Acral melanomas (as melanomas occurring on the extremities are termed) present like most other melanomas, as a slow growing pigmented lesion. The presence of a satellite lesion is uncommon but almost diagnostic, and is the result of spread through the dermal lymphatics. A history of bleeding, increase in size and being raised all point to this being a malignant melanoma.
3. j. Implantation dermoid. Typically occurring as a consequence of a puncture wound, such as a rose thorn, implantation dermoids are nests of epidermis that grow deep to the dermis and present as a lump usually on the pulp of a finger or toe.
4. g. Kaposi's sarcoma. Common in patients with HIV infection, Kaposi's sarcoma also occurs more commonly in patients who are immunosuppressed for organ transplantation. Typically the lesions present 18 months after transplant, and are more common in people of Mediterranean descent. The causative agent is thought to be the human herpes virus 8 (HHV8), and in the transplant setting they often respond to withdrawal of immunosuppression or switching to the immunosuppressant sirolimus, which inhibits the actions of vascular endothelial growth factor (VEGF) and causes the lesion to regress.
5. d. Sequestration dermoid. In contrast to implantation dermoids, sequestration dermoids are rests of dermal cells that have been deposited during embryological development along epithelial fusion lines. They are common in the midline under the chin, and the inner and outer angles of the eyes (external angular dermoid). Erosion of the underlying skull is common, and occasionally they may communicate deeply through the skull.

8

1. j. Fibroadenoma. Typically highly mobile, small, discrete, firm lumps, they commonly appear in the third decade. Although formal triple assessment is indicated to exclude malignancy, they are benign and may be left *in situ*.
2. f. Galactocoele. Commonly occurring shortly after cessation of breastfeeding, galactocoeles are benign cysts containing milk.
3. b. Carcinoma of the breast. A previous history of mantle radiotherapy for Hodgkin's is associated with a much higher incidence of carcinoma of the breast. This tumour is fixed to skin and is most likely to be a carcinoma.
4. i. Breast abscess. Most breast abscesses occur in the context of lactation, but occasionally they can occur

spontaneously and are more common in patients with diabetes. In the absence of fluctuance to suggest pus the treatment involves intravenous antibiotics. In patients who develop breast inflammation while not lactating, the possibility of an inflammatory carcinoma should be borne in mind. However, the history is usually longer than in this case.

5. h. Duct ectasia. Postmenopausal involutional changes to the breast ducts result in the terminal ducts becoming dilated. They fill with serous secretions, which discharge periodically from multiple sites on the nipple.

9

1. d. Renal cell carcinoma. Adenocarcinoma of the kidney, also called renal cell carcinoma, hypernephroma and Grawitz's tumour, is twice as common in men as in women and presents after the age of 40 with painless haematuria. The tumour typically spreads along the renal vein into the vena cava, from where it may embolize into the lungs, as here. Polycythaemia and hypercalcaemia may occur due to ectopic production of erythropoietin and parathyroid hormone, respectively.
2. h. Polycystic kidney disease. Adult polycystic kidney disease is an autosomal dominant condition that is associated with berry aneurysms, which may present with subarachnoid haemorrhage or sudden death. It generally manifests with episodic haematuria, loin pain, hypertension and ultimately renal failure. Symptoms are rare before middle age.
3. e. Transitional cell carcinoma of the bladder. Transitional cell carcinoma of the bladder is more common in smokers (two-fold) and in workers in the aniline dye industry and rubber industry. It presents as painless haematuria. Tumours arising near the ureteric orifice at the base of the bladder may occlude the ureter, producing asymptomatic unilateral hydronephrosis.
4. j. Nephroblastoma. Nephroblastoma, or Wilms' tumour, usually occurs in children under the age of 5 years, and may be bilateral. It presents as a rapidly enlarging loin mass, with haematuria as a late feature since invasion of the renal pelvis tends to be late.
5. f. Ureteric calculus. Colicky loin pain radiating to the groin suggests ureteric colic. While in a 28-year-old it is likely to be due to a calculus, the same symptoms can occur in older patients with tumour debris or blood clots entering the ureter, or fragments of renal papillae in diabetic patients with papillary necrosis.

10

1. a. Abdominal ultrasound. The story is suggestive of biliary colic and the likely diagnosis is gallstones, either obstructing Hartmann's pouch or within the cystic duct. Gallbladder disease is best investigated with ultrasound, from which you will expect to determine the presence of gallstones, the thickness of the gallbladder wall (thickened suggests inflamed), and the diameter of the common bile duct. If the bile duct is dilated it suggests stones in the duct; ultrasound is not good at excluding bile duct stones, since duodenal gas obscures the lower bile duct where they may be hiding.
2. e. Abdominal CT scan. A history of pain radiating from the loin to groin is typical of ureteric colic. However, in this age group a ruptured aortic aneurysm is more likely, and the history of fainting would be compatible with bleeding. Ureteric colic tends to occur in the young or middle aged, and patients tend to walk about trying to get comfortable. A CT scan will confirm the presence of an aneurysm and whether it has leaked. Modern spiral CT scanners are also the best way to detect renal calculi.
3. g. Laparoscopy. Young women with right iliac fossa pain might have appendicitis but can also have a gynaecological emergency such a ruptured ectopic pregnancy, bleeding corpus luteal cyst or torted ovary. This history is more typical of a twisted ovarian cyst. This is best confirmed by laparoscopy, by which other diagnoses can be excluded. Ultrasound, while possibly detecting the presence of an ovarian cyst, is not very good at detecting torsion or appendicitis.
4. f. Serum amylase. The history is typical of acute pancreatitis, presumably due to his known gallstones. This would be best confirmed by a raised serum amylase. If the interval between the onset of pain and presentation was longer, 48 h for example, then a CT scan might be a better test since the amylase will have started to fall.
5. h. Erect chest X-ray. Alcohol and cigarette smoking are risk factors for peptic ulcer formation. The history is suggestive of a perforated peptic ulcer,

with sudden onset pain becoming generalized as peritoneal soiling occurs from the gastric contents. Rigidity is a feature of peritonitis. Diagnosis of a perforated viscus is confirmed by free intraperitoneal gas, traditionally detected on erect chest X-ray. However, not all perforations manifest on a chest X-ray, and CT is more sensitive in detecting free intraperitoneal gas.

SAQs Answers

1

a. • The condition being screened for has an early stage at which point intervention can stop the outcome, e.g. rupture in aortic aneurysm or cancer in cervical screening.

• The condition being screened for is serious enough to warrant screening, such as cancer and aneurysm.

• Prevalence – the condition should be common enough to justify the cost of population screening.

• Acceptability – the test should be acceptable to the subjects being tested, e.g. abdominal ultrasound.

• Sensitivity – the test should be able to detect subjects who have the condition being looked for; ultrasound is a sensitive test for aortic aneurysm.

• Specificity – the test should only detect patients with the condition and not those without it.

b. • Repair when the risk of death from rupture outweighs the risk of death from repair.

• Asymptomatic – for an aneurysm under 5.5 cm, the mortality is greater from operative repair than the risk of rupture and death; aortic aneurysms less than 5.5 cm in diameter are unlikely to rupture.

• Tender or otherwise symptomatic aneurysms need urgent repair regardless of size.

c. • *Endovascular repair*:

Less invasive

Requires a length of normal aorta below the renal artery origins to anchor the graft

Less suited to ruptured aneurysms.

• *Open repair*:

Suitable for aneurysms not amenable to endovascular repair

Suitable for ruptured aneurysms.

d. Rupture

Fistula formation – aorto-caval and aorto-enteric

Thrombosis

Distal embolization

• Infection

• Pressure effects – back pain.

2

a. Prehepatic

Hepatic

Posthepatic (obstructive).

b. • *General*:

Weight loss – malignancy or liver failure

Fevers/rigors – suggestive of cholangitis

Previous history of malignancy – liver secondaries

Recent diagnosis of diabetes – pancreatic neoplasm.

• *Prehepatic*:

Previous history of gallstones – pigment stones if haemolysis

Family history of anaemia or splenectomy.

• *Hepatic*:

Recent drugs, e.g. acute paracetamol poisoning, cholestatic jaundice due to chlorpromazine, some antibiotics

Liver toxins, e.g. halothane, chloroform

Alcohol history

Viral infection risk – hepatitis A, B and C

Non-viral infections – Weil's disease (sewage workers, farmers).

• *Obstructive*:

Pale stools and dark urine

Pain – colicky is suggestive of gallstones

Biliary surgery – strictures.

c. • *General*:

Nutrition

Colour – haemolytic jaundice is said to produce a lemon tinge.

• *Systemic features of liver disease*:

Leuconychia

Palmar erythema

Dupuytren's contractures

Metabolic flap

Bradycardia (feature of jaundice in general)

Spider naevi
Bruising and purpura
Gynaecomastia and small testes
Hypogonadism.

- *Abdominal examination*:
  Distension suggestive of ascites
  Caput medusae – indicating portosystemic shunts due to portal hypertension
  Palpable liver edge – hard/irregular is suggestive of malignancy
  Impalpable – shrunken due to cirrhosis
  Palpable gallbladder – if painless it is suggestive of a cause other than gallstones
  Splenomegaly (in portal hypertension due to cirrhosis).
- *Rectal examination*:
  Pale stools
  Anorectal varices in portal hypertension.

d. • Ultrasound – to confirm the presence of gallstones, liver tumours and dilated biliary tree due to pancreatic neoplasm.
• Reticulocyte count – raised in haemolysis, and haptoglobin reciprocally falls.
• Liver biopsy – will reveal the presence of parenchymal liver disease.

There are many other tests that are performed, such as liver biochemistry, prothrombin time, viral serology, and conjugated and unconjugated bilirubin, but the above three tests are likely to be the most discriminating in determining the cause of jaundice.

3

a. Acute pancreatitis, proved by the serum amylase. A CT scan may be indicated if presentation is delayed since the amylase falls after a few hours. Other possible diagnoses are acute gastritis and peptic ulcer disease.

b. Gallstones and alcohol are the two common causes. Others include:
Postoperative: cardiopulmonary bypass, partial gastrectomy, splenectomy
Endoscopic retrograde cholangio-pancreatography
Carcinoma of the ampulla or head of pancreas
Infection – mumps, cytomegalovirus, coxsackie
Trauma
Drugs
Hypothermia
Hypercalcaemia
Hyperlipidaemia
Vascular.

c. Clinically, looking at the patient's general appearance. A scoring system such as Ranson's or the Glasgow (Imrie) criteria may predict the likelihood of a patient developing severe pancreatitis. C-reactive protein is an independent predictor of severity.

d. Salivary gland disease – calculi, parotitis, mumps
Metabolic disease – diabetic ketoacidosis
Morphine administration – sphincter of Oddi spasm
Impaired renal excretion – macroamylasaemia and renal failure
Abdominal pathology:
perforated peptic ulcer
acute cholecystitis
intestinal obstruction
afferent loop obstruction post Pólya gastrectomy
ruptured abdominal aortic aneurysm
ruptured ectopic pregnancy
mesenteric infarction
pancreatic trauma.

4

a. • *Increased intra-abdominal pressure*:
Coughing
Lifting heavy objects
Straining at stool
Straining during micturition
Obesity.
• *Gender*: More common in men than women.

b. Nature of the hernia – sliding hernias are more difficult to repair.
Poor surgical technique – currently the best results are obtained using non-absorbable prosthetic mesh
Wound infection
Wound haematoma
Obesity
Diabetes – a risk factor for wound infection and poor healing.

c. • *Nature of the procedure.*
• *Technique to be used*: Open versus laparoscopic.
• *Procedure-specific risks*:
Recurrence
Damage to structures in the spermatic cord, especially the vas and arterial supply to the testis

Nerve damage – the ilioinguinal, iliohypogastric and genital branches of the genitofemoral nerves are all prone to damage
Chronic groin pain – occurs in up to 15% of patients
Urinary retention.

- *General risks of any procedure*:
  Anaesthetic complications
  Wound infection
  Wound haemorrhage
  Chest infection
  Thromboembolic disease.

d. • *Local anaesthetic repair*: There is less risk of complications since there is no need for fasting.

- *General anaesthetic*:
  Conversion from insulin injections to an insulin infusion and omit his subcutaneous insulin on the day of the operation
  Regular blood glucose monitoring
  Placed first on list.

5

a. • *Full thickness burns*:
They involve the whole dermis, which is destroyed
They are anaesthetic
They are often pale or white, with little blistering
Heal with scarring and contracture.

- *Partial thickness burns*:
  They are superficial
  Sensation is present
  They are erythematous with prominent blistering
  Heal completely since the underlying germinal layer is intact.

b. • *Fluid replacement requirement*: This is based on the surface area of the burn. The burn surface area is calculated using Wallace's rule of nines or, more appropriately in a child, a Lund and Browder chart.

- *Nature of fluid*: Hartmann's (Ringer's lactate) solution is used in the first 24 h, followed by a colloid infusion (e.g. albumen).
- *Rate of infusion*: This is based on the Parkland formula. Half the required volume, calculated from the surface area of the burn, is given in the first 8 h, the other half in the next 16 h.

c. Burnt skin and soot around the face, especially the mouth and nostrils
Difficulty breathing
Hypoxia
Pulmonary oedema.

d. Management involves both management of the burns themselves, and general supportive treatment.

- *Local treatment*:
  Debridement of necrotic tissue
  Cover full thickness burns after debridement with skin grafts, with priority to the eyelids, face, hands and joint flexures
  Escharotomy of full thickness, circumferential limb burns, to prevent contractures and impairment of limb blood flow
  Ventilatory support/tracheostomy if there are inhalational burns.
- *General treatment*:
  Analgesia
  Antibiotics – local application of sulfadiazine cream and systemic broad spectrum cover, covering streptococci, staphylococci and *Pseudomonas*, as well as fungal cover with fluconazole
  Tetanus prophylaxis – passive immunization if not previously immunized
  Nutrition – enteral nutrition wherever possible, parenteral when it is not.

e. • Prognosis depends on:
Depth and extent of the burn
Age, with a poorer outcome in the elderly and children.

- Factors contributing to the outcome are the occurrence of complications such as:
  Peptic ulceration
  Renal failure, due to hypovolaemia or myoglobinaemia, or nephrotoxic antibiotics
  Sepsis
  Airway involvement.

6

a. • *Infection*:
Intraperitoneal:
leak from appendix stump
interloop abscess – abscess between loops of intestine
subphrenic abscess
sub-hepatic abscess
pelvic abscess
intrahepatic abscess secondary to portal pyaemia
Wound
Chest
Urinary tract, especially if catheterized.

- *Drug reaction*: Antibiotics.
- *Thromboembolism*: Deep vein thrombosis/pulmonary embolism.
- *Infected venous cannula site.*
- *Antibiotic-induced colitis* (pseudomembranous colitis).

b. A thorough history and examination, looking for symptoms of chest and urinary infection, and abdominal examination including rectal examination (reveals a pelvic abscess). Investigations would include:
Chest X-ray (for chest infection)
Ultrasound of liver and diaphragm (for subphrenic, subhepatic and intrahepatic abscess)
Pelvic ultrasound for pelvic abscess
Abdominal CT for intraperitoneal abscess
Blood gases and CT pulmonary angiography to exclude pulmonary embolism
Duplex ultrasound scan of femoral and iliac veins for deep vein thrombosis
Urinary microscopy and culture
Stool culture
Sputum culture
Culture of any indwelling central venous cannulae, which would be removed when infection presents.

c. • *Prophylactic treatments*:
Antithrombotic:
low molecular weight heparin
thromboembolic stockings
intermittent calf compression intraoperatively
Antimicrobial:
metronidazole, 1 g given rectally prior to surgery and repeated once, if there is no intra-abdominal infection (unlike this case)
if there is evidence of infection within the peritoneum, broad spectrum antibiotics such as metronidazole and ciprofloxacin should be used.
- *Good operative technique*: Washing out the peritoneum.
- *Aseptic technique* in catheterization.
- *Early mobilization* and adequate analgesia to prevent chest sepsis.

d. • *Specific to the condition*:
Intra-abdominal adhesions – these are more common with intraperitoneal sepsis
Impaired fertility has been suggested following perforated appendicitis
Recurrent appendicitis – reported to occur occasionally if a long appendix stump is left; something that occurs more commonly with laparoscopic appendicectomy.
- *General, relating to any abdominal procedure*: Incisional hernia.

7

a. Simply, any infection acquired in a hospital. The infecting agents tend to be more resistant to antimicrobials than community-acquired infections.

b. • Surgery, where the normal skin barrier to infection is breached.
- Antibiotic use, predisposing to colonization with resistant organisms.
- Use of indwelling cannulae, which act as a portal of entry into the blood stream for skin organisms.
- Use of indwelling urinary catheters.
- Prosthetic use, such as hip prostheses, which are prone to infection.

c. Chest infection
Wound infection
Urinary infection
Antibiotic-associated colitis (pseudomembranous colitis).

d. • Removal of unnecessary cannulae and catheters.
- Antimicrobial prophylaxis: A short course or single dose to cover likely organisms, such as flucloxacillin to prevent *Staphylococcus aureus* infection of hip prostheses.
- Limited use of antibiotics: Prolonged courses result in the growth of resistant organisms.
- Good surgical technique:
Antisepsis
Removal of all devitalized tissue that might act as a focus for infection.

8

Classify the uses:
- *A means of retaining a tube*:
Urinary catheter, such as a Foley catheter
Sengstaken–Blakemore tube
Gastrostomy.
- *Sustained pressure*:
Sengstaken–Blakemore tube – this has two balloons, a distal one that anchors the tube in the stomach, and a more proximal sausage-shaped balloon that is inflated to tamponade bleeding oesophageal varices

Helmholz balloon – inflated in the bladder to cause pressure necrosis of the bladder mucosa in the treatment of bladder malignancy. This is no longer in common use.

- *Angioplasty*:
  Intravascular – to open occluded or stenosed arteries
  Endoluminal – to stretch a stenosis of, for example, the pyloric sphincter
  Adjuvant to stenting, where the balloon is used to expand a collapsed metal stent.
- *Embolectomy catheter*: Fogarty catheter where the catheter is pushed beyond a thrombus, before inflating the balloon and withdrawing the catheter, with the balloon pulling the clot before it.
- *Embolus*: Detachable balloons have been used to embolize arteries feeding organs, arteriovenous fistulae or aneurysms.
- *Aid to the placement of a catheter*:
  A Swan–Ganz catheter uses the inflated balloon to allow the catheter to travel with the blood from the right atrium into the right ventricle and on to the pulmonary artery. The balloon is then inflated and deflated to measure left atrial (pulmonary capillary wedge pressure) and pulmonary artery pressure, respectively.
  Endoluminal intestinal catheters, such as the Jones tube and Baker tube, are passed through a hole in the stomach or jejunum and fed through the small bowel into the caecum. Once in the lumen, the balloon is inflated to enable the surgeon to manipulate it along the intestine into the caecum, where it may be deflated. Such tubes are used to prevent adhesions forming and kinking the intestine, since the lie of the intestine is dictated by the semirigid tube which can be removed after 3 weeks or so.

9

a. The most likely diagnosis is testicular cancer and the differential diagnosis is epididymo-orchitis.

b. • Seminoma.
• Non-seminomatous germ cell tumours, of which teratoma is the most common.

c. Both tend to present as smooth swellings of the testis.
• A seminoma cut surface is likened to a cut potato.
• A teratoma cut surface is cystic, sometimes likened to a colloid goitre.

d. • *Diagnosis*: This is best achieved with ultrasound of the scrotum.
• *Staging of a tumour*: Spread is via lymphatics and blood, so cross-sectional imaging such as CT of the abdomen and chest is required.
• *Tumour markers*: Alpha-fetoprotein is produced by teratomas; β-human gonadotrophin is produced by pure seminomas. If present such markers are useful in the follow-up of a patient, where recurrence of tumour can be detected as a rise in the serum tumour marker.

e. • *Radical orchidectomy*: The orchidectomy must be via an inguinal approach, not via the scrotum. Lymphatic drainage is via the iliac nodes to the para-aortic nodes. Exploring through the scrotum exposes a new lymphatic field to the tumour, which drains to the inguinal nodes, and may also necessitate scrotal irradiation to prevent local spread.
• *Adjuvant therapy*:
Irradiation – seminomas are very radio-sensitive.
Chemotherapy – platinum compounds, such as cisplatin and carboplatin have transformed the treatment of non-seminomatous germ cell tumours.

f. The prognosis is very good. In the absence of nodal spread there is a nearly 100% 5-year survival rate; even with abdominal nodal disease a 95% 5-year survival is achieved.

10

a. • *Congenital*: Bicuspid aortic valve.
• *Acquired*: Rheumatic valve disease.

b. There are two principal types of valve, the xenograft, made from a pig valve suspended on a metal frame, or a prosthetic valve, such as a bileaflet valve comprising two semicircular tilting leaflets.
A 55-year-old would be most likely to have had a prosthetic valve.
• *Xenograft*:
Shorter life, not suitable for circumstances where the valve may need to be replaced
Does not need anticoagulation
Most suited to older patients.
• *Prosthetic valve*:
Longer life
Requires anticoagulation
More suitable for younger patients.

c. Xenograft valves do not usually require anticoagulation. For prosthetic valves, there are two possible ways to manage her anticoagulation:

- *Heparinization*: Replace the warfarin with heparin so that if bleeding occurs the anticoagulation can be easily reversed.
- *Stop anticoagulation*: Prosthetic valves in the aortic position have a lower risk of thrombosis than valves in the mitral position. It is possible to stop anticoagulation completely for a period of hours, before restarting with heparin.
- Warfarin has a long half-life, so treatment should be stopped 3 days prior to surgery and replaced with heparin.

d. A low rectal carcinoma like this can be treated either by low anterior resection, with restoration of continuity by a low anastomosis, or by abdomino-perineal resection where the proximal colon is brought out as an end colostomy and the distal rectum is removed completely and the perineum closed.

A low anastomosis may be 'covered' by a proximal defunctioning stoma, such as a loop ileostomy, such that if the anastomosis leaks there will not be bowel contents leaking intraperitoneally. Once healing has occurred a barium enema is performed to rule out a leak, following which the loop ileostomy can be reversed.

e. Cuthbert Esquire Dukes (1890–1977) was a pathologist at St Mark's Hospital in London who classified rectal cancers according to their depth of invasion and the presence or absence of lymph node spread, as follows:

A: Tumour confined to the mucosa and submucosa

B: Invasion of the muscle wall

C: Regional lymph node involvement.

Index of cases by diagnosis

Index

Note: page numbers in *italics* refer to figures, those in **bold** refer to tables